Governors State University
Library
Hours:
Monday thru Thursday 8:30 to 10:30
Friday and Saturday 8:30 to 5:00
Sunday 1:00 to 5:00 (Fall and Winter Trimester Only)

DEMCO

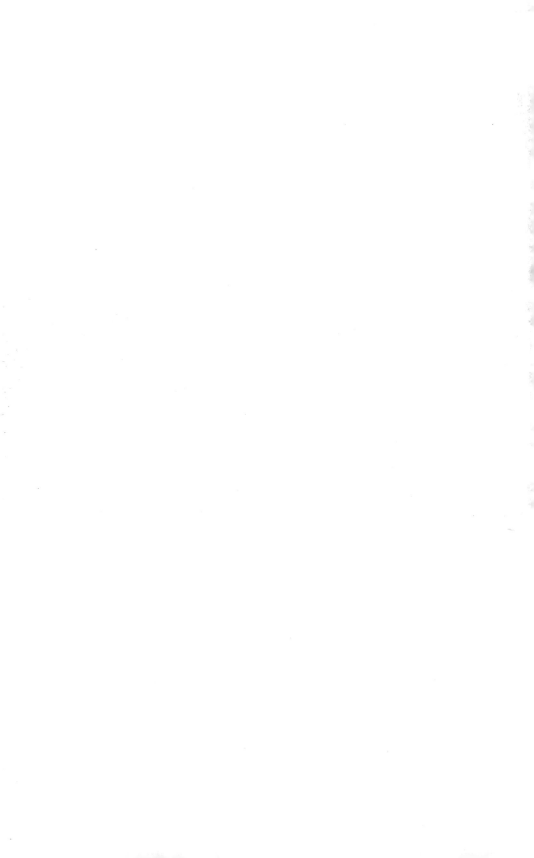

Recognition and Prevention of Major Mental and Substance Use Disorders

Recognition and Prevention of Major Mental and Substance Use Disorders

Edited by

Ming T. Tsuang, M.D., Ph.D., D.Sc.

William S. Stone, Ph.D.

Michael J. Lyons, Ph.D.

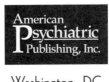

American Psychiatric Publishing, Inc.

Washington, DC
London, England

Note: The authors have worked to ensure that all information in this book is accurate at the time of publication and consistent with general psychiatric and medical standards, and that information concerning drug dosages, schedules, and routes of administration is accurate at the time of publication and consistent with standards set by the U.S. Food and Drug Administration and the general medical community. As medical research and practice continue to advance, however, therapeutic standards may change. Moreover, specific situations may require a specific therapeutic response not included in this book. For these reasons and because human and mechanical errors sometimes occur, we recommend that readers follow the advice of physicians directly involved in their care or the care of a member of their family.

Books published by American Psychiatric Publishing, Inc., represent the views and opinions of the individual authors and do not necessarily represent the policies and opinions of APPI or the American Psychiatric Association.

If you would like to buy between 25 and 99 copies of this or any other APPI title, you are eligible for a 20% discount; please contact APPI Customer Service at appi@psych.org or 800-368-5777. If you wish to buy 100 or more copies of the same title, please e-mail us at bulksales@psych.org for a price quote.

Manufactured in the United States of America on acid-free paper
11   10   09   08   07   5   4   3   2   1
First Edition

Typeset in Adobe's Jenson and Geometric231BT.

American Psychiatric Publishing, Inc.
1000 Wilson Boulevard
Arlington, VA 22209-3901
www.appi.org

Library of Congress Cataloging-in-Publication Data
Recognition and prevention of major mental and substance use disorders / edited by Ming T. Tsuang, William S. Stone, Michael J. Lyons.—1st ed.
        p. ; cm.
    Includes bibliographical references and index.
    ISBN 1-58562-308-3 (pbk. : alk. paper)
    1. Mental illness—Prevention. 2. Substance abuse—Prevention. 3. Mental illness—Diagnosis. 4. Substance abuse—Diagnosis. I. Tsuang, Ming T., 1931– II. Stone, William S. III. Lyons, Michael J., 1949–
    [DNLM: 1. Mental Disorders—prevention & control. 2. Substance-Related Disorders—prevention & control. WM 140 R311 2006]
    RA790.R39 2006
    616.89—dc22
                                                                        2006027485

British Library Cataloguing in Publication Data
A CIP record is available from the British Library.

CONTENTS

Contributors ix

Introduction xv
Ming T. Tsuang, M.D., Ph.D., D.Sc., William S. Stone, Ph.D., and
Michael J. Lyons, Ph.D.

Part I
Etiology of Major Mental and
Substance Use Disorders

1   Genetic Risk Factors for Mental Disorders: General Principles
and State of the Science. 3
Stephen J. Glatt, Ph.D., Stephen V. Faraone, Ph.D., and
Ming T. Tsuang, M.D., Ph.D., D.Sc.

2   Environmental Determinants of Psychosis:
A Focus on Drug Abuse. 21
Armin Raznahan, M.B.B.S.(Hons), M.R.C.P.C.H., M.R.C.Psych.,
Owen G. O'Daly, M.Sc., Evangelina Maria Tsapakis, B.Sc.(Hons),
M.B.B.S., M.R.C.Psych., and Robin M. Murray, D.Sc., F.R.C.Psych.

3   Social Environment and Psychiatric Disorders: A Historical
Review Presented on Receipt of the Paul H. Hoch Award. 53
Jane M. Murphy, Ph.D.

Part II
Vulnerability to Major Mental and Substance Use Disorders

4 Psychobiology of Resilience to Stress: Implications for
   Prevention of Anxiety 77
      Antonia S. New, M.D., Kathryn A. Keegan, B.A., and
      Dennis S. Charney, M.D.

5 Cognitive Vulnerability to Depression:
   Implications for Prevention. 97
      Lauren B. Alloy, Ph.D., Lyn Y. Abramson, Ph.D., Alex Cogswell, M.A.,
      Megan E. Hughes, M.A., and Brian M. Iacoviello, M.A.

6 Vulnerability to Alcohol and Drug Use Disorders. 115
      Deborah Hasin, Ph.D., Mark L. Hatzenbuehler, B.A.,
      Katherine Keyes-Wild, M.S., and Elizabeth Ogburn, M.S.

Part III
Prevention: Lessons From Schizophrenia

7 Treatment of the Schizophrenia Prodrome 159
      Barbara A. Cornblatt, Ph.D., Todd Lencz, Ph.D.,
      Christopher Smith, M.A., and Andrea Auther, Ph.D.

8 Adolescent Neurodevelopment: A Critical Period for
   Preventive Intervention 187
      Elaine F. Walker, Ph.D., Amanda McMillan, B.A.,
      Kevin Tessner, M.A., Vijay Mittal, M.A., and
      Hanan Trotman, B.A.

9 Toward Prevention of Schizophrenia: Early Detection and
   Intervention. 213
      Ming T. Tsuang, M.D., Ph.D., D.Sc., William S. Stone, Ph.D., and
      Michael J. Lyons, Ph.D.

Part IV
NIH Perspectives on Prevention

10 Prospects for the Prevention of Mental Illness:
Integrating Neuroscience and Behavior 241
Cheryl A. Boyce, Ph.D., Robert Heinssen, Ph.D.,
Courtney B. Ferrell, Ph.D., and Richard K. Nakamura, Ph.D.

11 Drugs and Alcohol: Treating and Preventing Abuse,
Addiction, and Their Medical Consequences 263
Nora D. Volkow, M.D., Ph.D., and Ting-Kai Li, M.D.

12 Alcoholism: Developmental Patterns of Drinking and
Prevention of Alcohol Use Disorders 297
Ting-Kai Li, M.D., Ellen Witt, Ph.D., and
Brenda G. Hewitt, B.A.

Part V
Challenges for the Near Future

13 Prevention of Alzheimer's Disease: Principles and Prospects . . . 319
John C.S. Breitner, M.D., M.P.H.

14 Five Facts About Preventing Drug Dependence 329
James C. Anthony, Ph.D.

15 Prevention of Aggressive Behavior Through Middle School
Using a First-Grade Classroom-Based Intervention 347
C. Hendricks Brown, Ph.D., Sheppard G. Kellam, M.D.,
Nick Ialongo, Ph.D., Jeanne Poduska, Sc.D., and Carla Ford, Ph.D.

16 Conceptually Driven Pharmacological Approaches to
Acute Trauma 371
Roger K. Pitman, M.D., and Douglas L. Delahanty, Ph.D.

Index 389

Contributors

Lyn Y. Abramson, Ph.D.
Sigmund Freud Professor of Psychology, Department of Psychology, University of Wisconsin, Madison, Wisconsin

Lauren B. Alloy, Ph.D.
Professor and Joseph Wolpe Distinguished Faculty Fellow in Psychology, Department of Psychology, Temple University, Philadelphia, Pennsylvania

James C. Anthony, Ph.D.
Professor and Chairman, Department of Epidemiology, College of Human Medicine, Michigan State University, East Lansing, Michigan

Andrea Auther, Ph.D.
Department of Psychiatry Research, The Zucker Hillside Hospital of the North Shore–Long Island Jewish Health System, Glen Oaks, New York

Cheryl A. Boyce, Ph.D.
Associate Director for Pediatric Research Training and Career Development, Division of Mental Disorders, and Chief, Abuse and Neglect Program, National Institute of Mental Health Division of Pediatric Translational Research and Treatment Development, Bethesda, Maryland

John C. S. Breitner, M.D., M.P.H.
Director, Geriatric Research Education and Clinical Center, VA Puget Sound Health Care System; Professor and Head, Division of Geriatric Psychiatry, Department of Psychiatry and Behavioral Sciences, University of Washington School of Medicine, Seattle, Washington

C. Hendricks Brown, M.D.
Professor, Department of Epidemiology and Biostatistics, College of Public Health, University of South Florida, Tampa, Florida

Dennis S. Charney, M.D.
Dean for Academic and Scientific Affairs for Mount Sinai School of Medicine, Senior Vice President for Health Sciences of The Mount Sinai Medical Center, Anne and Joel Ehrenkranz Professor, Departments of Psychiatry, Neuroscience, and Pharmacology and Biological Chemistry, New York, New York

Alex Cogswell, M.A.
Doctoral Student, Department of Psychology, Temple University, Philadelphia, Pennsylvania

Barbara A. Cornblatt, Ph.D.
Professor of Psychiatry, Department of Psychiatry Research, The Zucker Hillside Hospital of the North Shore–Long Island Jewish Health System, Glen Oaks, New York

Douglas L. Delahanty, Ph.D.
Associate Professor, Department of Psychology, Kent State University, Kent, Ohio

Stephen V. Faraone, Ph.D.
Director, Medical Genetics Research Program; Professor, Department of Psychiatry; Professor, Department of Neuroscience and Physiology; Director, Child and Adolescent Psychiatry Research, SUNY Upstate Medical University, Syracuse, New York

Courtney B. Ferrell, Ph.D.
Program Chief, Individual Fellowships Program, NIMH Division of Pediatric Translational Research and Treatment Development, Bethesda, Maryland

Carla Ford, Ph.D.
American Institutes for Research, Center for Integrating Education and Prevention in Schools, Baltimore, Maryland

Stephen J. Glatt, Ph.D.
Assistant Professor, Department of Psychiatry, University of California, San Diego, La Jolla, California; Research Associate, Veterans Medical Research Foundation, San Diego, California

Deborah Hasin, Ph.D.
Professor of Clinical Public Health, Departments of Epidemiology and Psychiatry, Columbia University, and New York State Psychiatric Institute, New York, New York

Mark L. Hatzenbuehler, B.A.
Assistant Research Scientist, New York State Psychiatric Institute, New York, New York

Robert Heinssen, Ph.D.
Program Officer, Psychotic Disorders Research Program, Adult Psychopathology and Prevention Research Program, National Institute of Mental Health Division of Mental Disorders, Behavioral Research and AIDS, Bethesda, Maryland

Brenda G. Hewitt, B.A.
Special Assistant to the Director, National Institute on Alcohol Abuse and Alcoholism, National Institutes of Health, Bethesda, Maryland

Megan E. Hughes, M.A.
Doctoral Student, Department of Psychology, Temple University, Philadelphia, Pennsylvania

Brian M. Iacoviello, M.A.
Doctoral Student, Department of Psychology, Temple University, Philadelphia, Pennsylvania

Nick Ialongo, Ph.D.
Professor, Bloomberg School of Public Health, Johns Hopkins University, Baltimore, Maryland

Kathryn A. Keegan, B.A.
Research Associate, Department of Psychiatry, Mount Sinai School of Medicine, New York, New York

Sheppard G. Kellam, M.D.
Senior Research Fellow, Director, Center for Integrating Education and Prevention Research in Schools, American Institutes for Research, Baltimore, Maryland

Katherine Keyes-Wild, M.S.
Assistant Research Scientist, New York State Psychiatric Institute, New York, New York

Todd Lencz, Ph.D.
Assistant Professor of Psychiatry, Department of Psychiatry Research, The Zucker Hillside Hospital of the North Shore–Long Island Jewish Health System, Glen Oaks, New York

Ting-Kai Li, M.D.
Director, National Institute on Alcohol Abuse and Alcoholism, National Institutes of Health, Bethesda, Maryland

Michael J. Lyons, Ph.D.
Professor and Director of Clinical Programs, Department of Psychology, Boston University; Chief of Twin Studies, Harvard Institute of Psychiatric Epidemiology and Genetics, Boston, Massachusetts

Amanda McMillan, B.A.
Research Coordinator, Department of Psychology, Emory University, Atlanta, Georgia

Vijay Mittal, M.A.
Graduate Student, Department of Psychology, Emory University, Atlanta, Georgia

Jane M. Murphy, Ph.D.
Professor of Psychiatry, Harvard Medical School; Professor in Epidemiology, Harvard School of Public Health; Epidemiologist, Massachusetts General Hospital, Boston, Massachusetts

Robin M. Murray, D.Sc., F.R.C.Psych.
Professor of Psychiatry, Department of Institute of Psychiatry, Division of Psychological Medicine and Psychiatry, Institute of Psychiatry, King's College London, London, England

Richard K. Nakamura, Ph.D.
Deputy Director, Office of the Director, National Institute of Mental Health, Bethesda, Maryland

Antonia S. New, M.D.
Associate Professor of Psychiatry, Mount Sinai School of Medicine and Bronx VA Medical Center, New York, New York

Owen G. O'Daly, M.Sc.
Doctoral Student, Department of Psychiatry, Division of Psychological Medicine and Psychiatry, Institute of Psychiatry, King's College London, London, England

Elizabeth Ogburn, M.S.
Assistant Research Scientist, New York State Psychiatric Institute, New York, New York

Roger K. Pitman, M.D.
Department of Psychiatry, Massachusetts General Hospital and Harvard Medical School, Boston, Massachusetts

Jeanne Poduska, Sc.D.
Principal Research Scientist, Deputy Director, Center for Integrating Education and Prevention Research in Schools, American Institutes for Research, Baltimore, Maryland

Armin Raznahan, M.B.B.S.(Hons), M.R.C.P.C.H., M.R.C.Psych.
Clinical Research Worker, Department of Child and Adolescent Psychiatry, Institute of Psychiatry, King's College London, London, England

Christopher Smith, M.A.
Department of Psychiatry Research, The Zucker Hillside Hospital of the North Shore–Long Island Jewish Health System, Glen Oaks, New York

William S. Stone, Ph.D.
Assistant Professor of Psychology in the Department of Psychiatry, Massachusetts Mental Health Center Academic Division of Public Sector Psychiatry; Assistant Professor, Department of Psychiatry, Beth Israel Deaconess Medical Center; Harvard Medical School Training Coordinator, Harvard Institute of Psychiatric Epidemiology and Genetics, Boston, Massachusetts

Kevin Tessner, M.A.
Graduate Student, Department of Psychology, Emory University, Atlanta, Georgia

Hanan Trotman, B.A.
Graduate Student, Department of Psychology, Emory University, Atlanta, Georgia

Evangelina Maria Tsapakis, B.Sc.(Hons), M.B.B.S., M.R.C.Psych.
Department of Psychiatry, Division of Psychological Medicine and Psychiatry, Institute of Psychiatry, King's College London, London, England

Ming T. Tsuang, M.D., Ph.D., D.Sc.
University Professor, University of California; Distinguished Professor of Psychiatry and Director, Center for Behavioral Genomics, Department of Psychiatry, University of California, San Diego, La Jolla, California; Adjunct Professor and Director, Harvard Institute of Psychiatric Epidemiology and Genetics, Department of Epidemiology, Harvard School of Public Health, Boston, Massachusetts; Senior Lecturer, Massachusetts Mental Health Center Academic Division of Public Psychiatry, Department of Psychiatry, Beth Israel Deaconess Medical Center, Harvard Medical School, Boston, Massachusetts

Nora D. Volkow, M.D., Ph.D.
Director, National Institute on Drug Abuse; Chief, Laboratory of Neuroimaging, National Institute on Alcohol Abuse and Alcoholism, National Institutes of Health, Bethesda, Maryland

Elaine F. Walker, Ph.D.
Samuel Candler Dobbs Professor of Psychology and Neuroscience, Department of Psychology, Emory University, Atlanta, Georgia

Ellen Witt, Ph.D.
Health Scientist Administrator, National Institute on Alcohol Abuse and Alcoholism, National Institutes of Health, Bethesda, Maryland

Introduction

Major mental disorders impose a great burden on the affected individuals, their families, and society. Despite significant advances in psychiatric diagnosis, treatment, and elucidation of etiological factors, obstacles to progress remain formidable. At least one consensual conclusion from research into many psychiatric disorders, however, points toward a common goal in the future: Better clinical outcomes are associated with earlier initiation of treatment. Actually preventing these disorders would provide immense benefit in terms of saving both money and human suffering. The 2005 meeting of the American Psychopathological Association addressed a number of key issues for making progress in preventing major mental disorders, ranging from the level of the DNA molecule to the level of governmental policy. Presentations addressed how prevention efforts should be informed by the knowledge of indicators of vulnerability and an understanding of the etiology. Approaches to prevention at the level of public policy were considered through presentations by representatives of the National Institutes of Health. Examples from areas of psychopathology that have already been the focus of considerable attention, such as schizophrenia, Alzheimer's disease, substance abuse, antisocial personality disorder, and posttraumatic stress disorder (PTSD), exemplified approaches to prevention. This volume retains the organization used in the meeting to address the current status of early intervention in, and prevention of, mental and substance abuse disorders.

The first section—"Etiology of Major Mental and Substance Use Disorders"—addresses issues that are critical precursors to efforts to prevent mental disorders. In general, efforts to prevent a disorder should be informed by an understanding of factors that contribute to the development of the disorder. Fortunately, although it is desirable to understand the etiology of a disorder in order to undertake preventive efforts, examples from other fields demonstrate that efficacious preventive efforts may be carried out on the basis of incorrect theories of etiology. For example, efforts to prevent malaria by draining swamps to reduce the "bad air" responsible for malaria actually did reduce the incidence of malaria, although the underlying rationale was completely misguided. In this section, Stephen Glatt and colleagues first review genetic methodologies and current findings in mental disorders, with an emphasis on schizophrenia. The next two chapters examine environmental variables, both biological and psychosocial, and how they may influence vulnerability. In the first of these, Robin Murray and colleagues present data on the role of substance abuse, particularly marijuana and psychostimulants, in increasing the vulnerability to developing schizophrenia. Jane Murphy then presents data on psychosocial factors that contribute to the etiology of psychiatric disorders.

The second section—"Vulnerability to Major Mental and Substance Use Disorders"—examines vulnerability factors for several relevant disorders. Dennis Charney and colleagues address how stress and its concomitant psychobiological responses may increase vulnerability to mental disorders. Lauren Alloy and colleagues then examine how cognitive factors may represent a major part of the vulnerability to depression, and Deborah Hasin and colleagues review evidence for factors associated with vulnerability to alcohol and drug use disorders.

The third section—"Prevention: Lessons From Schizophrenia"—addresses the disorder on which the most comprehensive and sophisticated research efforts have been focused. Barbara Cornblatt and colleagues discuss implications of prodromal studies for the prevention of schizophrenia, and Elaine Walker and colleagues describe relationships among stress, critical periods, and the development of schizophrenia. Both authors and their colleagues propose interesting and provocative neurodevelopmental theories of schizophrenia and provide promising frameworks for planning prevention efforts. Ming Tsuang and colleagues then present an intriguing approach for translating successful treatment methods into efforts to prevent the transition from the vulnerability, to the prodrome of the disorder, to the full-blown illness.

The fourth section—"NIH Perspectives on Prevention"—brings together contributions by leaders from the three institutes of the National Institutes of Health that are responsible for the United States' efforts to reduce the personal and societal burdens imposed by mental disorders—the National Institute of Mental Health (Richard Nakamura), the National Institute on Drug Abuse (Nora Volkow), and the National Institute of Alcohol Abuse and Alcoholism (Ting-Kai Li). In their presentations, these authors and their colleagues make a strong case for how basic scientific understanding of mental disorders can be translated into public policy.

The final section—"Challenges for the Near Future"—comprises four chapters that describe cutting-edge projects to prevent mental disorders. John Breitner discusses the status of prevention research for Alzheimer's disease; James Anthony focuses on the prevention of drug dependence; C. Hendricks Brown and colleagues discuss prevention of antisocial behavior, including a program that begins as early as the first grade; and Roger Pitman and Douglas Delahanty assess the status of secondary prevention efforts for PTSD, with a focus on pharmacological interventions. Each of these chapters provides compelling accounts of how knowledge that already exists can form the basis of extremely promising preventive efforts.

At the conclusion of each chapter, the editors have delineated or added a section on the clinical implications of the presented material. This represents our effort to enhance the value of the material in this volume by trying to identify the clinical relevance of the information. It is hoped that the multidimensional and interdisciplinary nature of early intervention and prevention efforts will benefit clinicians and researchers alike who share the goal of preventing mental and substance abuse disorders.

Ming T. Tsuang, M.D., Ph.D., D.Sc.
William S. Stone, Ph.D.
Michael J. Lyons, Ph.D.

Part I

Etiology of
Major Mental and
Substance Use Disorders

1

Genetic Risk Factors for Mental Disorders

General Principles and State of the Science

Stephen J. Glatt, Ph.D.
Stephen V. Faraone, Ph.D.
Ming T. Tsuang, M.D., Ph.D., D.Sc.

The purpose of this chapter is to provide a broad overview of what we know about the genetics of mental disorders, with special emphasis on evaluating our progress and prospects for using this information to prevent psychiatric illnesses. As the title suggests, we provide a brief review of the behavioral and molecular genetic methods and principles that guide the search for genes influencing these conditions. We also evaluate the evidence implicating familial and genetic factors in general, and specific genes and alleles in particular. As one of the most heritable—and most often studied—mental disorders, schizophrenia will be the focus of our review; however, general principles will be emphasized, and particularly successful efforts directed at other mental disorders will also be highlighted where appropriate. The chapter concludes with a series of recommendations to hasten the discovery of risk genes[1] for mental disorders and to foster the translation of these findings into effective early intervention and prevention protocols.

BEHAVIORAL GENETIC METHODS AND PRINCIPLES

Family Studies

The first question that must be asked and answered when attempting to delineate the genetic and environmental components of a complex mental disorder is "Does the phenotype run in families?" or "Is this phenotype familial?" This question can be answered through the use of family studies. The basic design of the family study begins with the ascertainment of a group of case subjects who are affected by the disorder and a comparable group of control subjects who do not have the disorder. Next, the biological relatives of these index subjects, or *probands*, are ascertained and evaluated for presence of the illness—or, in some cases, subthreshold forms of the illness. The rate of the disorder or of associated "spectrum conditions" among family members of affected probands is then compared with the rate of the disorder among family members of control probands to determine the familial risk or relative risk.

If a psychiatric disorder has a genetic etiology, then biological relatives of case subjects should have a higher likelihood than relatives of control subjects of carrying the gene or genes that influenced illness in their relative, and thus they should be at greater risk for the illness themselves. In addition, the risk to relatives of case subjects should be correlated with their degree of relationship to the proband, or the amount of genes they share in common. First-degree relatives, such as parents, siblings, and children, share 50% of their genes, on average, with the proband. Thus, first-degree relatives of case subjects should be at greater risk for the disorder than second-degree relatives (grandparents, uncles, aunts, nephews, nieces, and half-siblings), who share only 25% of their genes with the proband.

---

[1]Most psychiatric disorders exhibit complex, non-Mendelian inheritance patterns and thus are thought to result from the joint effects of multiple genes and environmental factors. For this reason, we refer to the genes for psychiatric disorders as "risk genes" rather than "disease genes," since none may be either necessary or sufficient to elicit illness.

Twin Studies

Once a disorder has been established as familial, it becomes necessary to determine whether that pattern is attributable to the inheritance of genes or to shared familial and other environmental factors. It is also important to quantify the contribution of genes relative to the contribution of environmental factors, as this may encourage or discourage future molecular genetic studies; it may also influence the decisions made by individuals seeking genetic counseling and the usefulness of family information in identifying high-risk individuals to target for early intervention and prevention protocols. These questions can be answered by both twin studies and adoption studies; however, our focus in this chapter will be twin studies, primarily because they are relatively easy to conduct and thus the most popular.

In twin study designs, identical (monozygotic [MZ]) and fraternal (dizygotic [DZ]) twin pairs are ascertained if at least one member of the pair is affected with a disorder. Twin pairs are deemed "concordant" if both members of the pair have the illness and "discordant" if only one member of the pair is affected. The ratio of concordant to discordant MZ twin pairs is then compared with the ratio of concordant to discordant DZ twin pairs.

MZ twins are derived from the same zygote and thus share 100% of their genetic material. By contrast, DZ twins result from separate fertilizations and thus share, on average, 50% of their genes—that is, no more or less than any other pair of siblings. Thus, a typical MZ twin pair will have 50% more genes in common than a typical DZ twin pair. However, the degree of similarity in environmental exposures between members of a MZ twin pair should be no different than that between members of a DZ twin pair. Thus, any difference in concordance for a mental illness between the two types of twin pairs can be attributed to the effects of the additional gene sharing in the MZ twins. In other words, sharing 50% more genes in common can be inferred to be responsible for any increased phenotypic similarity among MZ twin pairs relative to DZ twin pairs.

If the concordance for a mental illness is higher among MZ twin pairs than among DZ twin pairs, this is a good indication that there is a genetic contribution to the disorder; if MZ and DZ twin pairs have approximately equal concordance rates, environmental factors are more strongly implicated. Frequently, concordance rates among twin pairs are used to estimate the "heritability" of a disorder. *Heritability* refers to the degree to which genetic factors influence variability in the manifestation of the phenotype. Heritability in the broad sense is the ratio of genetic to phenotypic variances, or the proportion of variance in schizophrenia risk that is accounted for by variability in genetic factors. A heritability of 1.0 indicates that all variability in the phenotype is due to genetic factors alone. By contrast, a heritability of zero indicates that all phenotypic variation is attributable to environmental factors.

GENERAL FAMILIAL AND GENETIC FACTORS IMPLICATED IN MENTAL DISORDERS

Family Studies

As shown in Table 1–1, many disorders identified in the fourth edition of the *Diagnostic and Statistical Manual of Mental Disorders* (DSM-IV; American Psychiatric Association 1994) have been evaluated within the framework of a family study, thus yielding an estimate of the risk of illness to a sibling of an affected person (locus-specific relative recurrence risk ratio of disease for a sibling of the affected person, or ls). For the most part, familial risk estimates for psychiatric conditions have been found to range from 4 to 12, indicating that, depending on the disorder, a sibling of an affected individual is 4 to 12 times more likely to develop the disorder compared with an individual from the general population.

It is noteworthy, however, that most family studies of psychiatric disorders that have included second- and third-degree relatives of the proband have observed a nonlinear relationship between relative risk for illness and degree of relationship to the proband (i.e., expected proportion of shared genes). Thus, for example, the consensus from studies of schizophrenia is that second-degree relatives of schizophrenia patients are at an approximately two- to threefold increased risk of illness, but first-degree relatives are at a tenfold increased risk, despite a mere doubling of expected alleles shared with the proband. Furthermore, the risk to offspring of two schizophrenic parents, from whom the affected offspring received all of his or her genes, is not absolute (approximately 46%); this pattern is also observed in studies of most other psychiatric disorders. These results underscore the complexity of the genetic bases for psychiatric disorders and imply that gene–gene interactions (epistasis) as well as environmental factors must contribute to their etiologies.

Consistent with modern conceptualizations of schizophrenia and certain other mental illnesses as continuous—rather than discrete—entities, most evidence suggests that family members of an affected patient are at heightened risk for spectrum conditions in addition to their increased liability to the full disorder of interest. For example, approximately 9% of the relatives of a schizophrenia patient will have a psychotic disorder that does not meet criteria for schizophrenia (e.g., schizoaffective disorder, psychosis not otherwise specified). Aggregation of schizotypal personality disorder is also frequently observed in families affected by schizophrenia, with an incidence as high as 14.6% in relatives of a schizophrenia patient. These data are also consistent with a multidetermined etiology for these conditions, whereby possession of only one or a few risk factors increases risk for illness somewhat, but possession of a greater quantity of these factors can elicit a full-blown, diagnosable illness.

Collectively, the evidence from family studies suggests that psychiatric conditions do aggregate within families, that multiple genes and environmental factors may be involved in these illnesses, and that these disorders can present (even within families) with different degrees of severity. Despite this powerful evidence, it is important to recognize that familiality does not necessarily establish heritability. For example, religion and language are familial traits, as all members of the same family often practice the same religion and speak the same language. These facts do not reflect the transmission of "religion genes" or "language genes" through the family, but rather the common environment and upbringing shared by family members.

Twin Studies

The suggestions raised by these family studies can be formally evaluated through the use of twin studies, and as can be seen in Table 1–1, the heritability of many psychiatric disorders has already been examined. Indeed, perhaps due to the relative ease of ascertaining twin pairs as opposed to nuclear families or extended pedigrees, more psychiatric disorders have been subjected to a twin analysis than to a family study. Of those psychiatric disorders described in DSM-IV that have been the subject of a twin study, all but one was found to be significantly heritable. Estimates of the heritability of these disorders vary widely, from a high of more than 90% for autism (Bailey et al. 1995) to a low of 0% for dysthymia (Lyons et al. 1998). Thus, while some psychiatric disorders may have no genetic basis, most have a genetic component and several are predominantly attributable to genes.

Analogous to the results of family studies, MZ twins often have a rate of concordance for a psychiatric illness that is greater than twice that observed among DZ twins, despite the fact that their expected proportion of shared genes is only double that of DZ twins. For example, the best evidence from twin studies of schizophrenia suggests a rate of concordance of approximately 46%–53% for MZ twins and 14%–15% for DZ twins. These data further support the possibility of epistasis in the etiology of the disorder, and similar results have been observed in twin studies of other psychiatric conditions. Furthermore, MZ

Table 1–1. Results of family, twin, linkage, and association studies of psychiatric disorders

Psychiatric disorder	RR	Heritability	Linked loci	Associated genes
Autism	22	93	7q	GABRAB3, SLC6A4
Tourette's disorder	12	90	11q	SLITRK1, TBCD
Schizoaffective disorder	11	85	1q	DISC1
Bipolar disorder	8	84	6q, 8q	BDNF, DRD4, MAOA, SLC6A4
Schizophrenia	12	84	1q, 2q, 8p, 22q	DRD2, DTNBP1, HTR2A, NRG1, RGS4
Narcissistic personality disorder	—	79	—	—
Obsessive-compulsive personality disorder	—	78	—	—
Cannabis abuse	6	76	—	—
Attention-deficit/hyperactivity disorder	4	75	4p, 5p, 6q, 16p, 17p	DRD4, DRD5, SLC6A3, DBH, SLC6A4, HTR1B, SNAP25
Conduct disorder	—	74	9q, 17q	DRD4, SLC6A4
Anorexia nervosa	11	71	13q	BDNF, HTR2A, SLC6A2
Stuttering	5	70	12q, 18p	SOX3
Antisocial personality disorder	—	69	—	MAOA
Borderline personality disorder	—	69	—	—
Obsessive-compulsive disorder	4	68	17q, 13q, 11p	HTR2A, SLC6A4
Histrionic personality disorder	—	67	—	—
Stimulant abuse	—	66	—	—
Hallucinogen abuse	—	65	—	—
Gender identity disorder	—	62	—	—

Table 1–1. Results of family, twin, linkage, and association studies of psychiatric disorders *(continued)*

Psychiatric disorder	RR	Heritability	Linked loci	Associated genes
Oppositional defiant disorder	—	61	—	—
Nicotine dependence	—	60	5q, 9q, 20q	CYP2A6, GABRAB2
Sleepwalking	—	60	—	—
Sedative abuse	—	59	—	—
Alzheimer's disease	2	58	4p, 7q, 10q, 12p, 12q, 17q, 19p, 20p	A2M, ACE, APOE, APP, BCHE, LRP1, MAPT, NOS3
Dependent personality disorder	—	57	—	—
Bulimia nervosa	4	55	10p	BDNF
Dyslexia	—	53	1p, 2p, 3p, 6p, 15q, 18p, Xq	DCDC2
Dissociative identity disorder	—	48	—	—
Pathological gambling	4	46	—	—
Panic disorder	5	43	9q, 13q, 22q	ADORA2A
Suicide	10	43	—	SLC6A4, TPH
Nightmare disorder	—	41	—	—
Agoraphobia	4	38	3q	—
Opiate abuse	10	38	17q	DRD4, OPRM1
Postpartum psychosis	11	38	—	TNFA, TPH
Posttraumatic stress disorder	—	38	—	—
Major depression	4	37	13q, 12q, 15q	DRD4, SLC6A3, TH
Narcolepsy	—	37	4p, 17q, 21q	HLA-DBQ1

Table 1–1.   Results of family, twin, linkage, and association studies of psychiatric disorders *(continued)*

Psychiatric disorder	RR	Heritability	Linked loci	Associated genes
Alcohol abuse	2	36	13q, 4q, 4p	ALDH2, ADH2, ADH3
Cocaine abuse	4	32	9q	—
Generalized anxiety disorder	6	32	—	—
Insomnia	—	32	12q, 14q, 20p	—
Schizoid personality disorder	4	29	—	—
Seasonal affective disorder	—	29	—	HTR2A
Simple phobia	4	29	14q	—
Avoidant personality disorder	4	28	—	—
Paranoid personality disorder	4	28	—	—
Schizotypal personality disorder	5	28	—	—
Social phobia	4	25	16q	—
Enuresis	—	24	12q, 13q	—
Dysthymia	—	—	—	—

Note.   All values denote representative, replicated, or consensus estimates, but all available data relevant to each parameter may not be reflected in this table. RR = relative risk.

twins are not 100% concordant for any psychiatric disorder, confirming that environmental factors make a strong contribution to the overall risk, even for the most heritable mental disorders.

The results of behavioral genetic studies of psychiatric disorders have a clear bearing on the identification of individuals at risk for these conditions, which in turn informs the development of early intervention and prevention strategies. For example, the risk of an individual developing autism if they have an affected sibling can be quantified quite clearly from family study data (approximately 22-fold increased risk). This suggests that siblings of children with autism would be prime targets for the development and validation of effective early interventions. On the other hand, twin-study data have shown us that there is little or no genetic contribution to dysthymia and that environmental factors account for more than two-thirds of the risk for many disorders such as enuresis, some phobias, cocaine abuse, and several personality disorders. These results suggest that early intervention and prevention efforts focusing on behavioral interventions or environmental manipulations may have a heightened chance for success in modifying the risk for these illnesses.

MOLECULAR GENETIC METHODS AND PRINCIPLES

Linkage Studies

Knowing that genetic factors are involved in the etiology of a psychiatric disorder—and to what degree—is essential for designing optimal molecular genetic studies to reveal the chromosomal location of the responsible risk genes. Linkage analysis is a highly appropriate strategy for identifying regions of chromosomes that have a high likelihood of harboring risk genes for an illness. Families are ascertained for linkage analysis through a proband affected with the disorder of interest. Each individual in the family is then genotyped at a series of DNA markers (not necessarily in genes) spaced evenly throughout the genome, and the co-segregation of these DNA markers with the illness is tracked in each pedigree. Evidence for co-segregation at each marker locus is summed across pedigrees to derive an index of the likelihood of the obtained patterns of marker–phenotype co-segregation given the sampled pedigree structures.

Linkage analysis is made possible by the "crossing over" which takes place between two homologous chromosomes during meiosis, the process by which gametes are created. Genetic transmission occurs because we inherit one member of each pair of chromosomes from our mother and one from our father; however, these inherited chromosomes are not identical to any of the original parental chromosomes. During meiosis, the original chromosomes in a pair cross over each other and exchange portions of their DNA. After multiple crossovers, the resulting two chromosomes each consist of a new and unique combination of genes. The probability that two genes on the same chromosome will recombine during meiosis is a function of their physical distance from each other. We say that two loci on the same chromosome are "linked" when they are so close to each other that crossing over rarely or never occurs between them. Closely linked genes usually remain together on the same chromosome after meiosis is complete. The greater the distance between loci on the same chromosome, the more likely it is that they will recombine.

Although the DNA markers used for linkage analysis are not presumed to be actual risk genes for the disorder, they are numerous and dense enough to ensure that their co-inheritance with a nearby (but unobserved) risk gene could be inferred with reasonable certainty based on the co-inheritance of the marker with the phenotype that is influenced by that risk gene. In this design, the disorder serves as a proxy for the risk gene; thus, DNA markers that commonly co-segregate with the disorder are presumed to co-segregate commonly with its underlying risk gene. Because the probability of co-segregation of two pieces of DNA is inversely proportional to the distance between them, the regularity of the co-segregation of the DNA marker and the disorder gives an indirect indication of the genetic distance between the DNA marker and the unobserved risk gene.

The possible outcomes of a linkage analysis will vary according to the structure of families ascertained for analysis. For example, linkage analysis can be performed with affected sibling pairs, or with other affected relative pairs, or with small nuclear families, or with large extended pedigrees. Regardless of what family structure is the principal unit of analysis, the common output across methods is some index of the degree of phenotypic similarity of family members and the degree of genotypic similarity between those individuals at each DNA marker. These indices are summed across families to determine the overall evidence for linkage at a given locus in the full sample. If a given DNA marker co-segregates with illness through families more often than would be expected by chance, this indicates that the marker is "linked" (i.e., is in relatively close physical proximity) to a risk gene that influences expression of the disorder.

Association Studies

Once regions of certain chromosomes have been implicated from linkage analysis as harboring a risk gene for a disorder, the next step is to identify what specific gene is segregating through families to give rise to that linkage signal. A gene can be selected for such analysis subsequent to linkage analysis as a means to follow-up on evidence for increased genetic similarity at a locus among affected individuals in a family (i.e., a "positional candidate gene" approach). Alternatively, specific genes can be examined in the absence of linkage information if there is some compelling physiological reason to suspect that the gene influences risk for a given disorder (i.e., a "functional candidate gene" approach). For example, dopamine system genes, such as receptors and transporters, are commonly examined as functional candidates for schizophrenia. In contrast to linkage analysis, which uses random DNA markers as proxies for nearby risk genes, genetic association analysis is an appropriate method for determining if a particular gene variant has a direct effect on risk for an illness, or is in tight linkage disequilibrium with such a gene.

If a gene influences risk for a mental illness, this effect should be detectable as an increased frequency of the risk allele of the gene in case subjects compared with control subjects. Within the context of the family, such an effect would be detectable as an increased likelihood of an affected patient receiving the risk allele of the gene from his parent, even when both the risk and normal forms of the gene were present in the parent and should have been transmitted to offspring with equal frequency and likelihood.

In a case–control association study, we simply count the number of each type of allele of a gene that is found in case subjects and compare these counts with the allele distribution seen in the control group (this process can also be performed for genotypes). A simple statistical test can then be used to determine if the distribution of alleles observed in the group of case subjects is different from that seen in the control group. If it is different, then we have found evidence for a genetic association with the illness, where the allele that is overrepresented in the group of case subjects is considered the risk allele. The degree of overrepresentation of the risk allele in case subjects relative to control subjects can be used to derive an odds ratio, which gives a numeric indication of an individual's chance of being affected by a disorder if he or she possesses the risk allele. In family-based studies, we can use analogous statistics to determine whether any difference from the expected equal inheritance of risk and normal alleles of a gene is detected in affected probands who could have received either allele from their parent. In a family-based study, the odds ratio estimates the haplotype relative risk, which represents the increase in the probability of the affected offspring receiving the risk allele relative to the normal allele.

SPECIFIC CHROMOSOMAL LOCI AND GENES IMPLICATED IN MENTAL DISORDERS

Linkage Studies

For the most heritable psychiatric disorders, including schizophrenia, bipolar disorder, and autism, numerous independent genomewide linkage analyses have been performed (Table 1–1). In fact, each of these three disorders has been studied often enough by linkage analysis to allow for the quantitative combination of evidence across studies by meta-analysis. For autism, two meta-analyses have confirmed linkage to chromosome 7q, which was observed in several individual studies (Badner and Gershon 2002b; Trikalinos et al. 2006). Schizophrenia and bipolar disorder have also been subjected to more than one independent meta-analysis each, but with less agreement between the methods than has been observed for autism.

For schizophrenia, no less than 18 independent genomewide linkage analyses have been published to date. Each of these studies has identified at least one chromosomal region in which either significant or suggestive evidence for linkage was observed. Unfortunately, the major findings from these genomewide linkage scans do not, at first glance, appear to overlap to any great extent. Badner and Gershon (2002a) performed the first meta-analysis of these genomewide linkage scans, and the results of their pooled analysis identified loci on chromosomes 8p, 13q, and 22q as the best candidates for harboring schizophrenia risk genes. Other promising regions included 1q, 2q, 6q, and 15q, but evidence for linkage at these loci was weaker, indicating a need for further replication. Subsequently, Lewis et al. (2003) conducted a meta-analysis of these and additional studies using an alternate methodology. Their results were somewhat different, identifying chromosome 2q as the prime candidate linked locus, and revealing somewhat weaker evidence for linkage on chromosomes 1q, 3p, 5q, 6p, 8p, 11q, 14p, 20q, and 22q. However, both meta-analyses were consistent in identifying chromosomes 1q, 2q, 8p, and 22q as the most reliably linked loci across individual studies.

For bipolar disorder, the first meta-analysis (that of Badner and Gershon [2002a]) found the strongest evidence for significant linkage on chromosomes 13q and 22q. (Of note, these were two of the three loci these authors also identified as linked to schizophrenia.) In stark contrast, the meta-analysis of Segurado et al. (2003) found the strongest evidence for linkage at loci on chromosomes 9p, 10q, and 14q. Most recently, a combined analysis of primary genotype data (rather than pooled study-level results) from all 11 studies implicated chromosomes 6q and 8q as the strongest candidates for harboring risk genes for bipolar disorder, perhaps providing the best evidence to date on the topic.

Genomewide linkage analyses have thus provided some strong leads (but some ambiguous ones as well) in the search for loci harboring risk genes for some mental illnesses; however, the method is certainly not optimal for detecting genes with small effects on risk. For example, Risch and Merikangas (1996) illustrated that a locus conferring four times greater risk for a disorder could be detected by linkage analysis in 200–4,000 families; a reasonable number for today's large, multisite collaborative research studies. However, to detect a locus that increases risk by only 50%, a minimum of 18,000 families would be needed. This number of families is clearly unattainable by any single research group and, indeed, is beyond the reach of even the most effective research consortia. In fact, this number exceeds the total number of families studied to date in all published linkage analyses of schizophrenia, bipolar disorder, and autism combined. Therefore, for all practical purposes, we have reached an era in which linkage analysis may no longer be a feasible strategy to detect genes that have a small but reliable influence on risk for complex mental disorders, especially those disorders with less of a heritable component to their etiologies.

Association Studies

When reviewing the status of behavioral genetic studies of psychiatric disorders, we saw that fewer conditions had been subjected to family studies than to twin studies, even though the former have traditionally preceded the latter in the "chain of psychiatric genetic research" (Faraone et al. 1999). This may be due to the ease of ascertaining twins rather than entire families, as well as the enhanced inferential power afforded by the twin study method. Thus, whereas family studies give an indication of the familial aggregation of a disorder (which may or may not reflect genetic factors), a twin study can directly establish whether or not genes influence the disorder and to what degree. This same type of reversal is also true for molecular genetic studies, wherein linkage studies have recently become far outnumbered by association studies. Again, this may be due to the ease of ascertaining units of analysis for an association study (i.e., unrelated case and control subjects or, at most, small nuclear families with one affected individual) relative to a linkage study (i.e., affected sibling pairs or extended pedigrees). In addition, the information gleaned from an association study may be more direct than that from a linkage study, since the former can test for direct effects on risk for each studied polymorphism, while the latter only identifies linked loci which must then be subjected to further "fine mapping" to identify risk-conferring genes. Furthermore, in contrast to linkage analysis, association analysis should be more effective at detecting genes with small effects on liability. For example, Risch and Merikangas (1996) showed that a locus increasing risk for a complex disorder by 50% could be detected in as few as 950 subjects. This number of samples is more feasible than that needed to detect the same effect by linkage analysis (i.e., 18,000 families). In fact, many of the pooled association studies performed to date have attained such numbers of subjects.

Because of these favorable attributes of association methods, many studies (we estimate more than 2,700) of functional and positional candidate genes for psychiatric disorders have been conducted over the past two decades; however, only a handful of genes exhibit reasonably strong evidence for exerting reliable risk for one or more of these disorders (Table 1–1). The genes listed here are those that have been implicated by either 1) strongly significant evidence from a very large primary study, 2) significant evidence from two or more independent research groups, or 3) significant pooled evidence from meta-analysis. Although the genes listed in this table represent relatively strong candidates for these disorders, we must reiterate at this point that none of these genes are proven risk factors for an illness, and none is either necessary or sufficient for producing any psychiatric disorder. In fact, most have been found to increase risk less than twofold and account for only a small portion of the aggregate risk for the given mental illness in the population. In addition, the risk alleles and haplotypes identified in one sample are often not the same as those implicated in other studies. Thus, more work is needed to definitively specify the nature and magnitude of the influences of these genes on risk for the various mental disorders to which they have been associated.

Recently some progress has been made in identifying particular circumstances under which some of these genes more reliably influence risk. For example, Fanous et al. (2005) identified a stronger relationship between a high-risk haplotype of the dystrobrevin binding protein 1 gene (DTNBP1) and negative symptoms of schizophrenia, and Green et al. (2005) found a higher prevalence of certain neuregulin 1 gene (NRG1) variants in schizophrenia patients who had experienced a manic episode. Collectively, the results of association studies suggest that 1) both functional and positional candidate gene approaches can successfully identify risk genes, 2) only a fraction of the genes that influence risk for mental disorders has yet been discovered, and 3) examining alternative traits or subgroups of patients with mental disorders may be a fruitful means for parsing the heterogeneity of schizophrenia, increasing the genetic "signal to noise ratio," and discovering stronger associations.

Despite these successes, association studies remain plagued by some limitations, including their propensity for producing false-positive results (Lohmueller et al. 2003) and their limited breadth. Regarding the former, genes identified as associated with a mental illness in an initial study often overestimate the true effect size and subsequently fall victim to the winner's curse, wherein the same magnitude of an effect cannot be replicated (Glatt et al. 2003; Ioannidis et al. 2001). Regarding the latter, association methods have traditionally focused on one or at most a handful of genes at once, whereas linkage analysis constitutes a genomewide survey of (relatively) unselected markers. Unfortunately, the prior probability of selecting the right candidate gene (out of approximately 25,000 human genes) and the right polymorphism (out of more than 10 million in the human genome) for analysis is remote. Most candidate genes for mental disorders have been targeted on the basis of their expression within systems widely implicated in the disorder (e.g., functional candidate genes in the dopamine neurotransmitter systems in schizophrenia). This approach has thus far proven essential for clarifying the nature of dysfunction within these recognized candidate pathways; however, it may not be optimal for identifying additional novel risk factors outside of these systems. The recent advancement of laboratory and statistical methods for genomewide association analysis should allow for a more unbiased examination of association patterns throughout the genome and help resolve this dilemma in coming years (Thomas et al. 2005).

RECOMMENDATIONS FOR FUTURE RESEARCH

It is clear that the multifactorial polygenic etiologies and heterogeneity of psychiatric disorders obscure the discovery of their underlying genetic bases. The multifactorial polygenic nature of these diseases dictates that the "signals" obtained in linkage and association studies will be numerous and of very low intensity, while the heterogeneity of these disorders increases the "noise" against which these already-faint signals must be detected. Some of the most effective ways of combating these complexities are through the maximization of power, both by increasing sample size and by studying homogeneous groups of affected individuals. In identifying the numerous genes with small effects on risk for psychiatric illness, various data-pooling strategies, such as direct combination of primary data or combination of study-level data by meta-analysis, can be particularly effective. However, to overcome the obstacles introduced by heterogeneity, delineating and studying smaller, more homogeneous subgroups of affected individuals may have the greatest beneficial effects on power. When used in tandem, the practices of pooling and splitting will yield maximal power for genetic studies, and hasten the discovery of the full compendium of risk genes for each heritable psychiatric condition. Other promising avenues for elucidating risk genes include the analysis of gene–gene and gene–environment interactions. An often overlooked potential benefit of genetic research on mental disorders is that, once risk genes are identified, environmental risk factors may become easier to detect within subgroups of subjects who do or do not possess those risk genes.

CLINICAL IMPLICATIONS

Since the first draft of the human genome was produced in 2001 (Lander et al. 2001), scientists have been touting the promise of genetic analysis for identifying risk factors for common diseases and the development of personalized medicine. Yet, the vast potential of genetic studies to change the clinical practice of psychiatry remains almost entirely untapped. Presently, the results of behavior genetic analyses, such as the family and twin studies described in this chapter, can be useful in genetic counseling situations to inform individuals of their chances of becoming affected with a particular illness. In addition, this information can be used prospectively for family planning, and to help parents understand the risks for mental illnesses that may be carried by their children. However, families still cannot be examined for linkage at a particular locus to determine if they exhibit a particular pattern of marker transmission that suggests who in the family is at risk. Similarly, individuals in the population cannot be tested for the possession of particular genotypes to determine their cumulative risk of developing a particular disorder. The leads that have been generated from molecular genetic studies are simply not yet understood well enough to allow such uses. However, with continued advancement of laboratory and analytic methods, reliable risk genes for some psychiatric disorders are sure to emerge in the coming years.

Once genetic risk factors for psychiatric conditions become established and widely recognized, they can serve many purposes for early intervention and prevention efforts. For example, an objective, gene-based laboratory test could facilitate the arrival at a primary or differential diagnosis much more quickly than is presently possible. This in turn could speed the initiation of appropriate treatments, which consequently may promote better prognoses (McGlashan 1999). Ultimately, a panel of genetic markers for a mental illness might be administered to high-risk individuals from affected families or in the general population to determine their likelihood of progression toward illness even before any clinical symptoms are manifest, which would allow these individuals to be targeted for early intervention and prevention efforts as well. While recent successes in identifying specific risk genes for mental disorders are encouraging, much more work is needed to replicate and refine these results, and translate them into meaningful clinical applications.

REFERENCES

American Psychiatric Association: Diagnostic and Statistical Manual of Mental Disorders, 4th Edition. Washington, DC, American Psychiatric Association, 1994

Badner JA, Gershon ES: Meta-analysis of whole-genome linkage scans of bipolar disorder and schizophrenia. Mol Psychiatry 7:405–411, 2002a

Badner JA, Gershon ES: Regional meta-analysis of published data supports linkage of autism with markers on chromosome 7. Mol Psychiatry 7:56–66, 2002b

Bailey A, Le Couteur A, Gottesman I, et al: Autism as a strongly genetic disorder: evidence from a British twin study. Psychol Med 25:63–77, 1995

Fanous AH, Van Den Oord EJ, Riley BP, et al: Relationship between a high-risk haplotype in the DTNBP1 (dysbindin) gene and clinical features of schizophrenia. Am J Psychiatry 162:1824–1832, 2005

Faraone SV, Tsuang D, Tsuang MT: Genetics of Mental Disorders: A Guide for Students, Clinicians, and Researchers. New York, Guilford, 1999

Glatt SJ, Faraone SV, Tsuang MT: Meta-analysis identifies an association between the dopamine D2 receptor gene and schizophrenia. Mol Psychiatry 8:911–915, 2003

Green EK, Raybould R, Macgregor S, et al: Operation of the schizophrenia susceptibility gene, neuregulin 1, across traditional diagnostic boundaries to increase risk for bipolar disorder. Arch Gen Psychiatry 62:642–648, 2005

Ioannidis JP, Ntzani EE, Trikalinos TA, et al: Replication validity of genetic association studies. Nat Genet 29:306–309, 2001

Lander ES, Linton LM, Birren B, et al: Initial sequencing and analysis of the human genome. Nature 409:860–921, 2001

Lewis CM, Levinson DF, Wise LH, et al: Genome scan meta-analysis of schizophrenia and bipolar disorder, part II: schizophrenia. Am J Hum Genet 73:34–48, 2003

Lohmueller KE, Pearce CL, Pike M, et al: Meta-analysis of genetic association studies supports a contribution of common variants to susceptibility to common disease. Nat Genet 33:177–182, 2003

Lyons MJ, Eisen SA, Goldberg J, et al: A registry based twin study of depression in men. Arch Gen Psychiatry 55:468–472, 1998

McGlashan TH: Duration of untreated psychosis in first-episode schizophrenia: marker or determinant of course? Biol Psychiatry 46:899–907, 1999

Risch N, Merikangas K: The future of genetic studies of complex human diseases. Science 273:1516–1517, 1996

Segurado R, Detera-Wadleigh SD, Levinson DF, et al: Genome scan meta-analysis of schizophrenia and bipolar disorder, part III: bipolar disorder. Am J Hum Genet 73:49–62, 2003

Thomas DC, Haile RW, Duggan D: Recent developments in genomewide association scans: a workshop summary and review. Am J Hum Genet 77:337–345, 2005

Trikalinos TA, Karvouni A, Zintzaras E, et al: A heterogeneity-based genome search meta-analysis for autism-spectrum disorders. Mol Psychiatry 11:29–36, 2006

2

Environmental Determinants of Psychosis

A Focus on Drug Abuse

Armin Raznahan, M.B.B.S.(Hons), M.R.C.P.C.H., M.R.C.Psych.
Owen G. O'Daly, M.Sc.
Evangelina Maria Tsapakis, B.Sc.(Hons), M.B.B.S., M.R.C.Psych.
Robin M. Murray, D.Sc., F.R.C.Psych.

The importance of genetic factors in schizophrenia is well demonstrated (Cardno et al. 1999; Harrison and Owen 2003), and there is an extensive literature implicating a range of physical and social environmental factors. However, we only briefly touch on the latter in this chapter, as these have been extensively reviewed elsewhere, and instead we discuss the possible causal role of abuse of certain drugs. This is a particularly fruitful environmental factor on which to focus, because the neurobiological effects of substance abuse are relatively well understood.

BRIEF OVERVIEW OF OTHER ENVIRONMENTAL FACTORS

Prenatal and Perinatal Factors

An excess of winter and spring births among children who later develop schizophrenia exists in both the Southern and Northern Hemispheres, although it appears more noticeable, or at least better documented, in the latter (Adams and Kendell 1999; McGrath et al. 1995; Takei et al., in press). Maternal viral infection and malnutrition have been considered as possible explanations.

Elevated rates of schizophrenia were documented in individuals whose mothers were in their second trimester during influenza epidemics (O'Callaghan et al. 1991; Sham et al. 1992). However, these studies were ecological in nature and could not identify those pregnant mothers who were actually infected during the epidemics. Case–control studies that followed mothers known to have been infected with influenza generally failed to demonstrate an association (M. Cannon et al. 1994; Crow and Done 1992). Polio (Suvisaari et al. 1999) and rubella (Brown et al. 2000) have also been implicated. Recently, positive association has been claimed with maternal toxoplasmosis and herpes simplex from studies going back to examine maternal titers in serum collected from pregnant mothers whose offspring subsequently developed schizophrenia (Brown et al. 2005; Torrey et al. 1988). However, controversy continues over 1) whether maternal viral infection has any risk increasing effect on schizophrenia; 2) if it does, which viruses are implicated; and 3) whether the mechanism of any such effect is a specific one or whether the infection acts by simply impairing maternal health.

Susser and colleagues (Susser and Lin 1992; Susser et al. 1996) reported that individuals who were in utero during the Nazi blockade of the Netherlands were twice more likely to later develop schizophrenia. However, because of the fortunate rarity of whole population starvation, it has not been possible to replicate this study. Therefore, the role of prenatal malnutrition cannot be regarded as proven.

A historical review of research into obstetric events was carried out by M. Cannon et al. (2002), who concluded that, overall, obstetric complications had a relatively consistent but modest risk-increasing effect. A meta-analysis of case control studies that used the same measuring instrument (Geddes et al. 1999), found significant effects for maternal preeclampsia, premature rupture of membranes, and need for resuscitation. However, many of the studies included in this meta-analysis were small, the populations were heterogeneous, and the measure of obstetric events was retrospective maternal recall.

Fortunately, a number of larger and better-designed prospective cohort studies were published in the 1990s. T. D. Cannon et al. (2002), who carried out a meta-analysis of these, found robust associations between schizophrenia and complications of pregnancy, abnormal fetal growth and development, and complications of delivery. In short, there is a large measure of agreement that such obstetric hazards increase risk of schizophrenia but much less agreement over the mechanism of this effect, although hypoxia is favored by many (Gilmore and Murray 2006).

Urbanicity, Migration, and Social Factors

Psychosis is strongly associated with urbanicity (Sundquist et al. 2004), an effect that holds for both urban birth and urban upbringing. There is also a dose–response relationship, in that those born in larger towns or cities show proportionally greater risk, and the longer a child lives in an urban setting, the more the risk increases (Pedersen and Mortensen 2001). There is much debate as to what mediates this association, but the association cannot be explained away by neuropsychological impairment, obstetric complications, childhood socioeconomic status, household crowding, or excessive substance misuse. Van Os et al. (2004) have shown that urban birth acts synergistically with familial risk.

Rates of schizophrenia are increased in migrants (Sharpley et al. 2001). This risk is highest in those migrating from developing to developed countries and acts differentially across ethnic groups. Cantor-Graae and Selten (2005) argue, on the basis of this latter point, that psychosocial mechanisms may be involved. What such mechanisms might be is as yet uncertain, but social isolation and discrimination are currently being much researched (Boydell et al. 2004). Recent animal studies, which have shown that dopaminergic systems can be manipulated by means of isolation rearing or social defeat, have provided a theoretical framework as to how social factors might influence risk of psychosis (Selten and Cantor-Graae 2005).

Substance Misuse

Prevalence of Substance Misuse in Psychosis

Patients with schizophrenia have high levels of drug use (Table 2–1), although the rates vary considerably. This variation probably reflects both genuine differences in prevalence and also in the methodology employed. However, it is clear that there is an association between drug use in general and psychosis, both in patient populations and the general public (Johns et al. 2004; Murray et al. 2002).

The question of an association between schizophrenia and alcohol, opiates, and benzodiazepines remains open to debate (Miller and Guttman 1997; Murray et al. 2002; Phillips and Johnson 2001; Stimmel 1996). Furthermore, although nicotine is the drug most used by individuals with schizophrenia, there is little evidence to suggest that it plays a causal role in psychosis. Therefore, we concentrate here on the psychostimulants amphetamine, methamphetamine, and cocaine, which have long been known to produce at least short-term psychosis; the as-yet-relatively-understudied psychostimulant khat; and cannabis, whose putative causal role in schizophrenia has aroused much recent interest.

Psychostimulants.　The association between psychostimulant use and schizophrenia has been well supported (Boutros and Bowers 1996; Schneier et al. 1987). Thus, studies comparing psychostimulant abuse in subjects with schizophrenia and controls found more psychostimulant use in the former (Bartlett et al. 1997; Brady et al. 1990; Manschreck 1988). A review by Batel (2000) reported an average lifetime prevalence of stimulant use in schizophrenia patients of 26.5%, but individual reports have ranged up to 50% (Brady et al. 1990, 1991; Chen et al. 2003; DeQuardo et al. 1994; Lysaker et al. 1994; Mueser et al. 1990). Studies from Southeast Asia (Chen et al. 2003) and the Americas (SAMSHA 2000) suggest that in these regions, stimulant use among the general population is relatively common, and this common use is reflected in patient populations. For example, within a 2-year recruitment period in Taiwan, Chen et al. (2003) were able to identify 174 individuals presenting with methamphetamine-induced psychosis. Predictably, changing patterns of drug use in the general population are also reflected in patient populations. For example, in the U.S., cocaine abuse emerged in the 1980s as a major problem among schizophrenic patients, and methamphetamine abuse began rising dramatically in the late 1990s (Lysaker et al. 1994; Mueser et al. 1990; Ziedonis and Trudeau 1997). By contrast, in an epidemiological study of individuals with schizophrenia in London, the self-reported lifetime stimulant misuse was only 8.7% (Duke et al. 2001).

Cannabis.　Cannabis is the most widely used illicit substance worldwide (Bauman and Phongsavan 1999) and is the illicit drug most commonly used by people with psychosis (Fowler et al. 1998; Menezes et al. 1996). Thus, Hafner et al. (1999) found that among psychotic patients using illicit drugs in Germany, 88% actually used cannabis. Reports of a positive association between cannabis consumption and psychosis have come from many countries and cultures since the nineteenth century (Andreasson et al. 1987; Commission IHD 1894; Degenhardt et al. 2001; Linszen et al. 1994; Mueser et al. 2000). Studies of patients with schizophrenia have found the lifetime prevalence of cannabis abuse to range from

Table 2–1. Representative studies of drug use prevalence in patients with schizophrenia

Study	Country	Drug use prevalence
Blanchard et al. 2000	USA	Lifetime history of drug use in patients 40%–50%
Regier et al. 1988, 1990	USA	47% of patients met criteria for substance abuse compared with only 17% of the general population
Verdoux et al. 1996	France	43% of patients used drugs
Menezes et al. 1996	United Kingdom	36% of patients had used drugs within the past year
Modestin et al. 1997	Switzerland	54% of patients tested positive for substance use, 33% for alcohol or barbiturates, 25% for cannabis, and 20% for opiates and/or cocaine
Cassano et al. 1998	Italy	11.5% of patients with schizophrenia had comorbid substance abuse
Soyka et al. 1993	Germany	Lifetime prevalence estimated for two groups between 21.8% and 42.9%; 3 month prevalence of 21.3% and 29%
Fowler et al. 1998	Australia	26.8% of patients had used drugs within the past 6 months; however, lifetime prevalence for drug use was 59.8%
Jablensky et al. 2000	Australia	36% of men had psychotic illness; 16% of women used drugs

12% to 42% (Andreasson et al. 1987; Arndt et al. 1992; Dixon et al. 1991; Fowler et al. 1998; Linszen et al. 1994; Longhurst 1997; Mathers et al. 1991; Rolfe et al. 1993).

The prevalence of cannabis use in the general population and in patient groups is of course influenced by the availability of the drug. Nevertheless, a number of large cross-sectional national surveys have found that whatever the availability, patients with schizophrenia are approximately twice as likely to use cannabis as the general population (Hall and Degenhardt 2000; Regier et al. 1990; Robins and Regier 1991; Tien and Anthony 1990; van Os et al. 2002). This is supported by studies from as far a field as Malta (Grech 1998), South Africa (Rottanburg et al. 1982), and the West Indies (Knight 1976).

Hambrecht and Hafner (1996) found that one-third of patients with schizophrenia had used cannabis at least a year prior to the onset of their illness. A further one-third reported using cannabis during the development of symptoms. The final one-third of patients reported starting to use cannabis after their symptoms had developed.

In summary, patients with schizophrenia engage in substance abuse to a greater extent than the general population, and, apart from nicotine which is outside the scope of this review, the evidence of association is strongest for psychostimulants and for cannabis. The next logical questions are why this occurs and whether a plausible explanatory model can be constructed.

Nature of the Association Between Schizophrenia and Substance Use

The clear associations outlined in the previous subsection are of clinical significance as patients abusing psychostimulants and cannabis are known to have an earlier onset of psychosis, more symptomatic exacerbations, more frequent hospitalizations, poorer social functioning, and poorer compliance with treatment than non-drug abusers (Dixon et al. 1990; Margoles et al. 2004; Seibyl et al. 1993; Veen et al. 2004).

The many hypotheses put forward to explain the nature of the association between substance abuse and schizophrenia fall into three broad (though not necessarily mutually exclusive) groups: 1) those that suggest psychosis increases the risk of substance abuse, 2) those arguing for a shared common factor increasing the risk of both disorders and 3) those that argue explicitly for a causal role of substance abuse in the emergence of psychosis. We address each of these in turn.

Psychosis increases the risk of substance abuse. The independent-factor hypothesis sees substance misuse as a route to social identity and group membership among individuals with psychosis, who are prone to social isolation. There is little evidence in its favor.

The self-medication hypothesis argues that individuals with psychosis use illicit substances to ameliorate distressing symptoms and stems from observations that 1) many patients report subjective improvements after using illicit substances (Dixon et al. 1990), 2) amphetamines may improve negative symptoms (van Kammen and Boronow 1988), and 3) patients with schizophrenia who abuse cannabis report fewer symptoms of psychosis, depression, and anxiety than those who do not use cannabis (Dixon et al. 1990; Mueser et al. 2000). Several findings however, argue against such a hypothesis: Other psychiatric patients with distressing symptoms do not show the levels of substance abuse seen in psychosis (Glassman et al. 1992; Pohl et al. 1992), substance misuse in psychosis is associated with a poorer clinical outcome (Grech et al. 2005), and drug use by patients often precedes the manifestation of symptoms or the receipt of antipsychotic medication (Berti 1994; Buckley et al. 1998).

Substance abuse and psychosis are associated through shared causal factors. The common-factor hypothesis proposes common etiological factors for substance abuse and schizophrenia, be they genetic (Tsuang et al. 1982) or related to antisocial personality (Mueser et al. 1998). Chambers et al. (2001) presented a related model that has been dubbed the *primary addiction*. In this model, the underlying neuropathology of schizophrenia (which involves alterations in the neuroanatomical circuitry regulating positive reinforcement, incentive motivation, and behavioral inhibition) is seen as giving rise independently to both psychotic symptoms and a predilection to addiction. To date, there is little available data validating either of these hypotheses.

Substance misuse increases the risk of schizophrenia. This vulnerability hypothesis is supported by the observation that drug use often precedes the emergence of schizophrenia symptoms or the administration of medication and that earlier onset is observed in patients who abuse drugs (Allebeck et al. 1993; Andreasson et al. 1987; Rabinowitz et al. 1998; Tsuang et al. 1982). This model can sit comfortably with the common-factor and primary-addiction hypotheses, which argue for increased levels of substance abuse in individuals at risk of developing schizophrenia. The remainder of this chapter will be devoted to examining the evidence for the vulnerability proposal and to possible mechanisms.

CONTRIBUTION OF SUBSTANCE MISUSE TO PSYCHOSIS

Psychostimulants

In the late 1950s, Connell (1958) reported 36 amphetamine-using patients with schizophrenia-like symptoms, of whom 9 developed protracted symptoms lasting over 2 months and 3 had symptoms indefinitely. Amphetamines and cocaine both trigger brief psychotic episodes and intensify preexisting symptoms (Poole and Brabbins 1996; Turner and Tsuang 1990). Indeed, psychostimulant use is said to produce a syndrome indistinguishable from schizophrenia (Boutros and Bowers 1996; Flaum and Schultz 1996). A dose–response relationship has been reported between plasma levels of amphetamines and psychopathology in patients presenting to emergency departments with psychostimulant psychosis (Batki and Harris 2004). However, in most cases the psychostimulant-induced psychotic symptoms are only transient.

Among 60 patients admitted for amphetamine-related conditions who had been using oral or intravenous amphetamine for a mean of 3.7 years (Angrist and Gersheron 1969), 32% reported experiencing a paranoid hallucinatory psychosis. A smaller study (Bell 1973) elicited psychosis in 12 of 14 amphetamine-dependent patients, usually within 35–70 minutes of the start of an intravenous infusion of the drug. The picture was characterized primarily by paranoid delusions, which were observed in 12 of 14 subjects, although in most cases these delusions were of only mild intensity. The psychotic state lasted for 1–2 days in 9 cases and for 6 days in two cases, and 26 days in a patient who was actually found to be covertly ingesting more psychostimulants while in hospital.

Curran et al. (2004) recently conducted a systematic review of experimental, case–control, and longitudinal studies investigating psychostimulant use and psychosis in humans. The majority of experimental studies identified involved single doses of dexamphetamine or methylphenidate given intravenously to subjects with schizophrenia. A subset of studies also used a control group. A meta-analysis was performed to compare the differences in response between control subjects, subjects with schizophrenia in remission, and subjects with positive symptoms. The rates of increased positive symptoms were 10.2%, 28.3%, and 51.4%, respectively. Among individuals with schizophrenia, no significant effect of antipsychotic medication on the response to a single dose of stimulants was found. When subjects with psychotic disorders who abused psychostimulants were compared with similarly diagnosed individuals who did not, those abusing psychostimulants showed a lower age of illness onset, fewer negative symptoms, more paranoid themes, fewer first-rank symptoms, and more hallucinatory experiences (Dermatis et al. 1998; Lysaker et al. 1994; Rosse et al. 1994; Serper et al. 1995; Seibyl et al. 1993).

Some investigators have followed up individuals prescribed psychostimulants. Cherland and Fitzpatrick (1999) found that over a 5-year period, 9 of 192 children prescribed psychostimulants for ADHD developed mood-incongruent psychotic symptoms. Pawluck and Gorey (1995) reported that over 5 years, 2 of 11 adults receiving methylphenidate for narcolepsy developed psychotic symptoms. A Japanese study (Iwanami et al. 1994) described 104 patients; 16% of these displayed persistent psychotic behavior long after the methamphetamine and metabolites had been eliminated from the body; thus, while psychostimulant-induced psychosis is often transient, with chronic use the duration of illness may be prolonged.

There have been many reports of an association between the use of khat and psychosis. Khat is a shrub traditionally chewed in certain parts of East Africa and the Middle East whose leaves contain the amphetamine-like psychostimulant compound cathinone (Asuni and Pela 1986). Using a case–control design, Odenwald et al. (2005) investigated the association between khat use and psychotic symptoms in a Somalian population survey. They found that compared with control subjects, individuals with severe psychotic symptoms had significantly higher levels of khat use, and started using khat earlier in life. The amount of khat used prior to symptom onset correlated positively with certain positive symptoms, while the amount of khat used at the time of assessment, correlated negatively with negative symptoms. Despite potential selection and information bias and the confounding effect of "child soldiering," this study adds to existing data (Dhadphale and Omolo 1988; Numan 2004) in arguing for a significant association between khat use and psychosis.

Cannabis

Few would argue against the evidence that cannabis can exacerbate preexisting psychotic symptoms or trigger their reemergence (Mathers and Ghodse 1992; Negrete et al. 1986; Thornicroft 1990). Intravenous administration of tetrahydrocannabinol (THC) to normal subjects also produces transient symptoms, behaviors, and cognitive deficits that resemble those seen in non-substance-related psychosis (D'Souza et al. 2004). However, there has been controversy about whether the psychosis persists beyond cessation of cannabis use, and whether it can cause the onset of psychosis de novo (Johns 2001).

If cannabis has a causal effect on the development of schizophrenia, then there should be evidence of a dose–response relationship (Thornicroft 1990). A study of Swedish army conscripts found that cannabis use increased the likelihood of developing schizophrenia twofold (Andreasson et al. 1987), with the increased risk rising to six times greater in heavy users (Andreasson et al. 1987, 1988). The latter risk dropped to 2.9-fold once psychiatric diagnosis at conscription was controlled for, to eliminate any potential self-medication confounds. A more recent study of the same cohort again found a dose–response relationship, with heavy cannabis use increasing the risk of psychosis 6.9-fold, dropping to 3.1 times the risk after adjustment for confounders (Table 2–2). A similar study of Israeli army conscripts (Weiser et al. 2002) demonstrated that those who later received treatment for schizophrenia had previously reported higher levels of drug use (mainly cannabis) than had those not requiring later treatment (12.4% vs. 5.9%). This study, however, did not control for the confounding influence of other drug use and did not test for a dose–response relationship (see Table 2–2).

Findings from two New Zealand–based birth cohort studies have also been reported. The Dunedin study found that cannabis use at age 15 years increased the risk of schizophreniform disorder at age 26 years from 3% to 10% (Arseneault et al. 2002); this study controlled for preexisting psychotic symptoms, thus ruling out any explanation based on the self-medication hypothesis. The Christchurch study found that for individuals who met diagnostic criteria for cannabis dependence at age 18 and 21 years, the risk of psychosis was 3.7 and 2.3 times greater, respectively, than that for individuals without cannabis dependence (Fergusson et al. 2003). Both of these studies suggested that the earlier the cannabis use, the greater the risk of schizophrenia (see Table 2–2). Such findings clearly point to the public health hazards posed by the rise in cannabis use among adolescents.

A Dutch population-based study found that individuals using cannabis at the time of the baseline interview were three times more likely to manifest psychotic symptoms 3 years later (van Os et al. 2002); this result remained significant after investigators controlled for a range of potential confounds. Furthermore, a cannabis dose effect was observed, and lifetime use at the first assessment was a stronger predictor of psychosis at 3 years than cannabis use at follow-up, implying that the psychosis was not simply a reflection of current cannabis intoxication.

More recently, interest has grown in exploring the degree to which cannabis use influences the expression of psychosis when the latter is conceived of as a continuum (Johns and Van Os 2001). Stefanis et al. (2004) demonstrated in a cross-sectional survey that lifetime cannabis use among a community sample of 19-year-olds was positively associated with both positive and negative dimensions of psychosis. The greater the amount of cannabis used, the stronger the association with psychotic symptoms. Furthermore, a stronger effect was found in those subjects who had used cannabis earlier, regardless of the frequency with which they had used it (Stefanis et al. 2004).

Semple et al. (2005) conducted a timely systematic review of the rapidly growing number of studies investigating the association between cannabis exposure and psychosis. A meta-analysis of the odds ratios for cannabis exposure among individuals with psychosis generated by case–control designs (both cross sectional and nested within prospective cohorts) arrived at overall odds ratio of 2.9 (95% confidence interval = 2.3–3.6) with random effect modeling. No publication bias was detected. Studies comparing psychotic symptoms in groups with varying cannabis exposure were also reviewed; these studies were found to not only consistently report a significantly elevated number of individuals with psychotic symptoms among cannabis users, but also to demonstrate a dose–response relationship. These findings suggest that earlier exposure to cannabis is associated with an even higher risk of later psychosis.

Despite the repeatedly demonstrated and robust association between cannabis use and psychosis, legitimate questions have been asked about potential methodological limitations (Macleod et al. 2004), namely 1) could the observed association largely reflect the effects of residual confounding? and 2) could the observed association be accounted for by reverse causality? In attempting to provide answers, Fergusson et al. (2005) recently employed sophisticated statistical techniques in a further analysis of data from the Christchurch cohort. Their findings argue for a negative answer to both questions.

MECHANISMS BY WHICH SUBSTANCE MISUSE CAUSES PSYCHOSIS

The neurobiological mechanisms underlying psychosis consequent upon drug abuse have been extensively studied, and although much remains to be explained, an etiopathological framework is now starting to emerge that implicates anomalies in dopamine transmission in both the reinforcing effects of drugs of abuse and in schizophrenia.

Dopamine and Mechanisms of Drug Reward

The mesocorticolimbic system consists of dopamine neurons, which project from the ventral tegmental area (VTA) to the nucleus accumbens (NAc), the frontal cortex, the olfactory tubercle, the amygdala, and the septal area. Animal

Table 2–2. Longitudinal studies of the relationship between cannabis use and the development of schizophrenia

Study	Country	Population (size)	Follow-up period, years	Cannabis use defined as	Diagnostic criteria	Adjusted risk effect size (OR)	Dose–response relationship	Confounding factors
Andreasson et al. 1987, 1988	Sweden[a]	Conscript cohort (45,570)	15	Use >50 times at age 18 years	ICD-8	2.3	Yes	Psychiatric diagnosis at conscription, parents divorced
Zammit et al. 2002	Sweden[a]	Conscript cohort (50,053)	27	Use >50 times at age 18 years	ICD-8/9	3.1	Yes	Diagnosis at conscription, IQ, social integration, disturbed upbringing, cigarette smoking in place of upbringing
Van Os et al. 2002	Netherlands	Population-based (4,104)	3	Use at baseline (age 16–17 years)	BPRS	2.76	Yes	Age, gender, ethnic group, single marital status, education, urban dwelling
Fergusson et al. 2003	New Zealand	Birth cohort (1,011)	3	DSM-IV cannabis dependence at age 21 years	SCL-90	1.8	N/A	Use of other drugs between follow-ups; gender, IQ, parental criminality

Table 2–2. Longitudinal studies of the relationship between cannabis use and the development of schizophrenia *(continued)*

Study	Country	Population (size)	Follow-up period, years	Cannabis use defined as	Diagnostic criteria	Adjusted risk effect size (OR)	Dose–response relationship	Confounding factors
Arseneault et al. 2002	New Zealand	Birth cohort (759)	11	Use by age 15 years; continued at 18 years	DSM-IV		N/A	Gender, social class, psychotic symptoms prior to cannabis use
Weiser et al. 2002	Israel[a]	Conscript cohort (50,413)	4–15	Sporadic users not included	ICD-9	2.0	N/A	Use of other drugs

Note. BPRS = Brief Psychiatric Rating Scale; SCL-90 = 90-item Symptom Checklist.
[a]Males only.

studies suggest that this dopaminergic system underpins the reinforcing effect of drugs of abuse (Koob 1992; Milner 1991; Nestler 1992), and that psychostimulants increase extracellular dopamine concentration in the NAc (Di Chiara and Imperato 1988; Tanda et al. 1997). The active component of cannabis, delta-9-tetrahydrocannabinol (Δ9-THC), is also known to cause dopamine release in both the nucleus accumbens and the medial prefrontal cortex (Gardner et al. 1991; Tanda et al. 1997). Furthermore, studies in both animals and humans suggest that dopamine agonists induce craving for drugs such as cocaine and nicotine (Breiter et al. 1997; Chambers et al. 2001; Ito et al. 2000; Stein et al. 1998; Stewart 2000) by stimulating the NAc.

Functional magnetic resonance imaging studies conducted in humans during infusion of drugs of abuse (Breiter et al. 1997; Stein et al. 1998) and cue-induced cravings for such drugs (Garavan et al. 2000; Maas et al. 1998; Schnieder et al. 2001; Wexler et al. 2001) confirm that addictive drugs activate the dopaminergic mesolimbic pathway. Positron emission tomography studies in humans have shown that blockade of the dopamine transporter by psychostimulants elicits the increase of extracellular dopamine in the ventral striatum and the reinforcing effects of the drugs (Volkow et al. 1997, 1999).

Dopamine codes for reward, for reward-associated stimuli, and for the motivation to procure the reward (Schultz et al. 2000). However, there is evidence that dopamine can be released before the consummation of "pleasure" (Berridge and Robinson 1998; Kapur and Mann 1992; McClure et al. 2003), and that increased dopamine release may lead to greater "wanting or craving" rather than "liking" of a drug (McClure et al. 2003; Zink et al. 2003). In drug-addicted subjects, there is decreased expression of D_2 receptors in the striatum, a decrease in dopamine release, and reduced activity of the orbitofrontal cortex (Martinez et al. 2004; Volkow et al. 2004). However, when addicted patients are exposed to drug-related stimuli, these hypodopaminergic regions, and associated structures, become hyperactive (Volkow et al. 2004).

Dopamine Hypothesis of Schizophrenia

The dopamine hypothesis of schizophrenia derives from the evidence that 1) direct or indirect dopamine agonists elicit positive symptoms of schizophrenia and 2) all antipsychotics block dopamine D_2–like receptors (Carlsson 1988, 1995; Carlsson and Lindqvist 1963; Davis et al. 1991; Lieberman et al. 1997, 2001; Snyder 1976). In the original formulation of the dopamine hypothesis, schizophrenic symptoms were thought to be caused by excessive dopamine transmission within the brain as a whole (Carlsson and Lindqvist 1963). However, the current model suggests that positive psychotic symptoms are mediated by excessive mesolimbic (VTA-NAc) dopaminergic activity, with negative symptoms resulting from a hypodopaminergic state in the frontal cortex (Carlsson 1995; Davis et al. 1991; Weinberger 1987).

Evidence for the excessive mesolimbic transmission has come from radioligand imaging studies demonstrating exaggerated dopamine release in the ventral striatum of patients with schizophrenia, in response to an amphetamine challenge (Abi-Dargham et al. 1998; Breier et al. 1997; Laruelle et al. 1996). The extent of this dopamine release was correlated with the degree of symptomatic exacerbation elicited by the drug challenge (Laruelle 2000). Furthermore, dopamine D_2/D_3 receptors have been reported to be elevated in schizophrenia (Abi-Dargham et al. 2000; Weinberger and Laruelle 2001). Finally, a number of reports have suggested abnormalities of presynaptic dopamine function (as indexed by ^{18}F-DOPA uptake) in schizophrenia (Hietala et al. 1995, 1999; Lindstrom et al. 1999; McGowan et al. 2004; Meyer-Lindenberg et al. 2002; Reith et al. 1994), although not all studies agree (Dao-Castellana et al. 1997; Elkashef et al. 2000). Overall, however, there is good evidence for altered dopaminergic transmission in the ventral striatum (including the NAc) in schizophrenia.

Kapur (2003) links excessive dopamine release in the mesolimbic system with psychotic symptoms by postulating that the former produces dysfunction in the dopamine-mediated mechanism of salience attribution. In essence, he suggests that because one function of dopamine is to "grab the attention" of the individual and thus to convert neutral stimuli into emotionally salient ones, excessive mesolimbic dopamine can cause the individual to attribute salience to inappropriate perceptions or thoughts. In this way, the individual establishes apparently meaningful connections between coincident events. Furthermore, the mesocorticolimbic pathway has a well-defined role in mediating the behavioral effects of stress exposure (Deutch et al. 1990; Kalivas and Stewart 1991) and the initial emergence, and relapse, of schizophrenia is often precipitated by stressful events (Norman and Malla 1993a, 1993b).

Dopamine Sensitization as a Shared Neurochemical Mechanism

Thus, activation of mesolimbic dopaminergic neurons may play a critical role in the pathogenesis of both drug dependence and schizophrenia. Behavioral sensitization provides a possible mechanism by which the posited dopaminergic abnormalities may develop. Intermittent pharmacological (or environmental) stimulation produces a progressive and enduring enhancement of a behavioral response, rather than the expected decrease in response (tolerance). Sensitization has been proposed as a model of the establishment of cue-dependent crav-ing and the relapse to drug taking in humans (Robinson and Berridge 1993), and most drugs of abuse have been shown to induce behavioral sensitization (Gorriti et al. 1999; Hooks et al. 1992a, 1992b; Schulz and Herz 1997; Shuster et al. 1977; Vanderschuren and Kalivas 2000), contingent on stimulation of dopa-mine terminal fields within the NAc (Kalivas and Stewart 1991).

Dopamine sensitization has also been proposed for a critical role in the pro-duction of positive symptoms of schizophrenia. As noted earlier, patients show an increase of dopamine release after amphetamine, suggesting that schizophre-nia might be associated with a state of endogenous sensitization (Laruelle 2000). Similar findings among subjects with schizotypal personality disorder (SPD) (Abi-Dargham et al. 2004) suggest that dopamine dysregulation in schizophre-nia spectrum disorders might have a trait component, being present in remitted patients with schizophrenia and in SPD, and an additional state component, as-sociated with psychotic exacerbations. Patients with schizophrenia are also par-ticularly sensitive to the psychosis-inducing effects of Δ9-THC, which is again compatible with a sensitized dopaminergic state (D'Souza et al. 2004).

Interestingly, repeated cocaine exposure in humans results in short-term psychotic symptoms being triggered more rapidly and after smaller amounts of cocaine (Bartlett et al. 1997). Patients with schizophrenia who are acutely ill or close to relapse and have had no previous exposure to psychostimulants have transient worsening of psychotic symptoms upon initial administration of am-phetamine, returning to their previous level of symptoms within a few hours (Lieberman et al. 1997). Furthermore, patients with schizophrenia fail to display the expected enhanced response on repeated administration, leading to the sug-gestion that they are already "maximally sensitized" to the dopamine-releasing effects of amphetamine (Strakowski et al. 1997).

Dopamine exerts modulatory influence within a number of cortico-striato-thalamo-cortical circuits. Schizophrenia is associated with a dysfunction in these circuits (Carlsson 1995; Deutch 1993; Laruelle et al. 2003; Weinberger 1987). Furthermore, as prefrontal lesions can also lead to increased (disinhib-ited) striatal function (Pycock et al. 1980), the enhanced sensitivity to subcorti-cal dopamine reported in schizophrenia and in substance abuse may be the result of the loss of "buffering" effect of the prefrontal cortex (Laruelle et al. 2003; Tzschentke 2001).

In summary, it seems that interconnected limbic, cortical, and subcortical circuits are implicated in both substance abuse and schizophrenia, and dopamine sensitization may underlie both conditions. The neurotransmitter glutamate, a number of intracellular signaling cascades (Svenningsson et al. 2003), and the dopamine D_3 receptor (*DRD3*) (Guillin et al. 2000; Gurevich et al. 1997; Staley and Mash 1996) have attracted much attention in relation to the development of dopamine sensitization, but unfortunately a fuller exploration of these is beyond the bounds of this chapter; they are discussed in O'Daly et al. (2005).

GENE–ENVIRONMENT INTERACTION

Only a minority of individuals who use cannabis and/or psychostimulants develop psychosis. An important question, therefore, is why some drug abusers develop psychosis while others do not. Some light was shed on this question by Chen et al. (2003) and Chen and Murray (2004) who showed that 174 methamphetamine abusers who developed psychosis showed more familial/genetic loading for schizophrenia and more childhood schizoid and schizotypal traits than 271 methamphetamine abusers who were able to continue abuse without any such symptoms; the length of the psychosis was also predicted by the same familial and childhood factors (Chen and Murray 2004).

A similar spectrum of liability may influence the reaction to cannabis (Arseneault et al. 2004; Stefanis et al. 2004). Thus, McGuire et al. (1995) found that people with cannabis-related psychosis had an increased familial morbidity risk for schizophrenia. An interesting French study asked nonpsychotic cannabis users to complete a questionnaire to assess their proneness to develop psychosis (Verdoux et al. 2002). Those with low scores reported experiencing enhanced levels of pleasure when using cannabis, whereas those with high scores for psychosis proneness responded to cannabis with increased hostility and suspiciousness. One possibility is that differences in genes controlling the dopamine system may underlie these individual differences in response to psychostimulants and cannabis.

Dopamine D_2–Like Receptor Genes

Dopamine receptor genes present themselves as obvious candidate genes in an exploration of the genetic basis of psychostimulant use in general, and psychostimulant-induced psychosis in particular. A recent association study compared dopamine D_2–like receptor polymorphisms (*DRD2* Taq IA, *DRD3* Ser9Gly, and *DRD4* exon III variable tandem repeat) in methamphetamine abusers, methamphetamine abusers with methamphetamine-induced psychosis, and healthy control subjects (Chen et al. 2004). Compared with control subjects, methamphetamine abusers had a higher prevalence of the seven-repeat *DRD4* allele. However, none of the markers studied were associated with methamphetamine-induced psychosis.

Catechol-O-Methyltransferase

The catechol-O-methyltransferase (COMT) gene (*COMT*) is positioned on chromosome 22q11, a region that has been linked with schizophrenia in genome scans (Lewis et al. 2003) and on the basis of its deletion in the velocardiofacial syndrome, which carries a risk of schizophrenia 30 times that of the general population (Murphy et al. 1999). A functional Val/Met polymorphism of *COMT* determines activity of the resultant enzyme, and consequently COMT activity increases from those with the Met/Met genotype through Met/Val to those with Val/Val (Mannisto and Kaakola 1999). Some family studies suggest differential transmission of the high-activity Val allele to individuals with schizophrenia, although a meta-analysis of case–control studies failed to find a significant association (Glatt et al. 2003; Li et al. 1996).

The *COMT* Val allele and chronic cannabis use have both been independently linked to impaired frontal function in both neurocognitive and functional imaging studies (Block et al. 2002; Egan et al. 2001; Lundqvist et al. 2001; Solowijj et al. 2002), and also to decreased frontal but increased mesolimbic dopamine (Akil et al. 2003; Tanda et al. 1997; Voruganti et al. 2001). An obvious question is whether there is any interaction between the two in causing psychosis.

In a recent extension of the Dunedin cohort study previously discussed, Caspi et al. (2005) investigated the effect that variation in *COMT* has on the risk of adult schizophrenia in adolescents using cannabis. Eight hundred and three individuals were placed in one of three groups according to *COMT* genotype (Met/Met, Val/Met, Val/Val), and genotype was then examined in relation to adolescent cannabis use. At age 26 years, subjects with a lifetime diagnosis of schizophrenia or schizophreniform disorder were identified with DSM criteria, and dimensional measures of psychosis were also generated at this age. In the analysis, adult cannabis use, amphetamine or hallucinogen use at ages 21 and 22 years, psychotic symptoms at age 11 years, childhood IQ, and conduct disorder were all controlled for.

While adolescent cannabis use did not appear to increase the risk of schizophreniform psychosis in those with the Met/Met genotype, it had a modest risk-increasing effect in those with Met/Val, and it produced a striking increase in risk among those with the Val/Val genotype. Adolescent cannabis use also showed a significant positive association with dimensional measures of psychosis in those with the Val/Val (but not Met/Met), a finding that persisted after all of the confounders above were controlled for. In a preliminary report, Henquet et al. (2005) showed that in experimental studies, subjects with the Val/Val genotype show a greater decrease in verbal memory and more auditory hallucinations than those with the Met/Met genotype when given a cannabis cigarette to smoke.

CONCLUSION

It is clear from the evidence that we have reviewed above that abuse of psychostimulants and cannabis may influence many aspects of psychosis: inception, cross-sectional clinical profile (Kavanagh et al. 2004), and longitudinal course (Dixon et al. 1990; Seibyl et al. 1993). One must be careful to tease association and causation apart for each of these, and to recognize that causative roads are rarely one-way. Nevertheless it does seem that the abuse of both types of drugs can increase the risk of developing psychosis, and that they probably do so by inducing dopamine sensitization. We have suggested elsewhere (Murray et al. 2002) that there may exist a spectrum of liability to psychosis, from, at the one extreme, individuals who need to consume large quantities of drugs to induce transient psychosis to, at the other extreme, vulnerable individuals who are precipitated into chronic psychosis on minimal use; the latter group are likely to share more genetic and environmental risk factors for psychosis than the former.

CLINICAL IMPLICATIONS

The literature on substance abuse and psychosis makes a compelling argument for the clinically deleterious effects of drugs in people with an elevated vulnerability to psychosis. Although we cannot yet predict which individuals will develop psychosis and which will not, we can counsel individuals in high-risk categories (e.g., relatives of individuals with schizophrenia) to avoid engaging in behaviors (i.e., substance abuse) that will increase their risk of psychosis to levels that are many times higher than the risk in the general population. Moreover, although the current evidence for an association between substance abuse and psychosis is strongest for psychostimulants and cannabis, other drugs (e.g., opiates) also affect some of the same neurobiological systems (e.g., dopamine transmission and reinforcement mechanisms) and are likely to increase clinical vulnerability as well.

REFERENCES

Abi-Dargham A, Gil R, Krystal J, et al: Increased striatal dopamine transmission in schizophrenia: confirmation in a second cohort. Am J Psychiatry 155:761–767, 1998

Abi-Dargham A, Rodenhiser J, Printz D, et al: Increased baseline occupancy of D2 receptors by dopamine in schizophrenia. Proc Natl Acad Sci U S A 97:8104–8109, 2000

Abi-Dargham A, Kegeles LS, Zea-Ponce Y, et al: Striatal amphetamine-induced dopamine release in patients with schizotypal personality disorder studied with single photon emission computed tomography and [123I]iodobenzamide. Biol Psychiatry 55:1001–1006, 2004

Adams W, Kendell RE: Annual variation in birth rate of people who subsequently develop schizophrenia. Br J Psychiatry 175:522–552, 1999

Akil M, Kolachana BS, Rothmond DA, et al: Catechol-O-methyltransferase genotype and dopamine regulation in the human brain. J Neurosci 23:2008–2013, 2003

Allebeck P, Adamsson C, Engstrom A, et al: Cannabis and schizophrenia: a longitudinal study of cases treated in Stockholm County. Acta Psychiatr Scand 88:21–24, 1993

Andreasson S, Allebeck P, Engstrom A, et al: Cannabis and schizophrenia. A longitudinal study of Swedish conscripts. Lancet 2(8574):1483–1486, 1987

Andreasson S, Allebeck P, Engstrom A, et al: Cannabis and schizophrenia. Lancet 1(8592):1000–1001, 1988

Angrist BM, Gersheron S: Amphetamine abuse in New York City—1966 to 1968. Semin Psychiatry 1:195–207, 1969

Arndt S, Tyrrell G, Flaum M, et al: Comorbidity of substance abuse and schizophrenia: the role of premorbid adjustment. Psychol Med 22:379–388, 1992

Arseneault L, Cannon M, Poulton R, et al: Cannabis use in adolescence and risk for adult psychosis: longitudinal prospective study. BMJ 325:1212–1213, 2002

Arseneault L, Cannon M, Witton J, et al: Causal association between cannabis and psychosis: examination of the evidence. Br J Psychiatry 184:110–117, 2004

Asuni T, Pela OA: Drug abuse in Africa. Bull Narcotics 38:55–64, 1986

Bartlett E, Hallin A, Chapman B, et al: Selective sensitization to the psychosis-inducing effects of cocaine: a possible marker for addiction relapse vulnerability? Neuropsychopharmacology 16:77–82, 1997

Batel P: Addiction and schizophrenia. Eur Psychiatry 15:115–122, 2000

Batki SL, Harris DS: Quantitative drug levels in stimulant psychosis: relationship to symptom severity, catecholamines and hyperkinesia. Am J Addict 13:461–470, 2004

Bauman A, Phongsavan P: Epidemiology of substance use in adolescence: prevalence, trends and policy implications. Drug Alcohol Depend 55:187–207, 1999

Bell DS: The experimental reproduction of amphetamine psychosis. Arch Gen Psychiatry 29:35–40, 1973

Berridge KC, Robinson T: What is the role of dopamine in reward: hedonic impact, reward learning, or incentive salience? Brain Res Rev 28:309–369, 1998

Berti A: Schizophrenia and substance abuse: the interface. Prog Neuropsychopharmacol Biol Psychiatry 18:279–284, 1994

Blanchard JJ, Brown SA, Horan WP, et al: Substance use disorders in schizophrenia: review, integration, and a proposed model. Clin Psychol Rev 20:207–234, 2000

Block RI, O'Leary DS, Hichwa RD, et al: Effects of frequent marijuana use on memory-related regional cerebral blood flow. Pharmacol Biochem Behav 72(1–2):237–250, 2002

Boutros NN, Bowers MB Jr: Chronic substance-induced psychotic disorders: state of the literature. J Neuropsychiatry Clin Neurosci 8:262–269, 1996

Boydell J, van Os J, Murray RM: Is there a role for social factors in a comprehensive model for schizophrenia? in Neurodevelopment and Schizophrenia. Edited by Keshavan M, Kennedy J, Murray RM. Cambridge, UK, Cambridge University Press, 2004, pp 224–247

Brady K, Anton R, Ballenger JC, et al: Cocaine abuse among schizophrenic patients. Am J Psychiatry 147:1164–1167, 1990

Brady K, Casto S, Lydiard RB, et al: Substance abuse in an inpatient psychiatric sample. Am J Drug Alcohol Abuse 17:389–397, 1991

Breier A, Su TP, Saunders R, et al: Schizophrenia is associated with elevated amphetamine-induced synaptic dopamine concentrations: evidence from a novel positron emission tomography method. Proc Natl Acad Sci U S A 94:2569–2574, 1997

Breiter HC, Gollub RL, Weisskoff RM, et al: Acute effects of cocaine on human brain activity and emotion. Neuron 19:591–611, 1997

Brown AS, Cohen P, Greenwald S, et al: Nonaffective psychosis after prenatal exposure to rubella. Am J Psychiatry 157:438–443, 2000

Brown AS, Schaefer CA, Charles PQ, et al: Maternal exposure to toxoplasmosis and risk of schizophrenia in adult offspring. Am J Psychiatry 162:767–773, 2005

Buckley PF: Substance abuse in schizophrenia: a review. J Clin Psychiatry 59 (suppl 3): 26–30, 1998

Cannon M, Cotter D, Sham PC, et al: Schizophrenia in an Irish sample following prenatal exposure to the 1957 influenza epidemic: a case controlled, prospective follow-up study. Schizophr Res 11:95–104, 1994

Cannon M, Jones PB, Murray RM: Obstetric complications and schizophrenia: historical and meta-analytic review. Am J Psychiatry 159:1080–1092, 2002

Cannon TD, Rosso IM, Hollister JM, et al: A prospective cohort study of genetic and perinatal influences in the etiology of schizophrenia. Schizophr Bull 26:351–366, 2000

Cantor-Graae E, Selten JP: Schizophrenia and migration: a meta-analysis and review. Am J Psychiatry 162:12–24, 2005

Cardno AG, Marshall EJ, Coid B, et al: Heritability estimates for psychotic disorders. Arch Gen Psychiatry 56:162–168, 1999

Carlsson A: The current status of the dopamine hypothesis of schizophrenia. Neuropsychopharmacology 1:179–186,1988

Carlsson A: The dopamine theory revisited, in Schizophrenia. Edited by Hirsh S, Weinberger DR. Cambridge, UK, Blackwell, 1995, pp 379–400

Carlsson A, Lindqvist M: Effect of chlorpromazine or haloperidol on formation of 3-methoxytyramine and normetanephrine in mouse brain. Acta Pharmacol Toxicol (Copenh) 20:140–144, 1963

Caspi A, Moffitt TE, Cannon M, et al: Moderation of the effects of adolescent-onset cannabis use on adult psychosis by a functional polymorphism in the catechol-O-methyltransferase gene: longitudinal evidence of a gene X environment interaction. Biol Psychiatry 57:1117–1127, 2005

Cassano GB, Pini S, Saettoni M, et al: Occurrence and clinical correlates of psychiatric comorbidity in patients with psychotic disorders. J Clin Psychiatry 59:60–68, 1998

Chambers RA, Krystal JH, Self DW: A neurobiological basis for substance abuse co-morbidity in schizophrenia. Biol Psychiatry 50:71–83, 2001

Chen CK, Murray RM: How does drug abuse interact with familial and developmental factors in the etiology of schizophrenia? In Neurodevelopment and Schizophrenia. Edited by Keshavan MS, Kennedy JL, Murray RM. Cambridge, UK, Cambridge University Press, 2004, pp 248–269

Chen CK, Lin SK, Sham PC, et al: Premorbid characteristics and comorbidity of meth-amphetamine users with and without psychosis. Psychol Med 33:1407–1414, 2003

Chen CK, Hu X, Lin SK, et al: Association analysis of dopamine D2-like receptor genes and methamphetamine abuse. Psychiatr Genet 14:223–226, 2004

Cherland E, Fitzpatrick R: Psychotic side effects of psychostimulants: a five year review. Can J Psychiatry 44:811–881, 1991

Commission IHD: Report of the Indian Hemp Drugs Commission, 1893–1894. Simila, India, Government Central Printing Office, 1894

Connell PH: Amphetamine Psychosis. Glasgow, Scotland, Chapman Hall for the Institute of Psychiatry; 1958

Crow TJ, Done DJ: Prenatal exposure to influenza does not cause schizophrenia. Br J Psychiatry 161:390–393, 1992

Curran C, Byrappa N, McBride A: Stimulant psychosis: systematic review. Br J Psychiatry 185:196–204, 2004

Dao-Castellana MH, Paillere-Martinot ML, Hantraye P: Presynaptic dopaminergic function in the striatum of schizophrenic patients. Schizophr Res 23:167–174, 1997

Davis KL, Kahn RS, Ko G, et al: Dopamine in schizophrenia: a review and reconceptualization. Am J Psychiatry 148:1474–1486, 1991

Degenhardt L, Hall W, Lynskey M: Alcohol, cannabis and tobacco use among Australians: a comparison of their associations with other drug use and use disorders, affective and anxiety disorders, and psychosis. Addiction 96:1603–1614, 2001

Dermatis H, Galanter M, Egelko S, et al: Schizophrenia patients and cocaine use: antecedents to hospitalisation and course of treatment. Subst Abuse 19:169–217, 1998

DeQuardo JR, Carpenter CF, Tandon R: Patterns of substance abuse in schizophrenia: nature and significance. J Psychiatr Res 28:267–275, 1994

Deutch AY: Prefrontal cortical dopamine systems and the elaboration of functional corticostriatal circuits: implications for schizophrenia and Parkinson's disease. J Neural Transm Gen Sect 91:197–221, 1993

Deutch AY, Clark WA, Roth RH: Prefrontal cortical dopamine depletion enhances the responsiveness of mesolimbic dopamine neurons to stress. Brain Res 521:311–315, 1990

Dhadphale M, Omolo OE: Psychiatric morbidity amongst khat users. East African Medical Journal 65:355–359, 1988

Di Chiara G, Imperato A: Drugs abused by humans preferentially increase synaptic dopamine concentrations in the mesolimbic system of freely moving rats. Proc Natl Acad Sci U S A 85:5274–5278, 1988

Dixon L, Haas G, Weiden P, et al: Acute effects of drug abuse in schizophrenic patients: clinical observations and patients' self-reports. Schizophr Bull 16:69–79, 1990

Dixon L, Haas G, Weiden PJ, et al: Drug abuse in schizophrenic patients: clinical correlates and reasons for use. Am J Psychiatry 148:224–230, 1991

D'Souza DC, Perry E, MacDougall L, et al: The psychotomimetic effects of intravenous D-9-THC in healthy individuals: implications for psychosis. Neuropsychopharmacology 29:1558–1572, 2004

Duke PJ, Pantelis C, McPhillips MA, et al: Comorbid non-alcohol substance misuse among people with schizophrenia: epidemiological study in central London. British Journal of Psychiatry 179:509–513, 2001

Egan MF, Goldberg TE, Kolachana BS, et al: Effect of COMT Val108/158 Met genotype on frontal lobe function and risk for schizophrenia. Proc Natl Acad Sci U S A 98:6917–6922, 2001

Elkashef AM, Doudet D, Bryant T, et al: 6-(18)F-DOPA PET study in patients with schizophrenia. Positron emission tomography. Psychiatry Res 100:1–11, 2000

Fergusson DM, Horwood LJ, Swain-Campbell NR: Cannabis dependence and psychotic symptoms in young people. Psychol Med 33:15–21, 2003

Fergusson DM, Horwood LJ, Ridder EM: Tests of causal linkages between cannabis use and psychotic symptoms. Addiction 100:354–366, 2005

Flaum M, Schultz SK: When does amphetamine-induced psychosis become schizophrenia? Am J Psychiatry 153:812–815, 1996

Fowler IL, Carr VJ, Carter NT, et al: Patterns of current and lifetime substance use in schizophrenia. Schizophr Bull 24:443–455, 1998

Garavan H, Pankiewicz J, Bloom A, et al: Cue-induced cocaine craving: neuroanatomical specificity for drug users and drug stimuli. Am J Psychiatry 157:1789–1798, 2000

Gardner EL, Lowinson JH: Marijuana's interaction with brain reward systems: update 1991. Pharmacol Biochem Behav 40:571–580, 1991

Geddes JR, Verdoux H, Takei N, et al: Schizophrenia and complications of pregnancy and labour in individual patient data meta-analysis. Schizophr Bull 25:413–423, 1999

Gilmore JH, Murray RM: Prenatal and perinatal factors, in Textbook of Schizophrenia. Edited by Lieberman JA, Perkins DO, Stroup TS. Washington, DC, American Psychiatric Publishing, 2006, pp 71–85

Glassman AH, Covey LS, Dalack GW, et al: Cigarette smoking, major depression, and schizophrenia. Clin Neuropharmacol 15 (suppl 1, Pt A):560A–561A, 1992

Glatt SJ, Faraone SV, Tsuang MT: Association between a functional catechol-O-methyltransferase gene polymorphism and schizophrenia: meta-analysis of case-control and family based studies. Am J Psychiatry 160:469–476, 2003

Gorriti MA, Rodriguez de Fonseca F, Navarro M: Chronic (-)-delta9-tetrahydrocannabinol treatment induces sensitization to the psychomotor effects of amphetamine in rats. Eur J Pharmacol 365:133–142, 1999

Grech A: Comparison study of alcohol and illicit drug use in patients with recent-onset psychosis in London and Malta. Paper presented at the Ninth Bienniel Winter Workshop on Schizophrenia, Davos, Switzerland, February 1998

Grech A, Van Os J, Jones PB, et al: Cannabis use and outcome of recent onset psychosis. Eur Psychiatry 20:349–353, 2005

Guillin O, Diaz J, Carroll P, et al: BDNF controls dopamine D3 receptor expression and triggers behavioral sensitization. Nature 411:86–89, 2001

Gurevich EV, Bordelon Y, Shapiro RM, et al: Mesolimbic dopamine D3 receptors and use of antipsychotics in patients with schizophrenia. A postmortem study. Arch Gen Psychiatry 54:225–232, 1997

Hafner H, Maurer K, Loffler W, et al: Onset and prodromal phase as determinants of course, in Search for the Cause of Schizophrenia, Vol 4: Balance of the Century. Edited by Gattaz WH, Haffner H. Berlin, Germany, Springer Verlag, 1999, pp 35–38

Hall W, Degenhardt L: Cannabis use and psychosis: a review of clinical and epidemiological evidence. Aust N Z J Psychiatry 34:26–34, 2000

Hambrecht M, Hafner H: Substance abuse and the onset of schizophrenia. Biol Psychiatry 40:1155–1163, 1996

Harrison PJ, Owen MJ: Genes for schizophrenia? Recent findings and their pathophysiological implications. Lancet 361:417–419, 2003

Henquet C, Krabbendam L, Spauwen J, et al: Prospective cohort study of cannabis use, predisposition for psychosis, and psychotic symptoms in young people. BMJ 1:330, 2005

Hietala J, Syvalahti E, Vuorio K, et al: Presynaptic dopamine function in striatum of neuroleptic-naive schizophrenic patients. Lancet 346:1130–1131, 1995

Hietala J, Syvalahti E, Vilkman H, et al: Depressive symptoms and presynaptic dopamine function in neuroleptic-naive schizophrenia. Schizophr Res 35:41–50, 1999

Hooks MS, Colvin AC, Juncos JL, et al: Individual differences in basal and cocaine-stimulated extracellular dopamine in the nucleus accumbens using quantitative microdialysis. Brain Res 587:306–312, 1992a

Hooks MS, Jones GH, Liem BJ, et al: Sensitization and individual differences to IP amphetamine, cocaine, or caffeine following repeated intracranial amphetamine infusions. Pharmacol Biochem Behav 43:815–823, 1992b

Ito R, Dalley JW, Howes SR, et al: Dissociation in conditioned dopamine release in the nucleus accumbens core and shell in response to cocaine cues and during cocaine-seeking behavior in rats. J Neurosci 20:7489–7495, 2000

Iwanami A, Sugiyama A, Kuroki N, et al: Patients with methamphetamine psychosis admitted to a psychiatric hospital in Japan. A preliminary report. Acta Psychiatr Scand 89:428–432, 1994

Jablensky A, McGrath J, Herrman H, et al: Psychotic disorders in urban areas: an overview of the Study on Low Prevalence Disorders. Aust N Z J Psychiatry 34:221–236, 2000

Johns A: Psychiatric effects of cannabis. Br J Psychiatry 178:116–122, 2001

Johns A, Van Os J: The continuity of psychotic experiences in the general population. Clinical Psychology Review. 21:1125–1141, 2001

Johns LC, Cannon M, Singleton N, et al: The prevalence and correlates of self-reported psychotic symptoms in the British population. Br J Psychiatry 185:298–305, 2004

Kalivas PW, Stewart J: Dopamine transmission in the initiation and expression of drug- and stress-induced sensitization of motor activity. Brain Research Review 16:223–244, 1991

Kapur S: Psychosis as a state of aberrant salience: a framework linking biology, phenomenology, and pharmacology in schizophrenia. Am J Psychiatry 160:13–23, 2003

Kapur S, Mann JJ: Role of the dopaminergic system in depression. Biol Psychiatry 32:1–17, 1992

Kavanagh DJ, Waghorn G, Jenner L, et al: Demographic and clinical correlates of comorbid substance abuse in psychosis: multivariate analyses in epidemiological sample. Schizophr Res 66:115–124, 2004

Knight F: Role of cannabis in psychiatric disturbance. Ann N Y Acad Sci 282:64–71, 1976

Koob G: Dopamine, addiction and reward. Semin Neurosci 4:139–148, 1992

Laruelle M: The role of endogenous sensitization in the pathophysiology of schizophrenia: implications from recent brain imaging studies. Brain Res Rev 31:371–384, 2000

Laruelle M, Abi-Dargham A, van Dyck CH, et al: Single photon emission computerized tomography imaging of amphetamine-induced dopamine release in drug-free schizophrenic subjects. Proc Natl Acad Sci U S A 93:9235–9240, 1996

Laruelle M, Kegeles LS, Abi-Dargham A: Glutamate, dopamine, and schizophrenia: from pathophysiology to treatment. Ann N Y Acad Sci 1003:138–158, 2003

Lewis CM, Levinson DF, Wise LH, et al: Genome scan meta-analysis of schizophrenia and bipolar disorder, part II: schizophrenia. Am J Hum Genet 73:34–48, 2003

Li T, Sham PC, Vallada H, et al: Preferential transmission of the high activity allele of COMT in schizophrenia. Psychiatr Genet 6:131–133, 1996

Lieberman JA, Sheitman BB, Kinon BJ: Neurochemical sensitization in the pathophysiology of schizophrenia: deficits and dysfunction in neuronal regulation and plasticity. Neuropsychopharmacology 17:205–229, 1997

Lieberman JA, Perkins D, Belger A, et al: The early stages of schizophrenia: speculations on pathogenesis, pathophysiology, and therapeutic approaches. Biol Psychiatry 50:884–897, 2001

Lindstrom LH, Gefvert O, Hagberg G, et al: Increased dopamine synthesis rate in medial prefrontal cortex and striatum in schizophrenia indicated by L-(beta-11C) DOPA and PET. Biol Psychiatry 46:681–688, 1999

Linszen DH, Dingemans PM, Lenior ME: Cannabis abuse and the course of recent-onset schizophrenic disorders. Arch Gen Psychiatry 51:273–279, 1994

Longhurst JG: Cannabis and schizophrenia (letter). Br J Psychiatry 171:584–585, 1997

Lundqvist T, Jonsson S, Warkentin S: Frontal lobe dysfunction in long-term cannabis users. Neurotoxicol Teratol 23:437–443, 2001

Lysaker P, Bell M, Beam-Goulet J, et al: Relationship of positive and negative symptoms to cocaine abuse in schizophrenia. J Nerv Ment Dis 182:109–112, 1994

Maas LC, Lukas SE, Kaufman MJ, et al: Functional magnetic resonance imaging of human brain activation during cue-induced cocaine craving. Am J Psychiatry 155:124–126, 1998

Macleod J, Oakes R, Copello A, et al: Psychological and social sequelae of cannabis and other illicit drug use in young people: A systematic review of longitudinal, general population studies. Lancet 363: 1579–1588, 2004

Mannisto PT, Kaakola S: Catechol-O-methyltransferase (COMT): biochemistry, molecular biology, pharmacology and clinical efficacy of the new selective COMT inhibitors. Pharmacology Review 51: 593–628, 1999

Manschreck TC: Characteristics of freebase cocaine psychosis. Yale J Biol Med 61:115–122, 1988

Margoles HC, Malchy L, Negrete JC, et al: Drug and alcohol use among patients with schizophrenia and related psychoses: levels and consequences. Schizophr Res 67: 157–166, 2004

Martinez D, Broft A, Foltin RW, et al: Cocaine dependence and D(2) receptor availability in the functional subdivisions of the striatum: relationship with cocaine-seeking behavior. Neuropsychopharmacology 29:1190–1202, 2004

Mathers DC, Ghodse AH: Cannabis and psychotic illness. Br J Psychiatry 161:648–653, 1992

Mathers DC, Ghodse AH, Caan AW, et al: Cannabis use in a large sample of acute psychiatric admissions. Br J Addict 86:779–784, 1991

McClure SM, Daw ND, Montague PR: A computational substrate for incentive salience. Trends Neurosci 26:423–428, 2003

McGowan SW, Lawrence A, Sale T, et al: Presynaptic dopaminergic dysfunction in medicated schizophrenic patients. Arch Gen Psychiatry 61:134–142, 2004

McGrath J, Welham J, Pemberton M: Month of birth, hemisphere of birth and schizophrenia. Br J Psychiatry 167:783–785, 1995

McGuire PK, Jones P, Harvey I: Morbid risk of schizophrenia for relatives of patients with cannabis-associated psychosis. Schizophr Res 15:277–281, 1995

Menezes PR, Johnson S, Thornicroft G, et al: Drug and alcohol problems among individuals with severe mental illness in south London. Br J Psychiatry 168:612–619, 1996

Meyer-Lindenberg A, Miletich RS, Kohn PD, et al: Reduced prefrontal activity predicts exaggerated striatal dopaminergic function in schizophrenia. Nat Neurosci 5:267–271, 2002

Miller NS, Guttman JC: The integration of pharmacological therapy for co-morbid psychiatric and addictive disorders. J Psychoactive Drugs 29:249–254, 1997

Milner PM: Brain-stimulation reward: a review. Can J Psychology 45:1–36, 1991

Modestin J, Nussbaumer C, Angst K, et al: Use of potentially abusive psychotropic substances in psychiatric inpatients. Eur Arch Psychiatry Clin Neurosci 247:146–153, 1997

Mueser KT, Drake RE, Wallach MA: Dual diagnosis: a review of etiological theories. Addict Behav 23:717–734, 1998

Mueser KT, Yarnold PR, Levinson DF, et al: Prevalence of substance abuse in schizophrenia: demographic and clinical correlates. Schizophr Bull 16:31–56, 1990

Mueser KT, Yarnold PR, Rosenberg SD, et al: Substance use disorder in hospitalized severely mentally ill psychiatric patients: prevalence, correlates, and subgroups. Schizophrenia Bulletin 26:179–92, 2000

Murphy KC, Jones LA, Owen MJ: High rates of schizophrenia in adults with velocardiofacial syndrome. Arch Gen Psychiatry 56:940–945, 1999

Murray RM, Grech A, Phillips P, et al: What is the relationship between substance abuse and schizophrenia? In The Epidemiology of Schizophrenia. Edited by Murray R, Jones P, Susser E, et al. Cambridge, UK, Cambridge University Press, 2002, pp 317–342

Negrete JC, Knapp WP, Douglas DE, et al: Cannabis affects the severity of schizophrenic symptoms: results of a clinical survey. Psychol Med 16:515–520, 1986

Nestler EJ: Molecular mechanisms of drug addiction. J Neurosci 12:2439–2450, 1992

Norman RM, Malla AK: Stressful life events and schizophrenia, I: a review of the research. Br J Psychiatry 162:161–166, 1993a

Norman RM, Malla AK: Stressful life events and schizophrenia, II: conceptual and methodological issues. Br J Psychiatry 162:166–174, 1993b

Numan N: Exploration of adverse psychological symptoms in Yemeni khat users by the Symptom Checklist–90. Addiction 99:61–65, 2004

O'Callaghan E, Sham P, Takei N, et al: Schizophrenia after prenatal exposure to 1957 A2 influenza pandemic. Lancet 337:1248–1250, 1991

O'Daly OG, Guillin O, Tsapakis EM, et al: Schizophrenia and substance abuse co-morbidity: a role for dopamine sensitization? Journal of Dual Diagnosis 1:11–40, 2005

Odenwald M, Neuner F, Schauer M, et al: Khat use as risk factor for psychotic disorders: a cross-sectional and case-control study in Somalia. BMC Med 3:5, 2005

Pawluck DE, Gorey KM: Psychiatric morbidity in narcoleptics on chronic high dose methylphenidate therapy. J Nerv Ment Dis 183:45–48, 1995

Pedersen CB, Mortensen PB: Evidence of a dose-response relationship between urbanicity and schizophrenia risk. Arch Gen Psychiatry 58:1039–1046, 2001

Phillips P, Johnson S: How does drug and alcohol misuse develop among people with psychotic illness? A literature review. Soc Psychiatry Psychiatr Epidemiol 36:269–276, 2001

Pohl R, Yeragani VK, Balon R, et al: Smoking in patients with panic disorder. Psychiatry Res 43:253–262, 1992

Poole R, Brabbins C: Drug induced psychosis. Br J Psychiatry 168:135–138, 1996

Pycock CJ, Kerwin RW, Carter CJ: Effect of lesion of cortical dopamine terminals on subcortical dopamine receptors in rats. Nature 286:74–76, 1980

Rabinowitz J, Bromet EJ, Lavelle J, et al: Prevalence and severity of substance use disorders and onset of psychosis in first-admission psychotic patients. Psychol Med 28:1411–1419, 1998

Regier DA, Boyd JH, Burke JD, et al: One-month prevalence of mental disorders in the United States. Based on five Epidemiologic Catchment Area sites. Arch Gen Psychiatry 45:977–986, 1988

Regier DA, Farmer ME, Rae DS, et al: Comorbidity of mental disorders with alcohol and other drug abuse. Results from the Epidemiologic Catchment Area (ECA) Study. JAMA 264:2511–2518, 1990

Reith J, Benkelfat C, Sherwin A, et al: Elevated dopa decarboxylase activity in living brain of patients with psychosis. Proc Natl Acad Sci U S A 91:11651–11654, 1994

Robins LN, Regier DA (eds): Psychiatric Disorders in America: the Epidemiological Catchment Area Study. New York, Free Press, 1991

Robinson TE, Berridge KC: The neural basis of drug craving: an incentive-sensitization theory of addiction. Brain Res Rev 18:247–291, 1993

Rolfe M, Tang CM, Sabally S, et al: Psychosis and cannabis abuse in The Gambia. A case-control study. Br J Psychiatry 163:798–801, 1993

Rosse RB, McCarthy MV, Alim TN, et al: Phenomenological comparison of the idiopathic psychosis of schizophrenia and drug induced cocaine and phencyclidine psychosis: a retrospective study. Clin Neuropharmacol 17:359–369, 1994

Rottanburg D, Robins AH, Ben-Arie O, et al: Cannabis-associated psychosis with hypomanic features. Lancet 2(8312):1364–1366, 1982

Schneider F, Habel U, Wagner M, et al: Subcortical correlates of craving in recently abstinent alcoholic patients. Am J Psychiatry 158:1075–1083, 2001

Schneier FR, Siris SG: A review of psychoactive substance use and abuse in schizophrenia. Patterns of drug choice. J Nerv Ment Dis 175:641–652, 1987

Schultz W, Tremblay L, Hollerman JR: Reward processing in primate orbitofrontal cortex and basal ganglia. Cereb Cortex 10:272–284, 2000

Schulz R, Herz A: Naloxone-precipitated withdrawal reveals sensitization to neurotransmitters in morphine tolerant/dependent rats. Naunyn Schmiedebergs Arch Pharmacol 299:95–99, 1977

Seibyl JP, Satel SL, Anthony D, et al: Effects of cocaine on hospital course in schizophrenia. J Nerv Ment Dis 181:31–37, 1993

Selten JP, Cantor-Graae E: Social defeat: risk factor for schizophrenia? Br J Psychiatry 187:101–102, 2005

Semple DM, McIntosh AM, Lawrie SM: Cannabis as a risk factor for psychosis: systematic review. J Psychopharmacol 19:187–194, 2005

Serper MR, Alpert M, Richardson NA, et al: Clinical effects of recent cocaine use in patients with acute schizophrenia. Am J Psychiatry 152:1464–1469, 1995

Sham PC, O'Callaghan E, Takei N, et al. Schizophrenia following pre-natal exposure to influenza epidemics between 1936 and 1960. Br J Psychiatry 160:461–466, 1992

Sharpley M, Hutchinson G, McKenzie K, et al: Understanding the excess of psychosis among the African-Caribbean population in England. Review of current hypotheses. Br J Psychiatry Suppl 40:S60–S68, 2001

Shuster L, Yu G, Bates A: Sensitization to cocaine stimulation in mice. Psychopharmacology (Berl) 52:185–190, 1977

Snyder SH: The dopamine hypothesis of schizophrenia: focus on the dopamine receptor. Am J Psychiatry 133:197–202, 1976

Solowij N, Stephens RS, Roffman RA, et al: Cognitive functioning of long-term heavy cannabis users seeking treatment. JAMA 287:1123–1131, 2002

Soyka M, Albus M, Kathmann N, et al: Prevalence of alcohol and drug abuse in schizophrenic inpatients. Eur Arch Psychiatry Clin Neurosci 242:362–372, 1993

Staley JK, Mash DC: Adaptive increase in D3 dopamine receptors in the brain reward circuits of human cocaine fatalities. J Neurosci 16:6100–6106, 1996

Stefanis NC, Delespaul P, Henquet C, et al: Early adolescent cannabis exposure and positive and negative dimensions of psychosis. Addiction 99:1333–1341, 2004

Stein EA, Pankiewicz J, Harsch HH, et al: Nicotine-induced limbic cortical activation in the human brain: a functional MRI study. Am J Psychiatry 155:1009–1015, 1998

Stewart J: Pathways to relapse: the neurobiology of drug- and stress-induced relapse to drug-taking. J Psychiatry Neurosci 25:125–136, 2000

Stimmel GL: Benzodiazepines in schizophrenia. Pharmacotherapy 16:148S–151S; discussion 166S–168S, 1996

Strakowski SM, Sax KW, Setters MJ, et al: Lack of enhanced response to repeated d-amphetamine challenge in first-episode psychosis: implications for a sensitization model of psychosis in humans. Biol Psychiatry 42:749–755, 1997

Substance Abuse and Mental Health Services Administration (SAMHSA): National findings from the 1999 National Household Survey on Drug Abuse (DHHS Publication No. SMA 00-3466). Rockville, MD, Office of Applied Statistics, 2000

Sundquist K, Frank G, Sundquist J: Urbanisation and incidence of psychosis and depression. Br J Psychiatry 184:293–298, 2004

Susser ES, Lin SP: Schizophrenia after prenatal exposure to the Dutch hunger winter of 1944–1945. Arch Gen Psychiatry 49:983–988, 1992

Susser E, Neugebauer R, Hoek HW, et al: Schizophrenia after prenatal famine. Arch Gen Psychiatry 53:25–31, 1996

Suvisaari J, Haukka A, Tanskanene A, et al. Association between prenatal exposure to poliovirus infection and adult schizophrenia. Am J Psychiatry 156:110–110, 1999

Svenningsson P, Tzavara ET, Carruthers R, et al: Diverse psychotomimetics act through a common signaling pathway. Science 302:1412–1415, 2003

Tanda G, Pontieri FE, Di Chiara G: Cannabinoid and heroin activation of mesolimbic dopamine transmission by a common mu_1 opioid receptor mechanism. Science 276:2048–2050, 1997

Takei N, Kawai M, Murray RM, et al: Have recent studies of the seasonality of birth in schizophrenia added to our knowledge of the disease? in Neuropsychiatric Disorders and Infection. Edited by Fatemi SH. London, Taylor & Francis Medical Books, (in press)

Thornicroft G: Cannabis and psychosis. Is there epidemiological evidence for an association? Br J Psychiatry 157:25–33, 1990

Tien AY, Anthony JC: Epidemiological analysis of alcohol and drug use as risk factors for psychotic experiences. J Nerv Ment Dis 178:473–480, 1990

Torrey FE, Rawlings R, Waldman IN: Schizophrenic births and viral diseases in two states. Schizophr Res 1:73–77, 1988

Tsuang MT, Simpson JC, Kronfol Z: Subtypes of drug abuse with psychosis. Demographic characteristics, clinical features, and family history. Arch Gen Psychiatry 39:141–147, 1982

Turner WM, Tsuang MT: Impact of substance abuse on the course and outcome of schizophrenia. Schizophr Bull 16:87–95, 1990

Tzschentke TM: Pharmacology and behavioral pharmacology of the mesocortical dopamine system. Prog Neurobiol 63:241–320, 2001

Vanderschuren LJ, Kalivas PW: Alterations in dopaminergic and glutamatergic transmission in the induction and expression of behavioral sensitization: a critical review of preclinical studies. Psychopharmacology (Berl) 151:99–120, 2000 van Kammen DP, Boronow JJ: Dextro-amphetamine diminishes negative symptoms in schizophrenia. Int J Clin Psychopharmacol 3:111–121, 1988

van Os J, Bak M, Hanssen M, et al: Cannabis use and psychosis: a longitudinal population-based study. Am J Epidemiology 156:319–327, 2002

Van Os J, Pedersen CB, Mortensen PB: Confirmation of synergy between urbanicity and familial liability in the causation of psychosis. Am J Psychiatry 161:2312–2314, 2004

Veen ND, Selten JP, van der Tweel I, et al: Cannabis use and age at onset of schizophrenia. Am J Psychiatry 161:501–506, 2004

Verdoux H, Mury M, Besancon G, et al: Comparative study of substance dependence comorbidity in bipolar, schizophrenic and schizoaffective disorders. Encephale 22: 95–101, 1996

Verdoux H, Liraud F, Assens F, et al: Social and clinical consequences of cognitive deficits in early psychosis: a two-year follow-up study of first-admitted patients. Schizophr Res 56:149–159, 2002

Volkow ND, Wang GJ, Fischman MW, et al: Relationship between subjective effects of cocaine and dopamine transporter occupancy. Nature 386:827–830, 1997

Volkow ND, Wang GJ, Fowler JS, et al: Reinforcing effects of psychostimulants in humans are associated with increases in brain dopamine and occupancy of D(2) receptors. J Pharmacol Exp Ther 291:409–415, 1999

Volkow ND, Fowler JS, Wang GJ, et al: Dopamine in drug abuse and addiction: results from imaging studies and treatment implications. Mol Psychiatry 9:557–569, 2004

Voruganti LNP, Slomka P, Zabel P, et al: Cannabis induced dopamine release: an in vivo SPECT study. Psychiatr Res 107:173–177, 2001

Weinberger DR: Implications of normal brain development for the pathogenesis of schizophrenia. Arch Gen Psychiatry 44:660–669, 1987

Weinberger D, Laruelle M: Neurochemical and neuropharmacological imaging in schizophrenia, in Neuropsychopharmacology: The Fifth Generation of Progress. Edited by Davis KL, Charney DS, Coyle J, et al. Philadelphia, PA, Lippincott Williams & Wilkins, 2001, pp 833–855

Weiser M, Knobler HY, Noy S, et al: Clinical characteristics of adolescents later hospitalized for schizophrenia. Am J Med Genet 114:949–955, 2002

Wexler BE, Gottschalk CH, Fulbright RK, et al: Functional magnetic resonance imaging of cocaine craving. Am J Psychiatry 158:86–95, 2001

Zammit S, Allebeck P, Andreasson S, et al: Self reported cannabis use as a risk factor for schizophrenia: further analysis of 1969: historical cohort study. BMJ 325:1199, 2000

Ziedonis DM, Trudeau K: Motivation to quit using substances among individuals with schizophrenia: implications for a motivation-based treatment model. Schizophr Bull 23:229–238, 1997

Zink CF, Pagnoni G, Martin ME, et al: Human striatal response to salient nonrewarding stimuli. J Neurosci 23:8092–8097, 2003

3

Social Environment and Psychiatric Disorders

A Historical Review Presented on Receipt of the Paul H. Hoch Award

Jane M. Murphy, Ph.D.

This review concerns factors that have been variously called "psychosocial," "sociocultural," and "social environmental," and it deals with their role in research about the etiology of psychiatric disorders. In contrast to genetics and biology, the factors involved in these labels focus on life experiences in a social context.

ROLE OF THE NIMH

The review is based mainly on drawing together information from and about the National Institute of Mental Health (NIMH) which was created by President Truman in 1946. Although not operative until 1949, NIMH then became the governmental agency that is chiefly responsible for establishing the national research agenda. It does this not only by periodic commissions but also by being a main source of research funding.

53

As preface it is to be noted that the history of social environmental research is one not of steady growth but rather of abundant activity followed by a decline and then a recent resurgence. Social research had strong support from NIMH from 1949 until approximately 1975, when serious criticisms began to be leveled at it and much more attention was given to those disciplines that represented advances in brain research, psychopharmacology, and genetics. In the past few years, psychosocial research has begun to regain recognition.

The foremost reasons for the decline seem to have involved relevance and philosophy. Lack of relevance was seen in the tendency for some psychosocial research to focus on mental health rather than psychiatric disorders; for some to be concerned with basic research about psychosocial processes rather than potentially important etiological factors; and for some to have generated such high estimates of prevalence as to suggest that the phenomena being counted were transient periods of distress rather than serious mental illnesses. In terms of philosophy, different presidential administrations and different research orientations either favored or disfavored psychosocial research. In addition, some of the topics undertaken were so broad in scope—so little broken down into component parts—that implementation was impossible. The hallmark of the reemergence of social research is not only its practical relevance but its much improved methodology.

The first director of NIMH was Robert Felix, a psychiatrist who had been trained at the Colorado Psychopathic Hospital under Frank Ebaugh, a former student of Adolf Meyer (Cameron 1991). In the years before the Second World War, Meyer was a preeminent leader in American psychiatry, a promoter of "common-sense psychiatry," and an advocate for the influence of the social environment on human lives (Winters 1950). (Meyer was also the second president of the American Psychopathological Association.) In addition to psychiatric training in this tradition, Felix had also qualified in Public Health at Johns Hopkins.

Between 1946 when NIMH was created and 1949 when it actually began operating, Felix and Bowers (1948) published an article titled "Mental Hygiene and Socio-Environmental Factors" that described the programmatic approach and etiological philosophy of the new institute. The guiding premise was that "the impact of the social environment on the life history and the relevance of the life history to mental illness are no longer in serious question" and, further, that etiological cognizance of these facts would be fundamental to the research programs of the Institute. Social environment was defined in the broadest possible terms as the "knowledge, attitudes, and behavior patterns acquired through living with others," a definition that closely approximates the standard way of describing "culture" in the field of anthropology.

Among the studies cited were those by anthropologists Margaret Mead (1935) and Ruth Benedict (1934) that emphasized the molding force of culture on personality. Also cited was the work of Faris and Dunham (1939) that showed the concentration of schizophrenic patients in the poorest sections of Chicago, a study that contributed to the growing concern to understand the impact of socioeconomic status (SES). In view of the influence of these works, it is not surprising that Felix (1966) recommended that all psychiatric residents be well read in "social theory."

The plan for NIMH was to place the problem of the etiology of psychiatric disorders in "its full epidemiological context." The emphasis on epidemiology derived in part from the public health perspective that Felix had brought to his new position. It also came from his psychiatric training in the Meyerian tradition. Three of the first psychiatrists to apply epidemiological methods in their research had trained under Meyer: Paul Lemkau (1955), who formed the Department of Mental Hygiene in what was then called the Johns Hopkins School of Hygiene; Thomas A. C. Rennie, who headed the Midtown Manhattan Study until his death (Srole et al. 1962); and Alexander Leighton (1950, 1959), who in 1948 initiated the Stirling County Study, which I joined in 1951 and have directed since 1975 (Murphy 1980; Murphy et al. 2000).

Robert Felix was part of the Meyer legacy in regard to epidemiology, culture, and social structure. Where the nature of psychiatric disorders was concerned, however, Felix and Bowers (1948) drew on the Freudian approach, especially as articulated by Karl Menninger (1959), in seeing "mental health and mental illness as differing in degree rather than kind." This "antidiagnostic" approach was to have a profound influence on the next few decades of American psychiatric epidemiology through the Midtown Manhattan Study which, when it got under way, was partially supported by NIMH (Srole et al. 1962). Not only was the Midtown Study an epidemiological investigation that focused on life experience and social structure, but it also subscribed to the view that psychiatric illnesses vary more in degree than in kind and described the psychiatric findings as "mental health ratings." In contrast, the psychiatric approach of the Stirling County Study was "diagnostic" in its emphasis on discerning the different types of psychiatric syndromes. For various reasons to be suggested below, the diagnostic approach of the Stirling Study did not influence the surveys conducted over the next few decades either in the U.S. or in Canada, where the site of our study is located.

Other research that had formative influence at NIMH was work by Stouffer et al. (1949) conducted during the Second World War and published as a series of books under the general title of *The American Soldier*. The fourth volume (Stouffer et al. 1950), *Measurement and Prediction*, included as one of its authors John Clausen, a sociologist. Clausen was among the first to become part of the NIMH Intramural Program. He headed the Laboratory of Social Environmental Studies, one of the four laboratories created in those early years (Greenhouse 2003). The others were the Laboratories of Psychiatry, Psychology, and Clinical Sciences.

The current NIMH Intramural Programs are very different from the original programs. Where the social environment was a defining element at the beginning, it is represented by only one unit among the 33 that now exist, with most of the others emphasizing the biological and genetic underpinnings of human behavior. The most common concept conveyed in the titles of the programs is "neuro." Psychology is still present but it is qualified as "Neuropsychology."

HISTORICALLY SIGNIFICANT COMMISSIONS

The major change in focus that occurred, as discussed in the previous section, can be illustrated by the difference between two important commissions and the types of research they promoted. The first was the Joint Commission on Mental Illness and Health (1961), whose final report, *Action for Mental Health,* led to the Community Mental Health Centers program signed into effect by President Kennedy in 1963. The second was the President's Commission on Mental Health (1978) initiated by President Carter, an end product of which can, I suggest, be viewed as the first President Bush's establishment of the 1990s as the "Decade of the Brain."

Where the Joint Commission was concerned, several reports were sponsored that reflect a concern with the social environment. One dealt with community resources for mental health (Robinson et al. 1960); another with schools and mental health (Allinsmith and Goethals 1962); and still another with churches and mental health (McCann 1962). Also special attention was given to health in contrast to illness as in its report on positive mental health (Jahoda 1958).

One of the Commission's reports, *American's View their Mental Health* (Gurin et al. 1960), involved the first national sample study to be carried out regarding mental health. Conducted by members of the Michigan Survey Research Center in 1957, it was described as epidemiological and used questions from the Stirling and Midtown Studies. It was not, however, concerned with estimating prevalence. Rather it dealt with patterns of adjustment and the handling of emotional problems. The same approach was carried over to a new national sample study nearly 20 years later carried out by some of the same authors and reported in two volumes, *The Inner American* (Veroff et al. 1981a) and *Mental Health in America* (Veroff et al. 1981b). The authors of the second series indicated that the authors of the 1960 volume had been under considerable pressure to "classify a given proportion of the population as being especially needy of psychological help" but then went on to say that the earlier authors had refrained from such classification, "and that the authors of the new study were 'following suit'" (p. 8). Furthermore, the concept of "well-being" played a central role in these studies, thus reflecting the general stance of the Joint Commission in keeping mental health in the forefront and contributing to the antidiagnostic approach that had characterized the Midtown Study. It seems to me that the Joint Commission's disinterest in serious mental illness contributed substantially to the decline in support of social research.

Several other features of the research landscape during the 1960s and 1970s also contributed to dissatisfaction with psychosocial studies. The Midtown and Stirling Studies published their results during that period even though the research had been carried out earlier. A common reaction was that the estimates of prevalence were too high to be credible (Dohrenwend and Dohrenwend 1965). Despite their differences, the two studies indicated that the overall prevalence of clinically recognizable mental illness was about 20%. In the years since, most of the newer psychiatric epidemiological investigations have similarly suggested a figure of about 20% (Bland et al. 1988; Kessler et al. 1994a; Offord et al. 1996; Regier et al. 1988). In the 1960s and 1970s, however, the psychiatric community tended to think that the early studies were merely identifying the "worried well"—people who suffered from transient distress but who were not afflicted with serious mental illness.

Another feature was that most of the epidemiological studies carried out in the 1960s and 1970s, such as those of Phillips (1966) and Husaini et al. (1979), used short inventories of psychiatric questions, especially those derived from the Stirling and Midtown Studies (Langner 1962; Macmillan 1957). The use of such inventories made it possible to conduct studies that could be carried out quickly and without great cost. The ease of this type of research is one of the reasons that the much more time-consuming and costly diagnostic approach of the Stirling Study was not taken up by others during this period. Many of the surveys that used these short scales were carried out by sociologists and psychologists rather than by interdisciplinary teams directed by psychiatrists. Many of the surveys dealt with psychosocial and sociocultural concepts, and the scales were often interpreted as measuring "psychological distress."

NONEPIDEMIOLOGICAL SOCIAL MODELS

It would be misleading if the review of the 1960s and 1970s were limited to epidemiology. There were other approaches that also emphasized psychosocial factors and contributed to their diminished role in the national research agenda. One was the work of Gregory Bateson and co-workers (1956) on the "schizophrenogenic mother" with its strong emphasis on "double-bind communication" as an etiological source. This is not to say that communication lacks importance, but, as the work on expressed emotion seems to indicate, communication probably has more to do with the course of illness and outcome than with its etiology (Fallon et al. 1982).

Another approach was "labeling theory" as proposed by sociologists such as Becker (1963) and Scheff (1966). This approach was influenced by Thomas Szasz (1961) and R. D. Laing (1960), who promoted the view that the concept of mental illness is a myth in that what is termed mental illness is, in fact, simply behavior that is out of keeping with social norms. Labeling theory also drew heavily on the "self–other" theories of psychologist George Herbert Mead (1934). As with "double-bind communication," "self–other messages" are clearly important to human functioning and happiness. As bodies of theory about the relationship between psychosocial factors and psychiatric disorders, however, both the "schizophrenogenic mother" and "labeling" did much to discredit research on social factors (Murphy 1976).

DEVELOPMENTS AT NIMH

NIMH was not the funding agency for all of the aforementioned studies, nor was it responsible for the perceptions that developed about the existing research. Further, NIMH was continuing to include psychosocial research as an integral part of its mandate during these years. Felix stepped down as director and Stanley Yolles was appointed in 1964, the year President Johnson was elected. Encouraged by the philosophy of the Great Society and President Johnson's "pledge to apply scientific research to social problems," NIMH expanded its support on the mental health implications of poverty, crime, and other social ills (Judd 1998). This continued into the tenure of Bertram Brown, who became the director in 1970.

By the time that President Carter's Commission was established in 1977, NIMH had become part of an overarching institute named the Alcohol, Drug Abuse, and Mental Health Administration (ADAMHA) that also subsumed the National Institute on Alcohol Abuse and Alcoholism and the National Institute on Drug Abuse. Gerald Klerman was appointed the director of ADAMHA in 1977 and played a formative role in the development of the President's Commission on Mental Health (1978). The work of the Commission indicated that the Community Mental Health Act had not achieved adequate delivery of service to a large portion of the American population who needed such help. Those who were not being reached included the chronically mentally ill, children, adolescents, and the eldery. The Commission noted that "[r]acial and ethnic minorities, the urban poor, and migrant and seasonal farm workers continue to be underserved" (p. 4). The Commission pointed to the fact that since 1969, "our national research capacity has undergone substantial erosion" (p. 46) and indicated that the research areas requiring special attention were "long-term epidemiological and survey research" that would make it possible to understand the prevalence and incidence of psychiatric disorders in the U.S., as well as "expanded research on the ways mental health services are delivered" (p. 49).

Keenly aware of the need for new directions in mental health research, Klerman effected a transition of leadership in 1978 that brought Herbert Pardes to the post of director of NIMH. With Klerman's backing and building on the President's Commission on Mental Health, Pardes (1998) spearheaded a "reemergence of NIMH's scientific mission" (p. 14).

Also at this time, the construction and approval of the third revision of the *Diagnostic and Statistical Manual of Mental Disorders* (DSM-III; American Psychiatric Association 1980) revolutionized mental health research. For the first time, DSM provided an explicit stepwise procedure for making a diagnosis (essential features, associated symptomatology, and duration) as well as specific criteria for different types of diagnoses.

At NIMH, changes were taking place that began to highlight neuroscience and to lowlight psychosocial factors. The reemergence of NIMH's scientific mission was encapsulated in a reorganization that concentrated on five areas (Pardes 1998): 1) neuroscience and related brain and behavior research, 2) clinical research, 3) treatment research, 4) epidemiological research, and 5) mental health economics.

CHALLENGES TO PSYCHOSOCIAL RESEARCH

In terms of psychosocial factors, Pardes suggested that the lowlighting came from three sources. The first source was that some NIMH grants had received Senator Proxmire's Golden Fleece Awards for misuse of taxpayer money. However, of the approximately 100 Golden Fleece Awards currently described on the Internet (Taxpayers for Common Sense 2005), only two NIMH projects appear. One concerns "social relations in a Peruvian brothel" and the other explores "why bowlers, hockey fans, and pedestrians smile." Grants from the National Science Foundation far outnumber NIMH grants as recipients of these negative awards, but insofar as the awards pointed to topics of doubtful relevance to the mission of NIMH, criticism seems warranted even though these "fleeced" projects were not representative of most of the psychosocial research that had been carried out in the 1960s and 1970s. The second source of lowlighting was that the Reagan Administration, which came to office in 1981, was reluctant to support research of a broad social nature. While this was probably a powerful deterrent to advancing psychosocial research, it is not clear from the record what exactly was meant by "broad social issues." It seems likely, however, that the phrase referred to issues about the poor, the chronically ill, and the marginalized people—issues, in other words, that had been emphasized in the Carter Commission. The third source was the mixed views in academia about the quality of some of the extramural research. The examples of projects that received negative academic reaction were ones on "citizen empowerment" and "work performance in relation to cycles of the day" (Pardes 1998). Social research was clearly under serious attack, in some regards understandably so, and the survival of NIMH-sponsored psychosocial research was threatened.

BRIDGES TO THE PRESENT

Such research did not disappear, however, and I suggest that three circumstances have supported continuance, albeit without the same level of interest as pertains for neuroscience research. These circumstances can be thought of as "bridges" to the present.

One bridge was the worthwhile and rather obvious principle that social research funded by NIMH must focus specifically on psychiatric illness. For example, whereas earlier "work performance" had been studied in terms of morning, noon, and late afternoon, now it is being studied in terms of "depression" among workers (Wang et al. 2004).

Another bridge was the inclusion of the diagnosis posttraumatic stress disorder (PTSD) in DSM-III. At first I thought PTSD would put psychosocial research in a straitjacket because it specifically concerned stressors that are outside the range of usual human experience: combat, imprisonment, torture, major disasters, and physical violence. However, there has been, and continues to be, a great deal of trauma worldwide, and numerous useful studies have been carried out that document a link between stress and psychiatric status (North et al. 1999; Punämaki et al. 2005; Roussos et al. 2005). At the same time, some of the traumatic stressors considered as etiological to the disorder are more common than expected (Breslau 2002; Bromet et al. 1998). Our understanding of the nature of the disorder itself has been enriched by psychosocial research on the prevalence of trauma, the distribution of PTSD in community-based populations, vulnerabilities to both trauma and PTSD, and the comorbidity of PTSD with other psychiatric disorders (Breslau et al. 2002).

The third bridge was the support given to general-population epidemiology. In a special issue of the *Archives of General Psychiatry*, Myrna Weissman and Gerald Klerman (1978) pointed to the need for a new trend that would focus on discrete categories of psychiatric illness, and Lee Robins (1978) gave a history of psychiatric epidemiology that emphasized the need for a different direction. Also important was the fact that psychiatrists were taking an interest in epidemiology where earlier many, especially psychoanalysts, had looked upon the field as dealing only with superficial information about symptoms and impairment rather than intrapsychic dynamics.

The mandate from the President's Commission on Mental Health combined with the availability of DSM-III launched NIMH's Epidemiologic Catchment Area (ECA) Program. Psychiatrist Darrel Regier took a leading role in this program, with others, such as Jack Burke, John Helzer, and Dan Blazer, also being prominent. This does not mean that sociologists were not involved. Lee Robins played a major role, including in the construction of the Diagnostic Interview Schedule (DIS) as the data-gathering instrument to be used (Robins 1985; Robins et al. 1981). Similarly, William Eaton was responsible for many design features and later led the long-term follow-up of the Baltimore sample (Eaton et al. 1984, 2000). In the earlier studies there had been little involvement on the part of those formally trained in epidemiology. With the ECA, this situation changed through the collaboration of Myrna Weissman, for example, and because others, such as Regier and Burke, had received master's degrees in epidemiology over and above their psychiatric training. Although the contributors to the ECA are too numerous to name individually, the effort was a thoroughly interdisciplinary one and, in this, was more similar to the Midtown and Stirling studies than to most of the intervening investigations that used only psychiatric scales.

After publication of a large number of journal articles stemming from the ECA, the work was drawn together in a book titled *Psychiatric Disorders in America* (Robins and Regier 1991). Whereas the books that emanated from the Joint Commission (*Americans View Their Mental Health*, *The Inner American*, and *Mental Health in America*) had emphasized adjustment and well-being and specifically eschewed identifying the portion of the population that was in need of mental health care, the book that emanated from the Carter Commission addressed and carried out the very task rejected by the earlier workers.

The purpose of the ECA was to provide information which could be used in planning services as well as giving basic information about the prevalence and incidence of psychiatric disorders using diagnostic algorithms that distinguished between the different kinds of mental illnesses. A similar diagnostic approach pertained a decade later in the National Comorbidity Survey (NCS), which built on its forerunner by addressing the issue of how use of drugs and alcohol may combine with psychiatric disorders and how such comorbidity may influence service planning (Kessler et al. 1994a).

Both the ECA and the NCS have contributed materially to the continuance of psychosocial research in that they included information about the social issues outlined in the President's Commission on Mental Health (Bruce et al. 1991; Holzer et al. 1986; Kessler et al. 1995, 1998; Weissman et al. 1987).

As these bridges to survival began to be utilized, the way we talk about our work changed. "Mental health" has been replaced by "mental illness," or even more often by "psychiatric disorders." The broader designation of "sociocultural" has given way to the more narrow "psychosocial."

When the PTSD stressors specifically excluded "common experiences such as chronic illness, business losses, and marital conflict," it signaled what I believe is an unfortunate shift of attention. Over the years, the largest amount of psychosocial research has concerned precisely *those common events* that were excluded. In due course, research on life experiences had been coupled with investigation of social supports. Life stress and social support had become central to psychosocial research, and that feature of our tradition has been diminished.

Earlier, for example, the second volume of the Midtown Manhattan Study looked at a broad range of common events and found that it was not a matter of any one type but rather the accumulation of many negative events that made a difference (Langner and Michael 1963). A more recent example is the theoretical approach to life events developed by Brown and Harris (1978), which deals with the interrelationships and sequences of life events as they relate to depression among women. The model concerns background features, provoking agents, and vulnerabilities. The theory as a whole has not lent itself to easy replication, but individual components of it have been supported in numerous other studies.

ROLE OF SOCIAL CLASS

One of the psychosocial concepts that stands alone and yet involves life stress is social class. A major stride forward in the measurement of social class came from the work of Hollingshead and Redlich (1958) in their New Haven study of patients in treatment. Also, it became clear early on that an inverse relationship between SES and psychiatric prevalence was one of the most common findings in the growing number of community-based epidemiological studies (Dohrenwend and Dohrenwend 1969). This association carried the intriguing question of whether the relationship was due to social drift/selection or to social stress/causation. Strategies for studying the relationship have improved, as employed, for example, in a study in Israel carried out by Dohrenwend et al. (1992). The use of standardized interview methods and emphasis on diagnostic differences indicated that the association was probably due to selection in the case of schizophrenia and to stress in the case of depression.

In the Stirling Study, we investigated SES in relation to depression and anxiety by following subjects over time (Murphy et al. 1991). Anxiety tended to be a middle-class phenomenon while depression was strongly associated with low SES. The development of new cases of depression was more common among people in the low SES, a finding which seemed to support the stress hypothesis. But there was also a tendency for the depressed to move down in the social hierarchy, a finding that seemed to support the opposite hypothesis regarding drift.

While neither of these findings was significant, possibly due to the small numbers available when the samples had been broken down into various categories, the message of this study was that even with a disorder like depression a "little bit of both social causation and social drift" seemed to be involved. We concluded that answering the stress/drift question would require a much larger study: one that would begin with infants and children rather than adults, employ a much longer follow-up period, and entail much better evidence about both genetic vulnerability and different aspects of low SES. However, as far as our study went, the impact of "a little bit of both" was to maintain a tragically stable relationship between poverty and depression. Understanding this relationship is one of the vastly important tasks of psychiatric research, one that cries for a better integration of genetic and psychosocial evidence.

INTEGRATIVE APPROACHES

A number of new types of research strategies are beginning to involve integration of genetic and psychosocial evidence (e.g., twin studies that investigate social experiences as well as genetic influences) (Kendler et al. 2005). The emerging field of developmental epidemiology also has much to offer as a framework that makes the perspective of "cradle to the grave" seem old fashioned since it begins, not in the cradle, but rather with the genetic factors determined at conception as well as experiences in the mother's womb and through delivery. For example, it has been possible through this approach to assess the influence of a woman's use of nicotine during pregnancy on the child's subsequent likelihood of suffering from tobacco dependence (Buka et al. 2003).

In choosing the example of a pregnant woman's use of nicotine, I point to another new trend that involves the relationship between lifestyle behaviors and psychiatric disorders. Recently, for example, numerous studies have appeared that give information on the relationships of cigarette smoking or obesity to psychiatric disorders (Carpenter et al. 2000; Glassman et al. 1990; Murphy et al. 2003; Roberts et al. 2000). It is interesting, however, that life*style* has, to some extent, supplanted life *stress* as a focus of psychosocial research.

REEMERGENCE OF IMPORTANT THEMES

In addition, some of the ideas that were so prominent when NIMH was formed have now reappeared in new guises. For example, a prominent influence at that time was the Faris and Dunham (1939) study of the distribution of persons with schizophrenia in Chicago. Now we have the Project on Human Development in Chicago Neighborhoods, which, like the earlier study, is concerned with location of residence as one component of its multilevel strategy (Sampson et al. 1997). While violence has been a main focus of the new Chicago study, it also includes material about psychiatric disorders. Very importantly, it includes population-based data—both systematic and quantitative—on a large number of neighborhoods conceived as slices of the social environment.

Another influence at the beginning of NIMH was the cultural determinism of Margaret Mead and Ruth Benedict, including one of the oldest and continuingly popular ideas in our field—that is, that civilization causes psychiatric disorder and that higher rates of disorder are to be found in the most advanced cultures (Freud 1930/1961; Torrey 1980). During the past few decades, the question of how much disorder there is in different areas of the world has not commanded much attention. Rather, most of the psychiatric research on culture has concerned questions of whether a disorder like schizophrenia exists elsewhere and, if so, whether it exhibits the same symptom profile as in the West (World Health Organization 1973). Then later, the "new cross-cultural psychiatry" suggested, for example, that while depression seems to exist in most cultures, the somatic manifestations are likely to dominate the picture in non-Western areas (Kleinman 1977).

The World Health Organization (WHO) has, however, become genuinely concerned about prevalence, spurred in part by the message of the Global Burden of Disease that depression will shortly become one of the most common of the disease burdens (Murray and Lopez 1996). The World Mental Health Initiative in which Ronald Kessler plays a central role has reported noteworthy differences in rates of mood disorders, ranging from less than 1% in Nigeria to more than 9% in the U.S. based on national samples in 14 countries (WHO World Mental Health Survey Consortium 2004).

This initiative makes use of the Composite International Diagnostic Interview (CIDI) which was constructed with much attention to its appropriateness for research in different countries (Wittchen et al. 1991). Despite the use of such a common method of data gathering and other markedly improved procedures compared to earlier efforts, it seems very likely that part of the difference in rates is due to methodological problems. Such issues deserve and are being given further scrutiny. Even with perfected methods, however, there will very probably continue to be differences in rates across different areas of the world. Given that depression is an etiologically complex disorder, it would *not* be realistic to expect that all countries would show the same prevalence, and it *is* realistic to expect that some of the variability will be due to psychosocial experiences.

Thus for illustrative argument, let us assume that the findings in Table 3–1 are approximately correct. Insofar as these national samples reflect culture, culture seems to make a difference. Does the evidence indicate that "development" or "modernization" is noxious? If we accept the classification provided by the World Bank as to which of these countries is developed and which not, we see that the lowest rates (less than 1% to 2.5%) come from the less developed countries. But the more outstanding fact is that there is the broad range of rates for both the less and more developed areas. Further, it is not unreasonable to posit that some of the differences may relate to national strife, political upheaval, or to threats of war and terrorism rather than to culture per se.

In thinking about how cultural or national identity might make a difference, it is useful to have in mind an outline of human conditions that might vary in terms of cultural values and practices. What are the stress points as well as the sources of support that characterize different cultures? The importance of such an outline was in my mind when doing research among the Yupik-speaking Eskimos of Alaska and the Yorubas of Nigeria in the 1950s and 1960s as part of the cross-cultural extensions of the Stirling County Study (Murphy 1965, 1972, 1976). My outline of human conditions included the role of children in family life. The Eskimos had elaborate and effective cultural patterns for adopting children should a woman be barren; the Yorubas seemed to lack not only the institutions for adoption but also the concept of adoption itself. The role of the childless woman among the Yoruba was extremely stressful while not nearly so disadvantageous among the Eskimos. Thus the difference that culture makes may be especially understandable if it can be seen through the risks and protections offered in different cultural arrangements.

TEMPORAL CHANGES

In addition to the probability of differences in rates across nations and cultures, there is also the question of historical change within a single culture. In the late 1960s and early 1970s, several clinicians began to observe a change in the profile of patients seeking treatment (Klerman and Paykel 1970; Muncie 1963). Klerman (1976) observed that psychiatrists began to see "depressed patients who are younger, less severely ill, and more commonly neurotic than psychotic; and these patients presented in outpatient and ambulatory settings rather than at inpatient hospital facilities."

Drawing together data from the ECA as well as that from the family investigations in the Psychobiology of Depression Study, Klerman and Weissman (1989) pointed to evidence of an increase in the rate of depression through a "cohort effect" based on the fact that younger people had higher rates of disorder than older people. The same effect appeared later in the NCS (Kessler et al. 1994b). It also appeared in numbers of studies carried out in other nations where comparison was possible because of the investigations having used the DIS (Cross-National Collaborative Group 1992). While the actual rates of depression differed, as in the World Mental Health Initiative, the cross-cultural perspective strongly suggested that younger people in many parts of the world were at greater risk than older people, thereby heralding a general increase.

The evidence of a "cohort effect" was based on lifetime rates, which can be thought of as *retrospective incidence*. While this has led to speculation that the findings may have been influenced by recall bias, it is interesting that studies using other strategies have also reported an increasing rate of depression. For example, in the Lundby Study in Sweden, using *prospective incidence*, Hagnell et al. (1982) reported increases for both men and women but emphasized the increase among younger men. In the Stirling County Study, using *current prevalence*, we found that across independent samples selected in 1952, 1970, and 1992, the overall rate of depression remained stable (Murphy et al. 2000). There was, however, a redistribution of prevalence in the most recent sample with younger women showing a twofold higher rate than pertained for younger women in the earlier samples.

As with cultural and national differences in rates, the tracing of time trends in psychiatric disorders presents us with numerous methodological problems. Never-

Table 3–1. World Mental Health Initiative: 12-month prevalence of mood disorders

Less-developed countries	%	Developed countries	%
Nigeria	0.8	Japan	3.1
Shanghai	1.7	Germany	3.6
Beijing	2.5	Italy	3.8
Mexico	4.8	Spain	4.9
Lebanon	6.6	Belgium	6.2
Colombia	6.8	Netherlands	6.9
Ukraine	9.1	France	8.5
		United States	9.6

Source. Adapted from WHO World Mental Health Survey Consortium: "Prevalence, Severity, and Unmet Need for Treatment of Mental Disorders in the World Health Organization World Mental Health Surveys." *JAMA* 291:2581–2590, 2004, Table 2. Copyright 2004, American Medical Association. All rights reserved.

theless, studies concerned with the same goal but using different methods suggest that depression is increasing, at least in some segments of the population. It seems reasonable to begin to try to understand why there may be differences in rates over time as much as differences by place. As pertinent to the U.S., the increasing rate of depression has sometimes been referred to as the "bluing of America" (Glass 1990). The etiology of such "bluing," however, remains unknown. The possibility that psychosocial and sociocultural factors are implicated is compelling. One of the new challenges for research on the social environment is to build a profile of experiences and correlates that may throw light on the reasons for this increase.

In addition to cross-national differences in rates and changes in rates over time, there is a new NIMH initiative concerned with the psychiatric implications of cultural diversity within the United States called the Collaborative Psychiatric Epidemiology Surveys; these studies are specifically concerned with cultural and ethnic influences on psychiatric disorders (Colpe et al. 2004). One of the surveys involves not only African Americans but also blacks of Caribbean descent so that variations within the black population can be investigated (Jackson et al. 2004). A companion study focuses on Latino and Asian American populations (Alegria et al. 2004). In this multilevel study, "context" as well as social and cultural risk factors will be given full attention. These studies are being guided by the goal of filling out an outline of specific kinds of risks and protections such as family cultural conflict, neighborhood safety, everyday and perceived discrimination, and social cohesion.

CONCLUSION

In summary it can be noted that the earliest goals of NIMH involved the broad concepts of culture and social structure. In retrospect, I believe that the conceptual breadth got out of hand. The survival of the field was threatened at least partly because the broad concepts were not adequately broken down into outlines of researchable and comparable units of investigation. A narrowing of focus on specific types of psychosocial stress ensued, but now new strategies have come into play that involve integration of biogenetic and psychosocial evidence. At the same time, the broad concepts that gave orientation to NIMH have regained attention through initiatives enacted not only by NIMH but also by the WHO. These broad topics of "change over time" as well as "cultural, ethnic, and national differences" are being addressed in new ways that have a very good chance of avoiding the pitfalls of the past.

The fact remains, however, that at the present time neuroscience commands more attention and funding than research on the social environment. This increased attention relates materially to advances in brain research, thrusts forward in psychopharmacology, and the mapping of the human genome. Psychosociocultural research is clearly not the front runner in funding, but improvements in our methods, and the continuing evidence that much will remain unexplained if we do not provide answers, indicate that the field is alive and going forward.

CLINICAL IMPLICATIONS

It would be a serious mistake for clinicians to ignore the social and historical contexts in which their patients live. While much contemporary research on psychopathology emphasizes biological factors, recent demonstrations of important gene–environment interactions highlight the need for careful attention to the psychosocial environment. The understanding of clinical phenomena would be impaired if the purview failed to take account of the roles played, for example, by social class, lifestyle behaviors, and trauma, as well as by changes in the risks for and rates of disorders like major depression.

REFERENCES

Alegria M, Takeuchi D, Canino G, et al: Considering context, place and culture: the National Latino and Asian American Study. Int J Methods Psychiatr Res 13:208–220, 2004

Allinsmith W, Goethals GW: The Role of Schools in Mental Health (A Report to the Staff Director, Jack R. Ewalt, Joint Commission on Mental Illness and Health Monograph Series No 7). New York, Basic Books, 1962

American Psychiatric Association: Diagnostic and Statistical Manual of Mental Disorders, 3rd Edition. Washington, DC, American Psychiatric Association, 1980

Bateson G, Jackson D, Haley J, et al: Toward a theory of schizophrenia. Behav Sci 1:251, 1956

Becker HS: Outsiders: Studies in the Sociology of Deviance. New York, Free Press, 1963

Benedict R: Patterns of Culture. Boston, MA, Houghton Mifflin, 1934

Bland RC, Newman SC, Orn H (eds): Epidemiology of psychiatric disorders in Edmonton. Acta Psychiatr Scand 77 (suppl 338):1–80, 1988

Breslau N: Epidemiologic studies of trauma, posttraumatic stress disorder, and other psychiatric disorders. Can J Psychiatry 47:923–929, 2002

Breslau N, Chase GA, Anthony JC: The uniqueness of the DSM definition of posttraumatic stress disorder: implications for research. Psychol Med 32:573–576, 2002

Bromet E, Sonnega A, Kessler RC: Risk factors for DSM-III-R posttraumatic stress disorder: findings from the National Comorbidity Survey. Am J Epidemiol 147: 353–361, 1998

Brown GW, Harris T: Social Origins of Depression: A Study of Psychiatric Disorder in Women. New York, Free Press, 1978

Bruce ML, Takeuchi DT, Leaf PJ: Poverty and psychiatric status: longitudinal evidence from the New Haven Epidemiologic Catchment Area Study. Arch Gen Psychiatry 48:470–474, 1991

Buka SL, Shenassa ED, Niaura R: Elevated risk of tobacco dependence among offspring of mothers who smoked during pregnancy: a 30-year prospective study. Am J Psychiatry 160:1978–1984, 2003

Cameron DC: Robert Hanna Felix, MD, 1904–1990. Am J Psychiatry 148:7–9, 1991

Carpenter KM, Hasin DS, Allison DB, et al: Relationships between obesity and DSM-IV major depressive disorder, suicide ideation, and suicide attempts; results from a general population study. Am J Public Health 90:251–257, 2000

Colpe L, Merikangas K, Cuthbert B, et al: Guest Editorial: National Institute of Mental Health. Int J Methods Psychiatr Res 13:193–195, 2004

Cross-National Collaborative Group: The changing rate of major depression: cross-national comparisons. Review. JAMA 268:3098–3105, 1992

Dohrenwend BP, Dohrenwend BS: The problem of validity in field studies of psychological disorder. J Abnorm Psychol 70:52–69, 1965

Dohrenwend BP, Dohrenwend BS: Social Status and Psychological Disorder: A Causal Inquiry. New York, Wiley-Interscience, 1969

Dohrenwend BP, Levav I, Shout PE, et al: Socioeconomic status and psychiatric disorders: the causation-selection issue. Science 225:946–952, 1992

Eaton WW, Holzer CE, Von Korff M, et al: The design of the Epidemiologic Catchment Area surveys. Arch Gen Psychiatry 41:942–948, 1984

Eaton WW, Neufeld K, Chen LS, et al: A comparison of self-report and clinical diagnostic interviews for depression: Diagnostic Interview Schedule and Schedules for Clinical Assessment in Neuropsychiatry in the Baltimore Epidemiologic Catchment Area follow-up. Arch Gen Psychiatry 57:217–222, 2000

Fallon IR, Boyd JL, McGill CW, et al: Family management in the prevention of exacerbations of schizophrenia: a controlled study. N Engl J Med 306:1437–1440, 1982

Faris REL, Dunham HW: Mental Disorders in Urban Areas: An Ecological Study of Schizophrenia and Other Psychoses. Chicago, IL, University of Chicago Press, 1939

Felix RH: The preparation of a community-oriented psychiatrist. Am J Psychiatry 122 (suppl):2–7, 1966

Felix RH, Bowers RV: Mental hygiene and socio-environmental factors. Milbank Memorial Fund Quarterly 26:125–146, 1948

Freud S: Civilization and its discontents (1930), in Standard Edition of the Complete Psychological Works of Sigmund Freud, Vol 21. Translated and edited by Strachey J. London, Hogarth Press, 1961, pp 59–145

Glass RM: Blue mood, blackened lungs. Depression and smoking. JAMA 264:1583–1584, 1990

Glassman AH, Helzer JE, Covey LS, et al: Smoking, smoking cessation, and major depression. JAMA 264:1546–1549, 1990

Greenhouse SW: On psychiatry, epidemiology, and statistics: a view from the 1950s and 1960s. Stat Med 22:3311–3322, 2003

Gurin G, Veroff J, Feld S: Americans View Their Mental Health: A Nationwide Interview Survey (A Report to the Staff Director, Jack B. Ewalt; Joint Commission on Mental Illness and Health, Monograph Series No 4). New York, Basic Books, 1960

Hagnell O, Lanke J, Rorsman B, et al: Are we entering an age of melancholy? Depressive illnesses in a prospective epidemiological study over 25 years: the Lundby Study, Sweden. Psychol Med 12:279–289, 1982

Hollingshead AB, Redlich FC: Social Class and Mental Illness: A Community Study. New York, John Wiley & Sons, 1958

Holzer CE, Shea BM, Swanson JW, et al: The increased risk for specific psychiatric disorders among persons of low socioeconomic status. Am J Soc Psychiatry 6:259–271, 1986

Husaini BA, Neff JA, Stone RH: Psychiatric impairment in rural communities. J Community Psychol 7:137–146, 1979

Jackson JS, Torres M, Caldwell CH, et al: The National Survey of American Life: a study of racial, ethnic and cultural influences on mental disorders and mental health. Int J Methods Psychiatr Res 13:196–207, 2004

Jahoda M: Current Concepts of Positive Mental Health (A Report to the Staff Director, Jack R. Ewalt. Monograph Series No 1). New York, Basic Books, 1958

Joint Commission on Mental Illness and Health: Action for Mental Health: Final Report. New York, Basic Books, 1961

Judd LL: Historical highlights of the National Institute of Mental Health from 1946 to the present. Am J Psychiatry 155 (suppl 9):3–8, 1998

Kendler KS, Myers J, Prescott CA: Sex differences in the relationship between social support and risk for major depression: a longitudinal study of opposite-sex twin pairs. Am J Psychiatry 162:250–256, 2005

Kessler RC, McGonagle KA, Zhao S, et al: Lifetime and 12-month prevalence of DSM-III-R psychiatric disorders in the United States. Results from the National Comorbidity Survey. Arch Gen Psychiatry 51:8–19, 1994a

Kessler RC, McGonagle KA, Nelson CB, et al: Sex and depression in the National Comorbidity Survey, II: cohort effects. J Affect Disord 30:15–26, 1994b

Kessler RC, Foster CL, Saunders WB, et al: Social consequences of psychiatric disorders, I: educational attainment. Am J Psychiatry 152:1026–1032, 1995

Kessler RC, Walters EE, Forthofer MS: The social consequences of psychiatric disorders, III: probability of marital stability. Am J Psychiatry 155:1092–1096, 1998

Kleinman A: Depression, somatization, and the "new cross-cultural psychiatry." Soc Sci Med 11:3–10, 1977

Klerman GL: Age and clinical depression: today's youth in the twenty-first century. J Gerontol 31:318–323, 1976

Klerman GL, Paykel ES: Depressive pattern, social background and hospitalization. J Nerv Ment Dis 150:466–478, 1970

Klerman GL, Weissman MM: Increasing rates of depression. JAMA 261:2229–2235, 1989

Laing RD: The Divided Self: A Study of Sanity and Madness. Chicago, IL, Quadrangle Books, 1960

Langner TS: A twenty-two item screening score of psychiatric symptoms indicating impairment. J Health Hum Behav 3:269–276, 1962

Langner TS, Michael ST: Life Stress and Mental Health: The Midtown Manhattan Study (Thomas A. C. Rennie Series in Social Psychiatry, Vol 2). New York, Free Press of Glencoe, 1963

Leighton AH: A proposal for research in the epidemiology of psychiatric disorder, in Epidemiology of Mental Disorder: Papers Presented at a Round Table at the 1949 Annual Conference of the Milbank Memorial Fund, November 16–17, 1949. New York, Milbank Memorial Fund, 1950, pp 128–135

Leighton AH: My Name Is Legion: Foundations for a Theory of Man in Relation to Culture. New York, Basic Books, 1959

Lemkau PV: The epidemiological study of mental illnesses and mental health. Am J Psychiatry 111:801–808, 1955

Macmillan AM: The Health Opinion Survey: technique for estimating prevalence of psychoneurotic and related types of disorders in communities. Psychological Reports 3:325–339, 1957

McCann RV: The Churches and Mental Health (A Report to the Staff Director, Jack R. Ewalt, Joint Commission on Mental Illness and Health, Monograph Series No 8). New York, Basic Books, 1962

Mead GH: Mind, Self and Society. Chicago, IL, University of Chicago Press, 1934

Mead M: Sex and Temperament in Three Primitive Societies. New York, William Morrow, 1935

Menninger KA: Toward a unitary concept of mental illness, in A Psychiatrist's World: Selected Papers. Edited by Hall BH. New York, Viking Press, 1959, pp 516–528

Muncie W: Depression or depressions? Can Psychiatr Assoc J 8:217–224, 1963

Murphy JM: Social science concepts and cross-cultural methods for psychiatric research, in Approaches to Cross-Cultural Psychiatry. Edited by Murphy JM, Leighton AH. Ithaca, NY, Cornell University Press, 1965, pp 251–284

Murphy JM: A cross-cultural comparison of psychiatric disorder: Eskimos of Alaska, Yorubas of Nigeria, and Nova Scotians of Canada, in Transcultural Research in Mental Health. Edited by Lebra WP. Honolulu, University of Hawaii Press, 1972, pp 213–226

Murphy JM: Psychiatric labeling in cross-cultural perspective. Science 191:1019–1028, 1976

Murphy JM: Continuities in community-based psychiatric epidemiology. Arch Gen Psychiatry 37:1215–1223, 1980

Murphy JM, Olivier DC, Monson RR, et al: Depression and anxiety in relation to social status. A prospective epidemiologic study. Arch Gen Psychiatry 48:223–229, 1991

Murphy JM, Laird NM, Monson RR, et al: A 40-year perspective on the prevalence of depression the Stirling County Study. Arch Gen Psychiatry 57:209–215, 2000

Murphy JM, Horton NC, Monson RR, et al: Cigarette smoking in relation to depression; historical trends from the Stirling County Study. Am J Psychiatry 160:1663–1669, 2003

Murray CJL, Lopez AD (eds): The Global Burden of Disease: A Comprehensive Assessment of Mortality and Disability From Diseases, Injuries, and Risk Factors in 1990 and Projected to 2020 (Harvard School of Public Health on behalf of the World Health Organization and the World Bank). Cambridge, MA, Harvard University Press, 1996

North CS, Nixon SJ, Shariat S, et al: Psychiatric disorders among survivors of the Oklahoma City bombing. JAMA 282:755–762, 1999

Offord DR, Boyle MH, Campbell D, et al: One-year prevalence of psychiatric disorder in Ontarians 15 to 64 years of age. Can J Psychiatry 41:559–563, 1996

Pardes H: NIMH during the tenure of Director Herbert Pardes, M.D. (1978–1984): the President's Commission on Mental Health and the reemergence of NIMH's scientific mission. Am J Psychiatry 155 (suppl 9):14–19, 1998

Phillips DL: The "true prevalence" of mental illness in a New England state. Community Ment Health J 2:35–40, 1966

President's Commission on Mental Health: Report to the President from the President's Commission on Mental Health, Vol 1. Washington, DC, U.S. Government Printing Office, 1978

Punämaki RL, Komproe IH, Qouta S, et al: The role of peritraumatic dissociation and gender in the association between trauma and mental health in a Palestinian community sample. Am J Psychiatry 162:545–551, 2005

Regier DA, Boyd JH, Burke JD, et al: One-month prevalence of mental disorders in the United States: based on five Epidemiologic Catchment Area sites. Arch Gen Psychiatry 45:977–986, 1988

Roberts RE, Kaplan GA, Shema SJ, et al: Are the obese at greater risk for depression? Am J Epidemiol 152:163–170, 2000

Robins LN: Psychiatric epidemiology. Arch Gen Psychiatry 35:697–702, 1978

Robins LN: Epidemiology: reflections on testing the validity of psychiatric interviews. Arch Gen Psychiatry 42:918–924, 1985

Robins LN, Regier DA (eds): Psychiatric Disorders in America: The Epidemiologic Catchment Area Study. New York, Free Press, 1991

Robins LN, Helzer JE, Croughan J, et al: National Institute of Mental Health Diagnostic Interview Schedule: its history, characteristics and validity. Arch Gen Psychiatry 38:381–389, 1981

Robinson R, DeMarche DF, Wagle MK: Community Resources in Mental Health, Statistical Analysis of 3103 Counties by Hoover AC: A Report to the Staff Director, Jack R. Ewalt. Joint Commission on Mental Illness and Health (Monograph Series No 5). New York, Basic Books, 1960

Roussos A, Goenjian AK, Steinberg AM, et al: Posttraumatic stress and depressive reactions among children and adolescents after the 1999 earthquake in Ano Liosia, Greece. Am J Psychiatry 162:530–537, 2005

Sampson RJ, Raudenbush SW, Earls F: Neighborhoods and violent crime: a multilevel study of collective efficacy. Science 277:918–924, 1997

Scheff T. Being Mentally Ill: A Sociological Theory. Chicago, IL, Aldine, 1966

Srole L, Langner TS, Michael ST, et al: Mental Health in the Metropolis: The Midtown Manhattan Study. New York, McGraw-Hill, 1962

Stouffer SA, Lumsdaine AA, Lumsdaine MH, et al: The American Soldier: Combat and Its Aftermath, Vol 2. Princeton, NJ, Princeton University Press, 1949

Stouffer SA, Guttman L, Suchman EA, et al: Measurement and Prediction. Princeton, NJ, Princeton University Press, 1950

Szasz TS. The Myth of Mental Illness: Foundations of a Theory of Personal Conduct. New York, Hoeber-Harper, 1961

Taxpayers for Common Sense: Golden Fleece Awards: history of the Golden Fleece. Available at: http://www.taxpayer.net/awards/goldenfleece/history.htm. Accessed January 10, 2005.

Torrey EF. Schizophrenia and Civilization. New York, Jason Aronson, 1980

Veroff J, Douvan E, Kulka RA: The Inner American: A Self-Portrait From 1957 to 1976. New York, Basic Books, 1981a

Veroff J, Kulka RA, Douvan E: Mental Health in America: Patterns of Help-Seeking From 1957 to 1976. New York, Basic Books, 1981b

Wang PS, Beck AL, Berglund P, et al: Effects of major depression on moment-in-time work performance. Am J Psychiatry 161:1885–1891, 2004

Weissman MM, Klerman GL: Epidemiology of mental disorders: emerging trends in the United States. Arch Gen Psychiatry 35:705–712, 1978

Weissman MM, Leaf PJ, Bruce JL: Single-parent women: a community study. Soc Psychiatry 22:29–33, 1987

WHO World Mental Health Survey Consortium: Prevalence, severity, and unmet need for treatment of mental disorders in the World Health Organization World Mental Health Surveys. JAMA 291:2581–2590, 2004

Winters EE (ed): The Collected Papers of Adolf Meyer. Baltimore, MD, Johns Hopkins University Press, 1950

Wittchen HU, Robins LN, Cottler LB, et al: Cross-cultural feasibility, reliability and sources of variance of the Composite International Diagnostic Interview (CIDI) Multicentre WHO/ADAMHA field trials. Br J Psychiatry 159:645–653, 658, 1991

World Health Organization: Report of the International Pilot Study of Schizophrenia, Vol 1. Geneva, Switzerland, World Health Organization, 1973

Part II

Vulnerability to Major Mental and Substance Use Disorders

Psychobiology of Resilience to Stress

Implications for Prevention of Anxiety

Antonia S. New, M.D.

Kathryn A. Keegan, B.A.

Dennis S. Charney, M.D.

This chapter reviews neurobiological models associated with trauma exposure, with a focus on the varied response that individuals have following a traumatic event. While posttraumatic stress disorder (PTSD) is a clinically important problem that develops in some individuals following exposure to significant trauma, it has become clear that most individuals endure trauma exposure without developing symptoms of anxiety or depression. A growing interest in resilience has brought to light the response of some individuals who have the capacity to endure extremely stressful events without adverse sequelae, or even to demonstrate improved function, in response to extreme adversity.

The published literature suffers from the lack of a uniform definition of resilience. Some authors have described resilience as the absence of anxiety symptoms following exposure to a traumatic stress (King et al. 2003; Yehuda 2004), while others describe resilience as the ability to recover after developing symptoms of PTSD (Davidson et al. 2005). Still others argue that a more clinically relevant measure of resilience centers on the ability to function in a variety of domains after an unusually stressful experience, regardless of PTSD symptoms (Bonanno 2004; Luthar et al. 2000).

How common is resilience? Numerous studies have reported that while the U.S. population has a high rate of trauma exposure (DSM-III [American Psychiatric Association 1980] and DSM-III-R [American Psychiatric Association 1987]: 68.1%; by DSM-IV [American Psychiatric Association 1994], 89.6% of a community sample met criteria for trauma), only a minority of individuals subsequently develops PTSD (lifetime prevalence of PTSD is 5%–6% in men and 10%–14% in women). A 20-year longitudinal follow-up study of cases of childhood abuse and neglect verified in court (McGloin and Widom 2001) shows a 22% overall rate of functional resilience as demonstrated by the domains of successful employment/education, interpersonal and domestic stability, lack of psychiatric disorder or substance abuse, and lack of criminal arrests/behavior education/work. It appears from these data that more females than males were resilient, when the groups were matched for type and severity of trauma. A number of psychosocial factors have been associated with functional resilience to stressful life events (Updegraff and Taylor 2000), including positive adaptation and optimism in the face of stress (Andersson 1996), cognitive flexibility including reappraising negative events in a positive light, moral compass including religious disposition and spirituality (Pargament 1997), good social support (Cohen and Wills 1985) and social networks (Cohen et al. 1997), an active coping style (Aldwin 1991), and a sense of humor (Davidson et al. 2005). However, this chapter will focus on specific neurobiological models of response to stress and will identify the implications of these models in the prevention of clinical symptoms after trauma.

THE HPA AXIS IN STRESS-INDUCED DEPRESSION AND STRESS RESILIENCE

Normal Functions

Corticotropin-releasing hormone (CRH) is one of the most important mediators of the normal stress response. In response to acute and chronic stress, the paraventricular nucleus of the hypothalamus secretes corticotropin-releasing factor (CRF), which, in turn, stimulates the anterior pituitary gland to synthesize and release adrenocorticotropic hormone (ACTH) and locus coeruleus release of norepinephrine in the paraventricular nucleus, hippocampus, and prefrontal cortex (PFC) (Grammatopoulos and Chrousos 2002). ACTH then stimulates the synthesis and release of adrenal glucocorticoids. Cortisol mobilizes and replenishes energy stores, inhibits growth and reproductive systems, contains the immune response, and affects behavior through actions on multiple neurotransmitter systems and brain regions (reviewed in Hasler et al. 2004; Yehuda 2002).

Centrally administered CRH produces a number of symptoms and behaviors commonly seen in depression and anxiety, such as increased heart rate, increased blood pressure, decreased appetite, decreased sexual activity, increased arousal, and a reduction in reward expectations (Owens and Nemeroff 1991). Two subtypes of CRH receptors have been identified in human beings, CRH_1 and CRH_2 (Hsu and Hsueh 2001). Both receptors appear to play an important role in the stress response. Activation of CRH_1 receptors appears to be responsible for anxiety-like responses, while CRH_2 stimulation may produce anxiolytic responses (Bale et al. 2000, 2002). Psychological and physiological responses to stress may be determined, in part, by regulation of these two CRH receptor types in critical brain regions. Psychobiological resilience to stress-induced pathology may be related to the organism's ability to restrain the initial CRH response to acute stress and to prolong the CRH response to stress.

Impaired HPA Function

Alterations in hypothalamic-pituitary-adrenal (HPA) axis physiology and functioning have been reported consistently in patients diagnosed with mood disorders. In a subset of patients with depression (approximately 50%), the HPA axis appears to be hyperactive. Evidence of hyperactivity includes increased concentrations of CRH in the cerebrospinal fluid, increased urinary free cortisol, blunted ACTH response to CRH administration, and decreased tendency for the synthetic glucocorticoid dexamethasone (dexamethasone suppression test) to suppress cortisol. Antidepressants have been shown to normalize this excessive activation of the HPA axis in patients with major depression (reviewed by Nestler et al. 2002).

HPA abnormalities have also been demonstrated in PTSD by numerous studies. Specifically, elevated CRH has been seen in chronic PTSD (Baker et al. 1999; Bremner et al. 1997), suggesting hyperactivity of hypothalamic stress response, while studies have shown decreased peripheral stress response (Baker et al.

1999; Halbreich et al. 1989; Mason et al. 1986; Yehuda et al. 1991a, 1995b, 1996). This suggests an adrenocortical insufficiency in PTSD. Further support for this view comes from reported increased glucocorticoid receptor binding in peripheral mononuclear cells in combat PTSD (Yehuda et al. 1991b, 1993a), and hyper-suppression of cortisol in response to low-dose dexamethasone administration (Yehuda et al. 1993b, 1995a). Taken together, these findings suggest increased feedback inhibition in PTSD patients with enhanced secretion of CRH.

The role of CRH in stress response has implications for stress resilience and the prevention or reversal of stress-induced changes in neurobiological systems and behaviors. It may be possible to enhance stress resilience in at-risk or symp-tomatic individuals by providing pharmacological agents that stabilize HPA axis functioning. For example, blockade of CRH overdrive with CRH antago-nists might then serve as an anxiolytic, an antidepressant, and/or a preventive agent for the treatment of PTSD.

Dehydroepiandrosterone (DHEA) is another adrenal steroid that is released under stress. In response to fluctuating levels of ACTH, DHEA is released syn-chronously and episodically with cortisol. In the brain, DHEA's antiglucocorti-coid and antiglutaminergic activity may confer neuroprotection (reviewed in Charney 2004). Data supporting DHEA as a possible neurobiological resilience and stress protective factor include a negative correlation between DHEA reac-tivity (in response to ACTH administration) and severity of PTSD symptoms (Rasmusson et al. 2004) and a negative correlation between DHEA/cortisol and stress-induced levels of dissociation among elite special forces soldiers un-dergoing intense survival training (C.A. Morgan et al. 2004). Furthermore, DHEA administration has been shown to have antidepressant effects in patients with major depression (Wolkowitz et al. 1999).

NORADRENERGIC RESPONSE TO STRESS

During situations of danger, the sympathetic nervous system (SNS) releases epinephrine (E) and norepinephrine (NE) in order to protect the organism. The locus coeruleus (LC), the major NE cell-containing site, serves a critical role in the brain's alerting or vigilance system (Aston-Jones et al. 1998). Stress- and fear-related activation of the LC results in increased release of NE in a num-ber of brain regions that are involved in perceiving, evaluating, and responding to potentially threatening stimuli. Specifically, acute stress-related increases in NE have been found in the amygdala, hippocampus, striatum, and prefrontal cortex. Rapid activation of the LC/NE system appears to facilitate the organism's ability to respond effectively in dangerous situations (Charney and Deutch 1996). On the other hand, this rapid activation leads to exaggerated reactivity to internal or external trauma-associated cues. The magnitude of the sympathetic nervous system response to stress and danger varies from one person to the next. Some people have an unusually robust response to stress and in essence "overreact." Unchecked persistent sympathetic hyperresponsiveness may contribute to symptoms following a traumatic event. In contrast to PTSD patients, it is likely that physiologically resilient individuals maintain SNS activation within a window of adaptive elevation, high enough to respond to danger, but not so high as to produce incapacity, depression, anxiety, and fear (Charney 2004; C. A. Morgan et al. 2000a). A series of studies reviewed by Dienstbier (1989, 1991) suggests that performance is enhanced when this optimal level of SNS activation is characterized by relatively low levels of E and NE.

Evidence points to abnormalities in noradrenergic function in depression. Adult women with depression and a history of early childhood abuse demonstrate greater plasma cortisol response to psychological stress compared with depressed women without a history of abuse and healthy control subjects (Heim et al. 2000).

Considerable evidence also indicates that peripheral noradrenergic function is abnormal in PTSD. This has been observed both in the acute stages (De Bellis et al. 1999; Hawk et al. 2000) and upon provocation to remember the trauma (Bremner et al. 2003; Liberzon et al. 1999; Southwick et al. 1999a), whereas resting plasma NE levels in subjects with chronic PTSD are often normal (Hageman et al. 2001). Geracioti et al. (2001) reported that cerebrospinal fluid NE concentrations are abnormally elevated in PTSD.

Recent evidence suggests that α_2-adrenoreceptor gene polymorphisms may play a role in baseline catecholamine levels, intensity of stress-induced SNS activation, and rate of catecholamine return to baseline after stress. In a study of healthy subjects, homozygous carriers of the α_{2C}Del322-325-AR polymorphism had exaggerated total-body noradrenergic spillover at baseline, exaggerated yohimbine (an α_2-adrenergic receptor antagonist that increases the release of NE)–induced increases in anxiety and total-body noradrenergic spillover, and a slower-than-normal return of total-body noradrenergic spillover to baseline after yohimbine infusion (Neumeister et al. 2005). Such individuals may be more vulnerable to stress-related psychiatric disorders such as PTSD.

On the basis of the above-described animal and human studies, it is likely that noradrenergic activity is regulated within an optimal window in individuals who are resilient to stress and to the development of stress-related disorders such as PTSD. Additionally, one might predict that therapies and pharmacological agents that help contain stress-related noradrenergic responsivity would enhance stress re-silience and help to prevent stress-induced depression. Thus, pharmacological agents that reduce locus coeruleus firing rate—such as α_2-adrenergic agonists (e.g., clonidine, guanfacine), α_1 agonists (e.g., prazosin), β-adrenergic antago-nists (e.g., propranolol), and neuropeptide Y—might serve to foster stress resil-ience in at-risk individuals.

NEUROPEPTIDE Y MODULATION OF SYMPATHETIC RESPONSE

Neuropeptide Y (NPY) is an amino acid that is released with NE when the SNS is strongly activated (reviewed in Southwick et al. 1999a, 1999b). One of NPY's actions is to inhibit the continued release of NE so that the SNS does not "overshoot." NPY administration has also been shown to result in a decrease of HPA activation (Antonijevic et al. 2000). A number of studies by C. A. Morgan and colleagues (2000a, 2000b, 2001a, 2001b, 2002) confirmed that acute uncon-trollable stress results in increased levels of cortisol, NE, and plasma NPY. U.S. Army soldiers and U.S. Navy personnel who have participated in survival school training that included capture and interrogation demonstrated an increased level of plasma NPY positively correlated with elevation in plasma cortisol and NE. Interestingly, the stress-induced increase was significantly and negatively corre-lated with subjective reports of distress, which suggests that NPY might have had anxiolytic action in these subjects (Heilig and Murison 1987; Heilig et al. 1989).

C. A. Morgan et al. (2000b) also demonstrated that special operations forces had significantly higher levels of NPY secretion in response to acute stress than did soldiers who did not undergo special forces training. Furthermore, following survival training, NPY levels in special operations forces soldiers returned to baseline, whereas NPY returned to levels below baseline in non–special opera-tions soldiers. This study suggests that stress-related NPY secretion could re-flect a type of characteristic hardiness that may confer resilience during exposure to severe trauma. Taken together, the literature suggests that military personnel who exhibit decreased capacity for stress-induced NPY release and increased dissociation are at a greater risk for the development of stress-related illnesses such as PTSD. Further support for the role of stress resistance in PTSD comes from a study in male veterans showing the NPY levels were associated with de-gree of symptom recovery from PTSD (Yehuda et al. 2006).

EMOTIONAL MEMORIES AND MEMORY STORAGE

Differences in the memory encoding for emotional stimuli may also underlie individual differences in stress resistance. In healthy individuals, memory of newly learned information initially persists in a fragile state and consolidates over time (McGaugh 2000). Memory for emotionally salient aspects of traumatic events remains vivid and intact, while memory for other less salient information is often impaired. Gradual consolidation of memories may serve an adaptive function by enabling endogenous processes, activated by an experience, to modulate memory strength (McGaugh 2000).

Studies have demonstrated that memory for words from a word list is enhanced for emotionally salient words (e.g., "murder") and for visually salient words (e.g., "font") (Strange et al. 2003). In contrast to visually salient words, emotionally salient words diminish recall of the words immediately preceding the emotional words. The role of the catecholamines in this has been demonstrated by the administration of propranolol, a β-adrenergic receptor–blocking agent. Propranolol administration prior to memory encoding eliminates the memory enhancement of emotionally salient words but not of visually salient words (Strange et al. 2003). It also eliminates the relative amnesia for words preceding the emotionally salient words.

Similarly, memory for the emotional components of a story (narrative with slides) is also influenced by beta-blockers. In a study in which healthy subjects were asked to read and recall an emotional story prompted with slides, memory for an emotionally intense story was superior to memory for a nonemotional story during the placebo condition (Cahill et al. 1994). When administered before memory encoding, propranolol blocked the hyperamnesia elicited by the emotional story but did not alter the memory of the emotionally neutral story. This result was found specifically in response to propranolol but not to nadolol (a $\beta_{1,2}$-blocker that is much less capable of crossing the blood–brain barrier) (van Stegeren et al. 1998), suggesting that the reduced memory was a direct effect of the blockade of central β-adrenergic receptors. Animal studies suggest that contextual memory (a freezing reaction in the cage in which a shock occurred), but not cued memory (a bell the animal has been conditioned to associate with a shock) (Roozendaal et al. 2004), was impeded by propranolol administration. This effect of propranolol was seen when the drug was administered systemically and into the amygdala directly, but not when it was administered locally in alternate brain regions. This model of how emotional memories are laid down provides one mechanism by which hyperactivity of the NE response to stress in PTSD may predispose to an exaggeration of the overremembering of emotional memories, resulting in the prolonged intrusive traumatic memories seen in PTSD. The ability of central β-adrenergic antagonists to reduce the impact of emotionally salient information on memory may influence future treatment efforts in trauma-exposed populations, as the reduction of vivid forms of reexperiencing may decrease the chances of developing PTSD and increase levels of functionality posttrauma.

Studies have shown that the effect of beta blockade is specific to the amygdala. Specifically, functional magnetic resonance imaging (fMRI) studies have demonstrated that successful encoding of emotional—as compared with neutral—words is associated with amygdala activation. Administration of propranolol at encoding abolishes the enhanced amygdala activity. In addition, items that evoke amygdala activation at encoding evoke greater hippocampal responses at retrieval, despite the fact that propranolol is no longer present at retrieval. Thus, memory-related amygdala responses at encoding and hippocampal responses at recognition of emotional items depend on β-adrenergic engagement at encoding. This suggests that human emotional memory is associated with a β-adrenergic–dependent modulation of amygdala–hippocampal interactions (Strange and Dolan 2004).

PREVENTION OF PTSD: PROPRANOLOL

Pharmacological secondary prevention of PTSD (i.e., intervening after a traumatic event to forestall PTSD's development) is a topic of current medical interest that has received little investigation (Larkin 1999). Prospective, controlled pharmacological trials in patients with PTSD are under way (Brunet et al. 2005). Preliminary data suggest that the β-adrenergic blocker propranolol may be effective in the treatment of stress disorders. In a recent small-scale, prospective placebo-controlled trial, Pitman et al. (2002) administered propranolol to trauma survivors within 6 hours of exposure to the traumatic event, seeking to examine whether administration of propranolol could prevent evolution of PTSD. Despite poor dosage and compliance monitoring and a trial duration of only 10 days, results indicated that propranolol was more effective than placebo in preventing the development of PTSD at 1 and 3 months, although the difference did not reach statistical significance. However, none of the propranolol-treated subjects were psychophysiologically reactive, compared with 43% of the placebo-treated subjects, with "reactivity" defined according to an a priori discriminant function.

Open treatment trials of propranolol and acute PTSD were also conducted in children (Famularo et al. 1988) and reported a decrease in nightmares, explosiveness, exaggerated startle, insomnia, and hyperalertness. A recent case report (Taylor and Cahill 2002) described administration of propranolol (60 mg) orally, twice a day (1.75 mg/kg/day), to a woman with reemergent PTSD symptoms after multiple (six) motor vehicle accidents, the last three of which caused severe PTSD episodes lasting more than 6 months each, despite multiple pharmacotherapies. PTSD symptoms were rapidly and markedly reduced. The Clinician-Administered PTSD Scale score was reduced from an initial 86 to 56 by 11 days posttrauma. To our knowledge, this is the first report of the effects of propranolol treatment on PTSD. In an older open study, limited effects of propranolol were described in combat veterans with PTSD (Kolb et al. 1984). Propranolol's capacity to inhibit consolidation of emotionally laden memories makes it a particularly attractive potential agent for treatment of acute stress disorder and acute PTSD. Its capability to prevent or diminish LC sensitization and to reduce arousal could augment this effect by decreasing the subjective distress and emotional valence associated with traumatic memories.

BRAIN REGIONS IMPLICATED IN EMOTION REGULATION/ MODELS OF STRESS RESISTANCE

Role of the Amygdala in Mediating Fear and Anxiety

Brain-imaging studies further highlight the role of the amygdala in fear conditioning and in the development of emotional responses to environmental contexts (Charney 2004). The amygdala's role in mediating fear influences processing of the affective elements of social interactions. Rats and monkeys with amygdala lesions lose their fear of animals they would normally fear.

Studies in monkeys show that amygdala lesions not only reduce fear responses but also increase submissive behaviors. Various neuroimaging paradigms have confirmed amygdala activation in human subjects viewing fearful faces (Davidson 2002). Studies of amygdala activation in PTSD are mixed and are confounded by different behavioral paradigms of symptom provocation used in the various studies. Activation of the right amygdala was reported in combat-related PTSD in patients and control subjects exposed to traumatic imagery and combat pictures (Rauch et al. 1996; Shin et al. 1997), while activation of the left amygdala was found in response to combat sounds (Liberzon et al. 1999). Other studies that used similar paradigms, however, were unable to replicate the finding of greater amygdala activation in patients with PTSD (Bremner 1999; Bremner et al. 1999b; Zubieta et al. 1999). Additional evidence supporting the hypothesis of amygdala hyperactivity in PTSD comes from a recent positron emission tomography (PET) study that demonstrated increased left-amygdala activation during the fear-acquisition stage of a fear conditioning program (Bremner et al. 2005).

Early and transient activation of the amygdala can be missed by techniques such as PET or single photon emission computed tomography (SPECT), which have lower temporal resolution than do event-related fMRI studies. The greater temporal resolution of fMRI may clarify what underlies the mixed results on amygdala activation in both resiliency and PTSD. An fMRI study demonstrated activation of the amygdala when subjects viewed pictures of fearful faces presented below the level of awareness (Whalen et al. 1998). In contrast, the overt presentation of emotional faces resulted in significant medial PFC activation (Morris et al. 1999; Whalen et al. 1998). Exaggerated amygdala response to masked-fearful versus masked-happy faces has been demonstrated in patients with PTSD compared with combat veterans without PTSD, suggesting that PTSD patients exhibit exaggerated amygdala activation to general threat-related stimuli presented at the subliminal level (Rauch et al. 2000). A study of combat-related PTSD in male subjects showed exaggerated amygdala activation bilaterally in response to fearful versus happy faces (Shin et al. 2005).

Phelps et al. (2004) studied fear using a task involving "instructed fear." Although subjects do not actually receive an aversive stimulus, they are told that they will receive a shock under specific conditions and have what has been called "anticipatory anxiety." Instructed fear has been shown to result in fear responses similar to those observed in traditional fear conditioning, as measured by startle potentiation and skin conductance response (Grillon and Davis 1997; LaBar et al. 1998). One possible path to stress resistance is that subjects with less adverse outcomes after trauma simply have less amygdala activation responsivity to fear-inducing stimuli. In our paradigm, this would be demonstrated by a lower level of amygdala activation in response to the "threat" condition rather than the "safe."

PREFRONTAL MODULATION OF FEAR AND ANXIETY

A different model from the noradrenergically mediated overresponsiveness of the amygdala to stress is that even though all individuals experience intense fear in the face of trauma, stress-resistant subjects may be better able to manage their responses through effortful control of negative emotion. They may be able to reappraise a fearful situation through an enhanced capacity to recruit areas of PFC that modulate and dampen the fear response (Orr et al. 2000; Peri et al. 2000). On the basis of findings from several studies, Davidson (2002) suggested that the ventromedial and/or orbital PFC plays a central role in affective responding through modulating the time course of emotional responding, and particularly in recovery time. An additional brain region thought to play a central role in emotion processing is the subgenual anterior cingulate gyrus (ACG), often viewed as a component of the medial PFC. The subgenual ACG appears to underlie the cognitive process of determining salience of emotional stimuli. Evidence for this model relies on a number of lines of evidence, including the presence of extensive reciprocal connections between the amygdala and the PFC, particularly the medial and orbital zones of the PFC (Amaral and Insausti 1992) and ventral ACG (Devinsky et al. 1995; Paus 2001). Inputs from the PFC to the amygdala are thought to be predominantly inhibitory (Amaral and Insausti 1992). Another line of evidence (M.A. Morgan et al. 1993) shows that lesions of the medial PFC in rats extend the time until a conditioned aversive response is extinguished, suggesting that the medial PFC normally inhibits the amygdala as a component of extinction. In the absence of this normal inhibitory input, the amygdala remains unchecked and continues to maintain the learned aversive response. A third line of evidence comprises data indicating that individual differences in the degree of PFC cerebral blood flow significantly predict subjects' experience of negative emotion (Zald et al. 2002), and PET studies indicate that in healthy subjects, glucose metabolism in the left medial and lateral PFC is reciprocally associated with glucose metabolic rate in the amygdala (Abercrombie et al. 1998). Finally, a recent study showed that activity of the right PFC appears to be inversely correlated with amygdala activity (Hariri et al. 2000), suggesting an inhibitory influence of medial and perhaps dorsolateral PFC on limbic activity (Davidson and Irwin 1999). Furthermore, activation of the medial PFC, and the reciprocal relationship of the medial PFC with the amygdala, seem to underlie effortful cognitive control of negative emotion (Ochsner et al. 2004). These findings suggest that PFC plays an important role in top-down modulation of the amygdala and that the neural circuitry underlying extinction of fear conditioning in rodents is similar to that underlying subjective experience of negative emotion in human beings.

Studies evaluating medial PFC and ACG in PTSD have included both volumetric and functional studies. Volumetric studies of ACG in PTSD have shown that women with PTSD have significantly smaller ACG and ventromedial PFC compared with women with similar trauma histories without PTSD (Rauch et al. 2003). Another study of trauma victims of the Japanese subway sarin gas attack showed decreased ACG volume in victims who developed PTSD compared with those who did not develop PTSD (Yamasue et al. 2003). Together, these studies suggest that smaller PFC volume may be a vulnerability factor for PTSD.

Previous functional imaging studies in patients with PTSD have not included a non-PTSD trauma-exposed control group. However, a consistent finding among PET studies is the failure of activation of the ACG in response to personalized scripts of the abuse (Bremner et al. 1999a; Shin et al. 1999) or exposure to combat slides and sounds (Bremner et al. 1999b). An fMRI study of subjects with PTSD resulting from a variety of traumas demonstrated that in response to script-driven imagery, women with PTSD exhibited less activation of ACG, thalamus, and medial PFC in response to negative emotion than did control subjects (Lanius et al. 2002, 2003). In an fMRI study of emotional faces, men with combat-related PTSD showed a negative correlation between amygdala activation and signal changes in the medial PFC, suggesting a disconnect in the normal modulation of the amygdala by the medial PFC (Shin et al. 2005). In this study, PTSD symptom severity was also negatively related to signal changes in the medial PFC, suggesting that the diminished activation of the medial PFC in response to fearful versus happy faces was clinically significant.

Reappraisal is the deliberate conscious cognitive transformation of emotional experience. In both experimental and individual-difference studies, reappraising an aversive event in unemotional terms demonstrably reduces negative affect, and the ability to think about stressful events in a new way may play a key role in coping with trauma (Taylor 1983). Indeed, an ability to find meaning in or even benefit from major stressful experiences such as combat has been linked to reduced psychological distress and fewer PTSD symptoms (Aldwin et al. 1994; Davis et al. 1998). One study evaluating a cognitive reappraisal task showed that healthy individuals can reliably decrease their startle response to pictures that normally elicit negative emotions (Jackson et al. 2000). An fMRI study using a similar paradigm found that during active suppression of a memory, increased activation of the lateral and medial prefrontal regions and decreased activation of the amygdala and medial orbitofrontal cortex was observed (Ochsner et al. 2002); this finding was confirmed in a subsequent study, which showed activation of the dorsal PFC during conscious suppression, and also showed that activity of the medial PFC correlated with the magnitude of forgetting (Anderson et al. 2004). If the ability to activate reappraisal strategies in the face of aversive stimuli is related to reduced risk for developing PTSD, then stress-resistant individuals might show more activity during a reappraisal task in brain regions associated with reappraisal. This is an area under active study.

CLINICAL IMPLICATIONS

The models presented here are not mutually exclusive, but rather represent broad approaches to studying features of stress responsiveness that hold promise for the understanding of individual differences in response to stress. If we can understand what it is that leads some individuals to undergo extremely challenging and traumatic experiences and yet to continue to function well and to have a positive attitude, this might lead to a promising way to enhance stress resistance in those individuals who are vulnerable to posttraumatic symptoms. Although much work needs to be done, our current knowledge of the neurobiology of stress and psychological trauma underscores the importance of developing clinical treatments that both reduce the subjective experience of stress and improve function in brain regions that mediate stress and trauma. Fortunately, both cognitive (e.g., cognitive reappraisal) and psychopharmacological (e.g., propranolol administration) approaches are moving us closer to those goals.

REFERENCES

Abercrombie H, Schaefer SM, Larson CL, et al: Metabolic rate in the right amygdala predicts negative affect in depressed patients. Neuroreport 9:3301–3307, 1998

Aldwin CM: Does age affect the stress and coping process? Implications of age differences in perceived control. J Gerontol 46:P174–P180, 1991

Aldwin CM, Levenson MR, Spiro A 3rd: Vulnerability and resilience to combat exposure: can stress have lifelong effects? Psychol Aging 9:34–44, 1994

Amaral DG, Insausti R: Retrograde transport of D-[3H]-aspartate injected into the monkey amygdaloid complex. Exp Brain Res 88:375–388, 1992

American Psychiatric Association: Diagnostic and Statistical Manual of Mental Disorders, 3rd Edition. Washington, DC, American Psychiatric Association, 1980

American Psychiatric Association: Diagnostic and Statistical Manual of Mental Disorders, 3rd Edition, Revised. Washington, DC, American Psychiatric Association, 1987

American Psychiatric Association: Diagnostic and Statistical Manual of Mental Disorders, 4th Edition. Washington, DC, American Psychiatric Association, 1994

Anderson MC, Ochsner KN, Kuhl B, et al: Neural systems underlying the suppression of unwanted memories. Science 303:232–235, 2004

Andersson G: The benefits of optimism: a meta-analytic review of the Life Orientation Test. Personality and Individual Differences 21:719–725, 1996

Antonijevic IA, Murck H, Bohlhalter S, et al: Neuropeptide Y promotes sleep and inhibits ACTH and cortisol release in young men. Neuropharmacology 39:1474–1481, 2000

Aston-Jones G, Rajkowski J, Ivanova S, et al: Neuromodulation and cognitive performance: recent studies of noradrenergic locus ceruleus neurons in behaving monkeys. Adv Pharmacol 42:755–759, 1998

Baker DG, West SA, Nicholson WE, et al: Serial CSF corticotropin-releasing hormone levels and adrenocortical activity in combat veterans with posttraumatic stress disorder. Am J Psychiatry 156:585–588, 1999

Bale TL, Contarino A, Smith GW, et al: Mice deficient for corticotropin-releasing hormone receptor-2 display anxiety-like behaviour and are hypersensitive to stress. Nat Genet 24:410–414, 2000

Bale TL, Picetti R, Contarino A, et al: Mice deficient for both corticotropin-releasing factor receptor 1 (CRFR1) and CRFR2 have an impaired stress response and display sexually dichotomous anxiety-like behavior. J Neurosci 22:193–199, 2002

Bonanno GA: Loss, trauma, and human resilience: have we underestimated the human capacity to thrive after extremely aversive events? Am Psychol 59:20–28, 2004

Bremner JD: Alterations in brain structure and function associated with post-traumatic stress disorder. Semin Clin Neuropsychiatry 4:249–255, 1999

Bremner JD, Licinio J, Darnell A, et al: Elevated CSF corticotropin-releasing factor concentrations in posttraumatic stress disorder. Am J Psychiatry 154:624–629, 1997

Bremner JD, Narayan M, Staib LH, et al: Neural correlates of memories of childhood sexual abuse in women with and without posttraumatic stress disorder. Am J Psychiatry 156:1787–1795, 1999a

Bremner JD, Staib LH, Kaloupek D, et al: Neural correlates of exposure to traumatic pictures and sound in Vietnam combat veterans with and without posttraumatic stress disorder: a positron emission tomography study. Biol Psychiatry 45:806–816, 1999b

Bremner JD, Vythilingam M, Vermetten E, et al: Cortisol response to a cognitive stress challenge in posttraumatic stress disorder (PTSD) related to childhood abuse. Psychoneuroendocrinology 28:733–750, 2003

Bremner JD, Vermetten E, Schmahl C, et al: Positron emission tomographic imaging of neural correlates of a fear acquisition and extinction paradigm in women with childhood sexual-abuse-related post-traumatic stress disorder. Psychol Med 35:791–806, 2005

Brunet A, Orr SP, Tremblay J, et al: Post-retrieval propranolol weakens longstanding traumatic memories (abstract #60). Poster presented at: American College of Neuropsychopharmacology 44th Annual Meeting, Waikoloa, HI, December 11–15, 2005

Cahill L, Prins B, Weber M, et al: Beta-adrenergic activation and memory for emotional events. Nature 371(6499):702–704, 1994

Charney DS: Discovering the neural basis of human social anxiety: a diagnostic and therapeutic imperative. Am J Psychiatry 161:1–2, 2004

Charney DS: Psychobiological mechanisms of resilience and vulnerability: implications for successful adaptation to extreme stress. Am J Psychiatry 161:195–216, 2004

Charney DS, Deutch AY: A functional neuroanatomy of anxiety and fear: implications for the pathophysiology and treatment of anxiety disorders. Crit Rev Neurobiol 10 (3–4):419–446, 1996

Cohen S, Wills TA: Stress, social support, and the buffering hypothesis. Psychol Bull 98:310–357, 1985

Cohen S, Doyle WJ, Skoner DP, et al: Social ties and susceptibility to the common cold. JAMA 277:1940–1944, 1997

Davidson JR: Anxiety and affective style: role of prefrontal cortex and amygdala. Biol Psychiatry 51:68–80, 2002

Davidson JR, Irwin W: The functional neuroanatomy of emotion and affective style. Trends Cogn Sci 3:11–21, 1999

Davidson JR, Payne VM, Connor KM, et al: Trauma, resilience and saliostasis: effects of treatment in post-traumatic stress disorder. Int Clin Psychopharmacol 20:43–48, 2005

Davis CG, Nolen-Hoeksema S, Larson J: Making sense of loss and benefiting from the experience: two construals of meaning. J Pers Soc Psychol 75:561–574, 1998

De Bellis MD, Baum AS, Birmaher B, et al: A.E. Bennett Research Award. Developmental traumatology, part I: biological stress systems. Biol Psychiatry 45:1259–1270, 1999

Devinsky O, Morrell MJ, Vogt BA: Contributions of anterior cingulate cortex to behaviour. Brain 118(Pt 1):279–306, 1995

Dienstbier RA: Arousal and physiological toughness: implications for mental and physical health. Psychol Rev 96:84–100, 1989

Dienstbier RA: Behavioral correlates of sympathoadrenal reactivity: the toughness model. Med Sci Sports Exerc 23:846–852, 1991

Famularo R, Kinscherff R, Fenton T: Propranolol treatment for childhood posttraumatic stress disorder, acute type. A pilot study. Am J Dis Child 142:1244–1247, 1988

Geracioti TD Jr, Baker DG, Ekhator NN, et al: CSF norepinephrine concentrations in posttraumatic stress disorder. Am J Psychiatry 158:1227–1230, 2001

Grammatopoulos DK, Chrousos GP: Functional characteristics of CRH receptors and potential clinical applications of CRH-receptor antagonists. Trends Endocrinol Metab 13:436–444, 2002

Grillon C, Davis M: Effects of stress and shock anticipation on prepulse inhibition of the startle reflex. Psychophysiology 34:511–517, 1997

Hageman I, Andersen HS, Jorgensen MB: Post-traumatic stress disorder: a review of psychobiology and pharmacotherapy. Acta Psychiatr Scand 104:411–422, 2001

Halbreich U, Olympia J, Carson S, et al: Hypothalamo-pituitary-adrenal activity in endogenously depressed post-traumatic stress disorder patients. Psychoneuroendocrinology 14:365–370, 1989

Hariri AR, Bookheimer SY, Mazziotta JC: Modulating emotional responses: effects of a neocortical network on the limbic system. Neuroreport 11:43–48, 2000

Hasler G, Drevets WC, Manji HK, et al: Discovering endophenotypes for major depression. Neuropsychopharmacology 29:1765–1781, 2004

Hawk LW, Dougall AL, Ursano RJ, et al: Urinary catecholamines and cortisol in recent-onset posttraumatic stress disorder after motor vehicle accidents. Psychosom Med 62:423–434, 2000

Heilig M, Murison R: Intracerebroventricular neuropeptide Y suppresses open field and home cage activity in the rat. Regul Pept 19(3–4):221–231, 1987

Heilig M, Soderpalm B, Engel JA, et al: Centrally administered neuropeptide Y (NPY) produces anxiolytic-like effects in animal anxiety models. Psychopharmacology (Berl) 98:524–529, 1989

Heim C, Newport DJ, Heit S, et al: Pituitary-adrenal and autonomic responses to stress in women after sexual and physical abuse in childhood. JAMA 284:592–597, 2000

Hsu SY, Hsueh AJ: Human stresscopin and stresscopin-related peptide are selective ligands for the type 2 corticotropin-releasing hormone receptor. Nat Med 7:605–611, 2001

Jackson DC, Malmstadt JR, Larson CL, et al: Suppression and enhancement of emotional responses to unpleasant pictures. Psychophysiology 37:515–522, 2000

King LA, King DW, Salgado DM, et al: Contemporary longitudinal methods for the study of trauma and posttraumatic stress disorder. CNS Spectrums 8:686–692, 2003

Kolb LC, Burris BC, Griffiths S: Propranolol and clonidine in the treatment of the chronic post-traumatic stress disorders of war, in Posttraumatic Stress Disorder: Psychological and Biological Sequelae. Edited by van der Kolk BA. Washington, DC, American Psychiatric Press, 1984, pp 98–105

LaBar KS, Gatenby JC, Gore JC, et al: Human amygdala activation during conditioned fear acquisition and extinction: a mixed-trial fMRI study. Neuron 20:937–945, 1998

Lanius RA, Williamson PC, Boksman K, et al: Brain activation during script-driven imagery induced dissociative responses in PTSD: a functional magnetic resonance imaging investigation. Biol Psychiatry 52:305–311, 2002

Lanius RA, Williamson PC, Hopper J, et al: Recall of emotional states in posttraumatic stress disorder: an fMRI investigation. Biol Psychiatry 53:204–210, 2003

Larkin M: Can post-traumatic stress disorder be put on hold? Lancet 354:1008, 1999

Liberzon I, Lopez JF, Flagel SB, et al: Differential regulation of hippocampal glucocorticoid receptors mRNA and fast feedback: relevance to post-traumatic stress disorder. J Neuroendocrinol 11:11–17, 1999

Luthar SS, Cicchetti D, Becker B: The construct of resilience: a critical evaluation and guidelines for future work. Child Dev 71:543–562, 2000

Mason JW, Giller EL, Kosten TR, et al: Urinary free-cortisol levels in posttraumatic stress disorder patients. J Nerv Ment Dis 174:145–149, 1986

McGaugh JL: Memory—a century of consolidation. Science 287:248–251, 2000

McGloin JM, Widom CS: Resilience among abused and neglected children grown up. Dev Psychopathol 13:1021–1038, 2001

Morgan CA 3rd, Wang S, Mason J, et al: Hormone profiles in humans experiencing military survival training. Biol Psychiatry 47:891–901, 2000a

Morgan CA 3rd, Wang S, Southwick SM, et al: Plasma neuropeptide-Y concentrations in humans exposed to military survival training. Biol Psychiatry 47:902–909, 2000b

Morgan CA 3rd, Hazlett G, Wang S, et al: Symptoms of dissociation in humans experiencing acute, uncontrollable stress: a prospective investigation. Am J Psychiatry 158:1239–1247, 2001a

Morgan CA 3rd, Wang S, Rasmusson A, et al: Relationship among plasma cortisol, catecholamines, neuropeptide Y, and human performance during exposure to uncontrollable stress. Psychosom Med 63:412–422, 2001b

Morgan CA 3rd, Rasmusson AM, Wang S, et al: Neuropeptide-Y, cortisol, and subjective distress in humans exposed to acute stress: replication and extension of previous report. Biol Psychiatry 52:136–142, 2002

Morgan CA 3rd, Southwick S, Hazlett G, et al: Relationships among plasma dehydroepiandrosterone sulfate and cortisol levels, symptoms of dissociation, and objective performance in humans exposed to acute stress. Arch Gen Psychiatry 61:819–825, 2004

Morgan MA, Romanski LM, LeDoux JE: Extinction of emotional learning: contribution of medial prefrontal cortex. Neurosci Lett 163:109–113, 1993

Morris JS, Scott SK, Dolan RJ: Saying it with feeling: neural responses to emotional vocalizations. Neuropsychologia 37:1155–1163, 1999

Nestler EJ, Barrot M, DiLeone RJ, et al: Neurobiology of depression. Neuron 34:13–25, 2002

Neumeister A, Charney DS, Belfer I, et al: Sympathoneural and adrenomedullary functional effects of alpha2C-adrenoreceptor gene polymorphism in healthy humans. Pharmacogenet Genomics 15:143–149, 2005

Ochsner KN, Bunge SA, Gross JJ, et al: Rethinking feelings: an fMRI study of the cognitive regulation of emotion. J Cogn Neurosci 14:1215–1229, 2002

Ochsner KN, Ray RD, Cooper JC, et al: For better or for worse: neural systems supporting the cognitive down- and up-regulation of negative emotion. Neuroimage 23:483–499, 2004

Orr SP, Metzger LJ, Lasko NB, et al: De novo conditioning in trauma-exposed individuals with and without posttraumatic stress disorder. J Abnorm Psychol 109:290–298, 2000

Owens MJ, Nemeroff CB: Physiology and pharmacology of corticotropin-releasing factor. Pharmacol Rev 43:425–473, 1991

Pargament K: The Psychology of Religion and Coping: Theory, Research, Practice. New York, Guilford, 1997

Paus T: Primate anterior cingulate cortex: where motor control, drive and cognition interface. Nat Rev Neurosci 2:417–424, 2001

Peri T, Ben-Shakhar G, Orr SP, et al: Psychophysiologic assessment of aversive conditioning in posttraumatic stress disorder. Biol Psychiatry 47:512–519, 2000

Phelps EA, Delgado MR, Nearing KI, et al: Extinction learning in humans: role of the amygdala and vmPFC. Neuron 43:897–905, 2004

Pitman RK, Sanders KM, Zusman RM, et al: Pilot study of secondary prevention of posttraumatic stress disorder with propranolol. Biol Psychiatry 51:189–192, 2002

Rasmusson AM, Vasek J, Lipschitz DS, et al: An increased capacity for adrenal DHEA release is associated with decreased avoidance and negative mood symptoms in women with PTSD. Neuropsychopharmacology 29:1546–1557, 2004

Rauch SL, van der Kolk BA, Fisler RE, et al: A symptom provocation study of posttraumatic stress disorder using positron emission tomography and script-driven imagery. Arch Gen Psychiatry 53:380–387, 1996

Rauch SL, Whalen PJ, Shin LM, et al: Exaggerated amygdala response to masked facial stimuli in posttraumatic stress disorder: a functional MRI study. Biol Psychiatry 47:769–776, 2000

Rauch SL, Shin LM, Segal E, et al: Selectively reduced regional cortical volumes in posttraumatic stress disorder. Neuroreport 14:913–916, 2003

Roozendaal B, de Quervain DJ, Schelling G, et al: A systemically administered beta-adrenoceptor antagonist blocks corticosterone-induced impairment of contextual memory retrieval in rats. Neurobiol Learn Mem 81:150–154, 2004

Shin LM, Kosslyn SM, McNally RJ, et al: Visual imagery and perception in posttraumatic stress disorder. A positron emission tomographic investigation. Arch Gen Psychiatry 54:233–241, 1997

Shin LM, McNally RJ, Kosslyn SM, et al: Regional cerebral blood flow during script-driven imagery in childhood sexual abuse-related PTSD: a PET investigation. Am J Psychiatry 156:575–584, 1999

Shin LM, Wright CI, Cannistraro PA, et al: A functional magnetic resonance imaging study of amygdala and medial prefrontal cortex responses to overtly presented fearful faces in posttraumatic stress disorder. Arch Gen Psychiatry 62:273–281, 2005

Southwick SM, Bremner JD, Rasmusson A, et al: Role of norepinephrine in the pathophysiology and treatment of posttraumatic stress disorder. Biol Psychiatry 46:1192–1204, 1999a

Southwick SM, Paige S, Morgan CA 3rd, et al: Neurotransmitter alterations in PTSD: catecholamines and serotonin. Semin Clin Neuropsychiatry 4:242–248, 1999b

Strange BA, Dolan RJ: Beta-adrenergic modulation of emotional memory-evoked human amygdala and hippocampal responses. Proc Natl Acad Sci U S A 101:11454–11458, 2004

Strange BA, Hurlemann R, Dolan RJ: An emotion-induced retrograde amnesia in humans is amygdala- and beta-adrenergic-dependent. Proc Natl Acad Sci U S A 100:13626–13631, 2003

Taylor F, Cahill L: Propranolol for reemergent posttraumatic stress disorder following an event of retraumatization: a case study. J Trauma Stress 15:433–437, 2002

Taylor S: Adjustment to threatening events: a theory of cognitive adaptation. Am Psychol 38:1161–1173, 1983

Updegraff J, Taylor S: From vulnerability to growth: positive and negative effects of stressful life events, in Loss and Trauma: General and Close Relationships Perspectives. Edited by Harvey JH, Miller ED. Ann Arbor, MI, Edwards Brothers, 2000, pp 3–28

van Stegeren AH, Everaerd W, Cahill L, et al: Memory for emotional events: differential effects of centrally versus peripherally acting beta-blocking agents. Psychopharmacology (Berl) 138:305–310, 1998

Whalen PJ, Rauch SL, Etcoff NL, et al: Masked presentations of emotional facial expressions modulate amygdala activity without explicit knowledge. J Neurosci 18:411–418, 1998

Wolkowitz OM, Reus VI, Keebler A, et al: Double-blind treatment of major depression with dehydroepiandrosterone. Am J Psychiatry 156:646–649, 1999

Yamasue H, Kasai K, Iwanami A, et al: Voxel-based analysis of MRI reveals anterior cingulate gray-matter volume reduction in posttraumatic stress disorder due to terrorism. Proc Natl Acad Sci U S A 100:9039–9043, 2003

Yehuda R: Current status of cortisol findings in post-traumatic stress disorder. Psychiatr Clin North Am 25:341–368, vii, 2002

Yehuda R: Risk and resilience in posttraumatic stress disorder. J Clin Psychiatry 65 (suppl 1):29–36, 2004

Yehuda R, Giller EL, Southwick SM, et al: Hypothalamic-pituitary-adrenal dysfunction in posttraumatic stress disorder. Biol Psychiatry 30:1031–1048, 1991a

Yehuda R, Lowy MT, Southwick SM, et al: Lymphocyte glucocorticoid receptor number in posttraumatic stress disorder. Am J Psychiatry 148:499–504, 1991b

Yehuda R, Giller EL Jr, Mason JW: Psychoneuroendocrine assessment of posttraumatic stress disorder: current progress and new directions. Prog Neuropsychopharmacol Biol Psychiatry 17:541–550, 1993a

Yehuda R, Southwick SM, Krystal JH, et al: Enhanced suppression of cortisol following dexamethasone administration in posttraumatic stress disorder. Am J Psychiatry 150:83–86, 1993b

Yehuda R, Boisoneau D, Lowy MT, et al: Dose-response changes in plasma cortisol and lymphocyte glucocorticoid receptors following dexamethasone administration in combat veterans with and without posttraumatic stress disorder. Arch Gen Psychiatry 52:583–593, 1995a

Yehuda R, Kahana B, Binder-Brynes K, et al: Low urinary cortisol excretion in Holocaust survivors with posttraumatic stress disorder. Am J Psychiatry 152:982–986, 1995b

Yehuda R, Levengood RA, Schmeidler J, et al: Increased pituitary activation following metyrapone administration in post-traumatic stress disorder. Psychoneuroendocrinology 21:1–16, 1996

Yehuda R, Brand S, Yang RK: Plasma neuropeptide Y concentrations in combat-exposed veterans: relationship to trauma exposure, recovery from PTSD, and coping. Biol Psychiatry 59:660–663, 2006

Zald DH, Mattson DL, Pardo JV: Brain activity in ventromedial prefrontal cortex correlates with individual differences in negative affect. Proc Natl Acad Sci U S A 99: 2450–2454, 2002

Zubieta JK, Chinitz JA, Lombardi U, et al: Medial frontal cortex involvement in PTSD symptoms: a SPECT study. J Psychiatr Res 33:259–264, 1999

5

Cognitive Vulnerability to Depression

Implications for Prevention

Lauren B. Alloy, Ph.D.
Lyn Y. Abramson, Ph.D.
Alex Cogswell, M.A.
Megan E. Hughes, M.A.
Brian M. Iacoviello, M.A.

Imagine the following scenario. Two women are fired from their jobs at the same firm. One becomes upset and mildly discouraged for a couple of days and then picks herself up and begins searching the want ads for a new job. The other develops a serious episode of major depression lasting many months and never tries to find a new job. Why are some people vulnerable to depression while others never seem to become depressed or suffer only mild, short-lived dysphoria?

Investigators have attempted to understand vulnerability to depression in terms of individual differences in both biological processes and psychological characteristics that may modulate reactivity to stressful life events. In this chapter, we suggest that the way in which people typically construe events in their lives, or their "cognitive styles," is one factor that substantially affects their vulnerability to depression (Abramson et al. 2002; Alloy et al. 1999, 2006b). From the cognitive perspective, the meaning or interpretation that people give to their experiences influences whether or not they will become depressed and whether they will suffer repeated, severe, or long-lasting episodes of depression. Consequently, we review evidence from the Temple-Wisconsin Cognitive Vulnerability to Depression (CVD) Project (Alloy and Abramson 1999) that negative cognitive styles and the developmental antecedents of these styles, such as negative parenting practices and childhood maltreatment, increase vulnerability to clinically significant depression and suicidal behavior. We end with a brief discussion of the implications of the work on cognitive vulnerability to depression for prevention of this disorder.

To provide a context for our chapter, it is important to recognize that depression is one of the most common forms of psychopathology (Kessler 2002). Moreover, depression is highly recurrent (Judd 1997) and associated with significant impairment (e.g., Gotlib and Hammen 2002; Greenberg et al. 1996; Kessler et al. 2001; Roy et al. 2001; Sullivan et al. 2001). Indeed, given depression's unique combination of high lifetime prevalence, early age at onset, high chronicity, and great role impairment (Kessler 2000), the World Health Organization Global Burden of Disease Study ranked depression as the single most burdensome disease (Murray and Lopez 1996).

COGNITIVE VULNERABILITY THEORIES OF DEPRESSION

Two major cognitive theories of depression, the *hopelessness theory* (Abramson et al. 1989) and *Beck's theory* (Beck 1967, 1987), attempt to understand individual differences in people's vulnerability to depression in terms of a set of maladaptive cognitive styles. According to the hopelessness theory (Abramson et al. 1989), people who exhibit a negative inferential style are hypothesized to be more likely than people who do not exhibit such negative inferential styles to develop episodes of depression—in particular, the subtype of "hopelessness depression"—when they confront negative life events. A negative inferential style has three components: 1) a general tendency to attribute negative life events to stable (enduring) and global (widespread) causes (e.g., "It will last forever and affect everything I do"); 2) a tendency to infer that further negative consequences will follow from a current negative event or to "catastrophize"; and 3) a tendency to infer that the occurrence of a negative event in one's life means that one is deficient, flawed, or unworthy. In the hopelessness theory, individuals who exhibit negative inferential styles should be more likely to make negative inferences regarding the causes, consequences, and self-implications of any negative event they experience, thereby increasing the likelihood that they will develop hopelessness, the proximal cause of the symptoms of depression. Hopelessness, in turn, is defined as two jointly held expectations: 1) negative events will occur or desired events will not occur, and 2) there is nothing one can do to change this situation (i.e., "Bad things will keep happening to me, and there's nothing I can do about it").

Similarly, in Beck's (1967, 1987) theory, negative self-schemata revolving around themes of inadequacy, failure, loss, and worthlessness are hypothesized to provide cognitive vulnerability to depression. Such negative self-schemata are represented as a set of dysfunctional attitudes in which one believes that one's happiness and self-worth depend on being perfect and on other people's approval. When they encounter negative life events that impinge on their cognitive vulnerability, individuals exhibiting such dysfunctional attitudes are hypothesized to develop negatively biased construals of themselves, their personal worlds, and their futures (hopelessness) and, in turn, depressive symptoms. Although the hopelessness theory and Beck's theory differ in terms of some of their specifics, both hypothesize that negative cognitive styles increase vulnerability to depression through their effects on appraisals of personally relevant life events.

A particularly powerful strategy for testing the cognitive vulnerability hypothesis is the prospective "behavioral high-risk design" (e.g., Alloy and Abramson 1999; Alloy et al. 1992; Depue et al. 1981). The behavioral high-risk design involves studying individuals who do not currently have the disorder of interest, but who are hypothesized to be at high versus low risk for developing the disorder based on presence versus absence of the behavioral risk factor. For example, in testing the cognitive vulnerability hypotheses of depression, one would want to select nondepressed individuals who either exhibit or do not exhibit the hypothesized negative cognitive styles. These groups of cognitively high-risk (HR) and low-risk (LR) individuals can then be compared in regard to their likelihood of developing future episodes of depression. Recent studies using or approximating a behavioral high-risk design have provided substantial support for the cognitive vulnerability hypotheses as applied to depressive mood or symptoms (for a review, see Abramson et al. 2002). However, it is the CVD Project (Alloy and Abramson 1999), employing a prospective behavioral high-risk design, that provides the best evidence to date that negative cognitive styles act as vulnerability factors for clinically significant depressive disorders.

COGNITIVE VULNERABILITY TO DEPRESSION PROJECT: KEY FINDINGS

In the CVD Project, university freshmen who had no current Axis I psychiatric disorders at the outset of the study, but who were hypothesized to be at high risk (HR) or low risk (LR) for depression on the basis of their cognitive styles, were followed prospectively every 6 weeks for 2.5 years and then every 16 weeks for an additional 3 years with self-report and structured interview assessments of stressful life events, cognitions, and symptoms and diagnosable episodes of psychopathology. Participants were selected for the CVD Project with a two-phase screening procedure. In phase 1, the Dysfunctional Attitudes Scale (DAS; Weissman and Beck 1978) and Cognitive Style Questionnaire (CSQ; Alloy et al. 2000), which assesses inferential styles regarding the causes, consequences, and self-implications of negative life events, were administered to 5,378 freshmen at Temple University and the University of Wisconsin. Those participants who scored in the highest (most negative) quartile of the screening sample on both the DAS and CSQ composite for negative events formed a pool of potential HR participants, whereas those who scored in the lowest (most positive) quartile on both instruments formed a pool of potential LR participants. In phase 2, the Schedule for Affective Disorders and Schizophrenia—Lifetime Version (SADS-L; Spitzer et al. 1978), expanded to permit both Research Diagnostic Criteria (RDC; Spitzer et al. 1978) and DSM-III-R (American Psychiatric Association 1987) and DSM-IV (American Psychiatric Association 1994) diagnoses, was administered to a random subset of participants who met the phase 1 criteria. Participants who met RDC or DSM-III-R criteria for any current Axis I disorder at the time of the phase 1 screening were excluded from the study. Participants with a past unipolar mood disorder that had remitted for a minimum of 2 months were retained so as not to result in an unrepresentative sample of HR participants (for rationale, see Alloy and Abramson 1999; Alloy et al. 2000). The final CVD Project sample included 173 high-risk and 176 low-risk ethnically and socioeconomically diverse participants across the two sites (for sample demographic characteristics and representativeness, see Alloy et al. 2000).

During the first 2.5 years of follow-up, information regarding new onsets of depression and other disorders was obtained from expanded SADS—Change (SADS-C; Spitzer and Endicott 1978) interviews administered every 6 weeks. All diagnostic interviewers were unaware of participants' cognitive risk status. In addition to DSM-IV and RDC criteria being used, explicit diagnostic criteria for diagnosing hopelessness depression (HD) were developed. Interrater reliability was excellent, with kappas of 0.90 or greater for all project diagnoses.

Negative Cognitive Styles as Vulnerabilities for Depression and Suicidal Behavior

Do negative cognitive styles, in fact, confer risk for clinically significant depression? And, do they increase vulnerability to first lifetime onset of depression as well as to recurrences of depression? More than half of the CVD Project sample entered college with no prior history of clinically significant depression. Among these never-depressed individuals, HR participants were significantly more likely than LR participants to experience a first lifetime onset of major depression (16.2% vs. 2.7%, odds ratio [OR] = 7.4), minor depression (45.9% vs. 14.4%, OR = 5.6), and HD (35.1% vs. 3.6%, OR = 11.6) during the first 2.5 years of follow-up, controlling for initial depressive symptoms (Alloy et al. 2006a, 2006b). These findings provide especially strong support for the cognitive vulnerability hypothesis because they are based on a truly prospective test, uncontaminated by prior history of depression. Given that depression is a highly recurrent disorder, with up to 80% of individuals who have had one episode experiencing a recurrence (e.g., Judd 1997), it is also important to determine whether negative cognitive styles also confer risk for recurrences of depression as well as for first onset. Among participants with a prior depression, HR individuals also were significantly more likely than LR individuals to experience a recurrence of major depression (28.6% vs. 9.4%, OR = 3.8), minor depression (56.1% vs. 32.8%, OR = 3.1), and HD (50.0% vs. 18.8%, OR = 4.1) during the first 2.5 years of follow-up, controlling for initial depressive symptoms (Alloy et al. 2006a, 2006b). Thus, the cognitive vulnerability hypothesis was supported for recurrences of depression as well as for first onset, suggesting that similar cognitive vulnerability underlies the first and subsequent episodes of depression.

Do negative cognitive styles also predict onset of other disorders, or do they provide specific vulnerability to depression? In the full CVD Project sample, cognitive risk significantly predicted onset of any anxiety disorder (HR = 8.7%; LR = 2.3%; OR = 5.7); however, this association was entirely due to co-occurrence with depression (Alloy et al. 2006b). Participants with an onset of an anxiety disorder were divided into two groups: those with and without comorbid depression. Cognitive risk significantly predicted onset of anxiety disorder comorbid with depression (HR = 5.7%; LR = 0.6%; OR = 19.6), but not of anxiety disorder alone (HR = 2.9%; LR = 1.7%; OR = 1.4, $P < 0.80$). Cognitive risk also did not predict onset of any other disorders (Alloy et al. 2006b). These findings suggest that the risk conferred by negative cognitive styles may have considerable specificity to depressive disorders, insofar as there were no risk group differences in onset of anxiety or other disorders, unless they co-occurred with depression.

According to the cognitive theories of depression, negative cognitive styles should also confer vulnerability to suicidal behavior, ranging from suicidal ideation to completed suicides. Given that hopelessness has been found to be the best single psychological predictor of suicidal ideation, attempts, and completions (Abramson et al. 2000; Beck et al. 1985, 1990) and negative cognitive styles are hypothesized to increase risk for depression and suicide by increasing the likelihood of becoming hopeless (Abramson et al. 1989), levels of hopelessness should mediate the predictive association between negative cognitive styles and suicidal behavior. Consistent with this hypothesis, Abramson et al. (1998) found that HR participants in the CVD Project were more likely than LR participants to exhibit suicidal thinking and attempts over the first 2.5 years of prospective follow-up, and that this relation was mediated by participants' mean levels of hopelessness across the 2.5-year follow-up. Moreover, the predictive association between cognitive risk status and prospective levels of suicidal behavior was maintained even after statistically controlling for participants' prior history of suicidal behavior and for other risk factors for suicide (i.e., prior history of major and minor depression, borderline and antisocial personality dysfunction, and parental history of depression).

Rumination as an Additional Cognitive Vulnerability to Depression

According to another cognitive theory of depression, the response styles theory (Nolen-Hoeksema 1991), individuals who tend to ruminate in response to sad affect are at greater risk for experiencing prolonged and severe depressive episodes than are individuals who tend to distract themselves from dysphoria. Rumination is an emotion-regulation strategy that is recursive and persistent, involving perseverative self-focus on depressive symptoms and their causes and consequences. Several studies have found that depressive rumination is indeed associated with longer and more severe episodes of depression (for a review, see Spasojevic et al. 2003). In addition, prospective studies, including the CVD Project, have found that depressive rumination predicts onset of clinically significant major depression (Nolen-Hoeksema 2000; Spasojevic and Alloy 2001). Moreover, using CVD Project data, Spasojevic and Alloy (2001) found that a tendency to ruminate about one's dysphoria mediated the predictive association between negative cognitive styles and onset of major depressive episodes. Indeed, Abramson et al. (2002) argued that negative cognitive styles, by their very nature, should increase the likelihood of rumination because cognitively vulnerable individuals have difficulty disengaging their attention from the self-implications of negative life events.

Expanding upon the response styles theory, Robinson and Alloy (2003) hypothesized that individuals who exhibit negative cognitive styles and who also tend to ruminate about these negative cognitions in response to the occurrence of stressful life events ("stress-reactive rumination" as opposed to "emotion-focused rumination") may be more likely to develop episodes of depression in the first place. They reasoned that negative cognitive styles provide the negative content, but that this negative content may be more likely to lead to depression when it is "on one's mind" and recursively rehearsed than when it is not. Consistent with this hypothesis, Robinson and Alloy (2003) found that cognitive risk status and stress-reactive rumination measured at Time 1 of the CVD Project interacted to predict onset of major depression and HD. Among HR participants, those who were also high in stress-reactive rumination evidenced a higher prospective incidence of major depression and HD compared with those who did not tend to ruminate in response to stressors. LR participants exhibited low rates of major depression and HD, regardless of their levels of stress-reactive rumination. Thus, rumination may both mediate and moderate the risk for depression associated with negative cognitive styles.

Cognitive Vulnerability to Depression and the Role of Stressful Life Events

The findings from the CVD Project indicate that negative cognitive styles do, in fact, provide vulnerability to clinically significant depressive disorders and suicidal ideation and attempts. However, according to the cognitive theories of depression (Abramson et al. 1989; Beck 1967, 1987), the risk associated with negative cognitive styles is likely to culminate in depressive episodes when people experience negative life events, because individuals with negative cognitive styles are hypothesized to appraise the causes, consequences, and self-worth implications of stressful events they experience in a negative, maladaptive way. Thus, the cognitive theories of depression are vulnerability-stress theories in which negative cognitive styles are hypothesized to combine with the occurrence of negative life events to predict the onset of depressive episodes.

Life events were assessed in the CVD Project with a combination self-report and semistructured interview procedure. Every 6 weeks during the first 2.5 years of follow-up, participants completed the Life Events Scale (LES; Alloy and Clements 1992; Needles and Abramson 1990) containing 134 stressful events in a broad range of domains relevant to college students. The LES was followed by a Stress Interview (SI; Alloy and Abramson 1999), patterned after the Brown and Harris (1978) Life Events and Difficulties Schedule, conducted by interviewers who were unaware of participants' cognitive risk status and symptom status. The SI contained explicit criteria for defining what experiences counted as an instance of each event and those events reported on the LES that did not meet the event definition criteria on the SI were disqualified. Events were also rated on their objective severity and dated with accuracy on the SI (for SI reliability and validity data, see Safford et al., in press).

Preliminary analyses from the CVD Project indicated that cognitive risk status interacted with the number of negative life events participants experienced in the prior 6 weeks to predict onset of major or minor depressive episodes and of HD episodes significantly. HR participants who experienced high levels of recent negative events were significantly more likely to have an onset of major or minor depression and HD than HR participants who experienced low levels of recent stress or than LR participants regardless of their recent stress levels. Thus, consistent with the cognitive vulnerability–stress hypothesis, preliminary evidence suggests that negative life events are more likely to trigger depression among cognitively vulnerable than nonvulnerable individuals.

But what if HR individuals are more likely than LR individuals to become depressed not only because they interpret stressful events they encounter in a maladaptive fashion, but also because they are more likely to experience stressful events in the first place? Using the first 6 months of prospective follow-up data from the CVD Project, Safford et al. (in press) found that HR participants did indeed report significantly more total negative events than LR participants, controlling for current and past depression. Safford et al. considered the possibility that by virtue of their negative cognitive styles, HR individuals interpret even benign events as negative and thus exhibit an overreporting bias. If this is true, then HR participants would be expected to have a greater proportion of their reported events on the LES disqualified on the SI as not meeting the event definition criteria. However, HR and LR participants didn't differ in their proportion of disqualified events. A second possibility is stress generation (Hammen 1991; Monroe and Simons 1991). HR individuals may experience more stressful life events because they actively contribute to the cause of these events by virtue of the behaviors and characteristics associated with their vulnerability. If so, then HR participants should experience more life events that are at least partially dependent on their behavior, such as a breakup of a relationship, but not more events that are uncontrollable or independent of what they do, such as death of a loved one. Safford et al. found that HR participants did report significantly more events that were dependent on their behavior than did LR participants. Consequently, these findings suggest that negative cognitive styles may increase vulnerability to depression not only by leading to maladaptive interpretations of stressful events, but also by directly and indirectly increasing the likelihood of experiencing the negative events that trigger depression.

Origins of Cognitive Vulnerability to Depression

If negative cognitive styles and the tendency to ruminate indeed confer vulnerability to depression and suicidal behavior both by affecting individuals' exposure to and interpretation of negative life events, it becomes important to know how these styles develop. What are the origins of cognitive vulnerability to depression? (for a review, see Alloy et al. 2004). Such understanding may suggest relevant directions for research on potential preventive interventions for depression. Toward this end, as part of the CVD Project, the cognitive styles and parenting practices of 335 of the HR and LR participants' parents (217 mothers, 118 fathers) were assessed. Both participants and their parents reported on the parents' parenting behaviors and inferential feedback styles regarding the causes and consequences of negative events in their child's life. In addition, the HR and LR participants reported on their histories of childhood maltreatment from adults and peers.

History of Childhood Maltreatment

It is intriguing to consider the possibility that the negative cognitive styles of depressive individuals may, at least in part, be the internal representations of actual maltreatment that they experienced rather than cognitive distortions. For example, maybe the cognitively vulnerable freshman who infers that negative consequences will follow if he or she receives a low grade is a person who was abused as a child when he or she brought home low grades. Rose and Abramson (1992) proposed a developmental pathway by which childhood negative life events, especially maltreatment, may lead to the development of a negative cognitive style. They suggested that whereas a child may initially explain being beaten or verbally abused by his or her father by saying, "He was just in a bad mood today" (an external, unstable, specific attribution), repeated occurrences of abuse will disconfirm these more benign attributions, prompting the child to begin making hopelessness-inducing attributions about the abuse (e.g., "I'm a bad person who deserves all the bad things that happen to me"; an internal, stable, global attribution). Over time, the child's negative attributions may generalize to other negative events until a negative cognitive style develops. Rose and Abramson (1992) hypothesized that emotional maltreatment may be even more likely than either physical or sexual abuse to contribute to the development of negative cognitive styles because with emotional maltreatment, the abuser directly supplies the negative cognitions to the child (i.e., "You're so stupid; you'll never amount to anything").

In a qualitative and quantitative review of studies examining the relation between childhood maltreatment and cognitive vulnerability to depression, Gibb (2002) found that a history of both sexual and emotional maltreatment, but not physical abuse, was associated with negative cognitive styles. In the CVD Project, after controlling for participants' levels of depressive symptoms, researchers found that HR participants reported significantly higher levels of childhood emotional, but not physical or sexual, maltreatment than did LR participants, consistent with Rose and Abramson's hypothesis (Gibb et al. 2001a). In addition, participants' cognitive risk status fully or partially mediated the relationship between reported levels of emotional maltreatment and prospective onset of major depression and HD episodes (Gibb et al. 2001a) and levels of suicidal ideation (Gibb et al. 2001b) during the first 2.5 years of follow-up. Moreover, even when maltreatment by parents was statistically controlled, childhood emotional abuse from peers and romantic partners was still associated significantly with cognitive HR status (Gibb et al. 2004). These findings suggest that the relationship between childhood emotional maltreatment and cognitive vulnerability is not entirely attributable to genetic transmission or a negative family environment in general. Childhood history of maltreatment was also related to a ruminative response style in the CVD Project (Spasojevic and Alloy 2002). A reported history of childhood emotional abuse and, for women, of childhood sexual abuse were related to a ruminative response style and the tendency to ruminate fully or partially mediated the predictive association between these forms of abuse and prospective onset of major depression episodes.

Parental Inferential Feedback

Children may also learn their cognitive styles in part from inferential feedback they receive from parents regarding the causes and consequences of negative events in the child's life. Negative inferential feedback from parents and others (e.g., teachers) has consistently been associated with children's development of negative cognitive styles (for reviews, see Alloy et al. 2001, 2004). For example, in the CVD Project, Alloy et al. (2001) found that according to both participants' and parents' reports, both mothers and fathers of HR individuals provided more negative (stable, global) attributional feedback for negative events in their child's life than did mothers and fathers of LR individuals. In addition, mothers of HR participants also provided more negative consequence feedback for negative events in their child's life than did mothers of LR participants according to both respondents' reports, as did fathers according to the participants' reports. Moreover, mothers' inferential feedback predicted the likelihood of their child developing an episode of major, minor, or hopelessness depression over the 2.5-year prospective follow-up, mediated in part by the child's cognitive risk status (Alloy et al. 2001). Thus, there is some evidence that parents might contribute to the development of negative cognitive styles and vulnerability to depression in their offspring by providing negative inferential feedback to their child for negative events in the child's life.

Parenting Styles

In addition to maladaptive inferential feedback, other negative parenting practices may also contribute to the development of cognitive vulnerability to depression. In particular, a parenting style involving lack of emotional warmth or the presence of negative psychological control (criticism, intrusiveness, and guilt-induction), a pattern referred to as "affectionless control" by Parker (1983), has been most consistently implicated as a risk factor for depression (for reviews, see Alloy et al. 2001; Garber and Flynn 1998). Consistent with the lack of emotional warmth part of the "affectionless control" pattern, Alloy et al. (2001) found that both participants and their fathers reported that fathers of HR participants exhibited less warmth and acceptance than fathers of LR participants. There were no risk group differences for fathers' levels of psychological control or for mothers' parenting. In addition, low warmth or acceptance from fathers predicted prospective onset of major, minor, and hopelessness depression in their offspring during the 2.5-year follow-up, with the prediction of HD episodes mediated by the offspring's cognitive risk status. Negative parenting practices also were associated with a ruminative response style among CVD Project participants, but it was negative psychological control by both mothers and fathers, rather than lack of emotional warmth, that was related to depressive rumination (Spasojevic and Alloy 2002). In addition, rumination mediated the relationship between the over-controlling parenting and prospective onset of major depression in the college-aged offspring. Thus, both lack of emotional warmth and over-controlling parenting were related to offsprings' cognitive vulnerability to depression, through the alternative mechanisms of negative cognitive styles and rumination, respectively.

It's important to emphasize that the portion of the CVD Project regarding developmental antecedents of negative cognitive styles was retrospective. Thus, the developmental findings should be viewed as tentative. However, they provide an empirical rationale for more powerful prospective tests of the role that negative parenting practices, maladaptive inferential feedback regarding the causes and consequences of children's negative life events, and maltreatment may play in contributing to the development of negative cognitive styles and attendant vulnerability to depression and suicidal behavior.

CLINICAL IMPLICATIONS

Given that the findings from the CVD Project and other studies indicate that negative cognitive styles and a tendency to ruminate confer vulnerability to depression and suicidal behavior, interventions designed to prevent the formation of these vulnerabilities in the first place or remediate them, once formed, should decrease future depression and suicide. Recent work has indicated that the rates of clinical depression are quite low until mid to late adolescence; but then the rates skyrocket between the ages of 15 and 18 years (Hankin and Abramson 2001; Hankin et al. 1998). Of great interest, a growing body of work is beginning to suggest that cognitive vulnerability, in interaction with negative life events, may play an important role in contributing to this surge in depression in mid to late adolescence. Specifically, evidence suggests that cognitive vulnerability has developed and consolidated and is capable of participation in the causal chains featured in the cognitive theories of depression by early adolescence (Hankin and Abramson 2001). Thus, intervention efforts ideally should be directed at children before they reach early adolescence and puberty to prevent the formation and consolidation of cognitive vulnerability to depression. If successful on a large scale, such prevention efforts may help short-circuit the surge in depression that typically occurs in mid to late adolescence.

Cognitive-behavioral therapy (CBT) has been shown to be effective and recent findings suggest that it may also reduce risk for relapse and recurrence in adults (Hollon et al. 2002, 2005), in part by reducing the negativity of individuals' attributional styles (DeRubeis and Hollon 1995; Hollon and Beck 1994). Modifications of CBT for depression could be directed toward preadolescents before their cognitive styles have fully formed and consolidated. School-based CBT programs, such as the Penn Optimism Project (Gillham et al. 1995; Jaycox et al. 1994) and the Coping with Stress course (Clarke et al. 1995, 2001) are designed to directly train children and adolescents to challenge negative and irrational thoughts and to make more benign interpretations of stressful events, and have shown early signs of success. The Penn Optimism Project has been successful in reducing depressive symptoms, improving attributional style, and reducing classroom behavioral problems in diverse samples of children, including Caucasian and Latino samples in the United States and children in China (Cardemil et al. 2002; Jaycox et al. 1994; Yu and Seligman 2002). Importantly, a sample of low-income inner-city African American children found no benefit from the program (Cardemil et al. 2002). Clarke's program significantly reduced incidence rates of depression in at-risk adolescents, classified as such on the basis of both their parents' histories of major depression (Clarke et al. 2001) and their own elevated depressive symptoms at pretest (Clarke et al. 1995).

Given that negative cognitive styles may be especially likely to confer vulnerability to depression when exacerbated by rumination, depressogenic cognitive styles may also be altered indirectly by training individuals in more effective emotion-regulation strategies, such as effective problem-solving or active distraction, when appropriate. It may also be beneficial to teach cognitively vulnerable individuals with a childhood history of maltreatment to reinterpret their abusive histories. The reframing might target such individuals' beliefs that they were inherently bad and deserving of the abuse by introducing the corrective interpretation that they were raised by caretakers who, for whatever reason, did not have the psychological competence to raise them in a less abusive way.

Further, the findings on some of the potential developmental origins of depressogenic cognitive styles suggest that primary prevention efforts might be aimed at building positive cognitive styles in children. This could be accomplished by educating parents and teachers to provide feedback about more benign inferences for stressful events in children's lives, as well as through training parents in more emotionally supportive ways of interacting with their children (Rose and Abramson 1992). Such primary prevention efforts could contribute to the development of positive cognitive styles in youth that promote resilience in the face of stressful life events.

REFERENCES

Abramson LY, Metalsky GI, Alloy LB: Hopelessness depression: a theory-based subtype of depression. Psychol Rev 96:358–372, 1989

Abramson LY, Alloy LB, Hogan ME, et al: Suicidality and cognitive vulnerability to depression among college students: a prospective study. J Adolesc 21:473–487, 1998

Abramson LY, Alloy LB, Hogan ME, et al: The hopelessness theory of suicidality, in Suicide Science: Expanding Boundaries. Edited by Joiner TE, Rudd MD. Boston, MA, Kluwer Academic, 2000, pp 17–32

Abramson LY, Alloy LB, Hankin BL, et al: Cognitive vulnerability-stress models of depression in a self-regulatory and psychobiological context, in Handbook of Depression. Edited by Gotlib IH, Hammen CL. New York, Guilford, 2002, pp 268–294

Alloy LB, Abramson LY: The Temple-Wisconsin Cognitive Vulnerability to Depression (CVD) Project: conceptual background, design, and methods. J Cog Psychother: An International Quarterly 13:227–262, 1999

Alloy LB, Clements CM: Illusion of control: Invulnerability to negative affect and depressive symptoms after laboratory and natural stressors. J Abnorm Psychol 101: 234–245, 1992

Alloy LB, Lipman A, Abramson LY: Attributional style as a vulnerability factor for depression: validation by past history of mood disorders. Cog Ther Res 16:391–407, 1992

Alloy LB, Abramson LY, Whitehouse WG, et al: Depressogenic cognitive styles: predictive validity, information processing and personality characteristics, and developmental origins. Behav Res Ther 37:503–531, 1999

Alloy LB, Abramson LY, Hogan ME, et al: The Temple-Wisconsin Cognitive Vulnerability to Depression Project: lifetime history of Axis I psychopathology in individuals at high and low cognitive risk for depression. J Abnorm Psychol 109:403–418, 2000

Alloy LB, Abramson LY, Tashman NA, et al: Developmental origins of cognitive vulnerability to depression: Parenting, cognitive, and inferential feedback styles of the parents of individuals at high and low cognitive risk for depression. Cog Ther Res 25:397–423, 2001

Alloy LB, Abramson, LY, Gibb BE, et al: Developmental antecedents of cognitive vulnerability to depression: review of findings from the Cognitive Vulnerability to Depression Project. J Cog Psychother: An International Quarterly 18:115–133, 2004

Alloy LB, Abramson LY, Safford SM, et al: The Cognitive Vulnerability to Depression (CVD) Project: current findings and future directions, in Cognitive Vulnerability to Emotional Disorders. Edited by Alloy LB, Riskind JH. Hillsdale, NJ, Lawrence Erlbaum, 2006a, pp 33–61

Alloy LB, Abramson LY, Whitehouse WG, et al: Prospective incidence of first onsets and recurrences of depression in individuals at high and low cognitive risk for depression. J Abnorm Psychol 115:145–156, 2006b

American Psychiatric Association: Diagnostic and Statistical Manual of Mental Disorders, 3rd Edition, Revised. Washington, DC, American Psychiatric Association, 1987

American Psychiatric Association: Diagnostic and Statistical Manual of Mental Disorders, 4th Edition. Washington, DC, American Psychiatric Association, 1994

Beck AT: Depression: Clinical, experimental, and theoretical aspects. New York, Harper & Row, 1967

Beck AT: Cognitive models of depression. J Cog Psychother: An International Quarterly 1:5–37, 1987

Beck AT, Steer RA, Kovacs M, et al: Hopelessness and eventual suicide: a 10-year prospective study of patients hospitalized with suicidal ideation. Am J Psychiatry 142: 559–563, 1985

Beck AT, Brown G, Berchick RJ. et al: Relationship between hopelessness and ultimate suicide: a replication with psychiatric patients. Am J Psychiatry 147:190–195, 1990

Brown GW, Harris TO: Social Origins of Depression: A Study of Psychiatric Disorder in Women. New York, Free Press, 1978

Cardemil EV, Reivich KJ, Seligman MEP: The prevention of depressive symptoms in low-income minority middle school students. Preven and Treat 5: Article 8, 2002. Available at: http://journals.apa.org/prevention/volume5/pre0050008a.html. Accessed September 26, 2006.

Clarke GN, Hawkins W, Murphy M, et al: Targeted prevention of unipolar depressive disorder in an at-risk sample of high school adolescents: a randomized trial of a group cognitive intervention. J Am Acad Child Adolesc Psychiatry 34:312–321, 1995

Clarke GN, Hornbrook M, Lynch F, et al: A randomized trial of a group cognitive intervention for preventing depression in adolescent offspring of depressed parents. Arch Gen Psychiatry 58:1127–1134, 2001

Depue RA, Slater J, Wolfstetter-Kausch H, et al: A behavioral paradigm for identifying persons at risk for bipolar spectrum disorder: a conceptual framework and five validation studies (monograph). J Abnorm Psychol 90:381–437, 1981

DeRubeis RJ, Hollon SD: Explanatory style in the treatment of depression, in Explanatory Style. Edited by Buchanan GM, Seligman MEP. Hillsdale, NJ, Lawrence Erlbaum, 1995, pp 99–111

Garber J, Flynn C: Origins of the depressive cognitive style, in The Science of Clinical Psychology: Evidence of a Century's Progress. Edited by Routh D, DeRubeis RJ. Washington, DC, American Psychological Association, 1998, pp 53–93

Gibb BE: Childhood maltreatment and negative cognitive styles: A quantitative and qualitative review. Clin Psychol Rev 22:223–246, 2002

Gibb BE, Alloy LB, Abramson LY, et al: History of childhood maltreatment, depressogenic cognitive style, and episodes of depression in adulthood. Cog Ther Res 25:425–446, 2001a

Gibb BE, Alloy LB, Abramson LY, et al: Childhood maltreatment and college students' current suicidality: a test of the hopelessness theory. Suicide Life Threat Behav 31:405–415, 2001b

Gibb BE, Abramson LY, Alloy LB: Emotional maltreatment from parents, verbal peer victimization, and cognitive vulnerability to depression. Cog Ther Res 28:1–21, 2004

Gillham JE, Reivich KJ, Jaycox LH, et al: Prevention of depressive symptoms in school-children: two-year follow-up. Psychol Sci 6:343–351, 1995

Gotlib IH, Hammen C: Introduction, in Handbook of Depression, 3rd Edition. Edited by Gotlib IH, Hammen CL. New York, Guilford, 2002, pp 1–20

Greenberg P, Kessler RC, Nells T, et al: Depression in the workplace: an economic perspective, in Selective Serotonin Reuptake Inhibitors: Advances in Basic Research and Clinical Practice. Edited by Feighner JP, Boyer WF. New York, Wiley, 1996, pp 327–363

Hammen C: Generation of stress in the course of unipolar depression. J Abnorm Psychol 100:555–561, 1991

Hankin BL, Abramson LY: Development of gender differences in depression: an elaborated cognitive vulnerability-transactional stress theory. Psychol Bull 127:773–796, 2001

Hankin BL, Abramson LY, Moffitt TE, et al: Development of depression from preadolescence to young adulthood: emerging gender differences in a 10-year longitudinal study. J Abnorm Psychol 107:128–140, 1998

Hollon SD, Beck AT: Cognitive and cognitive-behavioral therapies, in Handbook of Psychotherapy and Behavior Change, 4th Edition. Edited by Bergin AE, Garfield SL. New York, Wiley, 1994, pp 428–466

Hollon SD, Thase ME, Markowitz JC: Treatment and prevention of depression. Psychol Sci Public Interest 3:39–77, 2002

Hollon SD, DeRubeis RJ, Shelton RC, et al:. Prevention of relapse following cognitive therapy vs. medications in moderate to severe depression. Arch Gen Psychiatry 62:417–422, 2005

Jaycox LH, Reivich KJ, Gillham J, et al: Prevention of depressive symptoms in school children. Behav Res Ther 32:801–816, 1994

Judd LL: The clinical course of unipolar major depressive disorders. Arch Gen Psychiatry 54:989–991, 1997

Kessler RC: Burden of depression, in Selective Serotonin Reuptake Inhibitors 1990–2000: A Decade of Developments. Edited by Kasper S, Carlsson A. Copenhagen, Denmark, H. Lundbeck A/S, 2000, pp 15–21

Kessler RC: Epidemiology of depression, in Handbook of Depression, 3rd Edition. Edited by Gotlib IH, Hammen CL. New York, Guilford, 2002, pp 23–42

Kessler RC, Avenovoli S, Merikangas KR: Mood disorders in children and adolescents: an epidemiological perspective. Biol Psychiatry 49:1002–1014, 2001

Monroe SM, Simons AD: Diathesis-stress theories in the context of life stress research: implications for the depressive disorders. Psychol Bull 110:406–425, 2001

Murray CJL, Lopez AD (eds): The Global Burden of Disease: A Comprehensive Assessment of Mortality and Disability From Diseases, Injuries, and Risk Factors in 1990 and Projected to 2020. Cambridge, MA, Harvard University Press, 1996

Needles DJ, Abramson LY: Positive life events, attributional style, and hopefulness: testing a model of recovery from depression. J Abnorm Psychol 99:156–165, 1990

Nolen-Hoeksema S: Responses to depression and their effects on the duration of the depressive episode. J Abnorm Psychol 100:20–28, 1991

Nolen-Hoeksema S: Ruminative responses predict depressive disorders. J Abnorm Psychol 109:504–511, 2000

Parker G: Parental "affectionless control" as an antecedent to adult depression. Arch Gen Psychiatry 34:138–147, 1983

Robinson MS, Alloy LB: Negative cognitive styles and stress-reactive rumination interact to predict depression: a prospective study. Cog Ther Res 27:275–291, 2003

Rose DT, Abramson LY: Developmental predictors of depressive cognitive style: research and theory, in Rochester Symposium on Developmental Psychopathology, Vol 4. Edited by Cicchetti D, Toth SL. Hillsdale, NJ, Lawrence Erlbaum, 1992, pp 323–349.

Roy K, Mitchell P, Wilhelm K: Depression and smoking: examining correlates in a subset of depressed patients. Aust N Z J Psychiatry 35:329–335, 2001

Safford SM, Alloy LB, Abramson LY, et al: Negative cognitive style as a predictor of negative life events in depression-prone individuals: a test of the stress generation hypothesis. J Affect Disord (in press)

Spasojevic J, Alloy LB: Rumination as a common mechanism relating depressive risk factors to depression. Emotion 1:25–37, 2001

Spasojevic J, Alloy LB: Who becomes a depressive ruminator? Developmental antecedents of ruminative response style. Journal of Cognitive Psychotherapy: An International Quarterly 16:405–419, 2002

Spasojevic J, Alloy LB, Abramson LY, et al: Reactive rumination: outcomes, mechanisms, and developmental antecedents, in Depressive Rumination: Nature, Theory and Treatment. Edited by Papageorgiou C, Wells A. New York, Wiley, 2003, pp 43–58

Spitzer R, Endicott J: Schedule for Affective Disorders and Schizophrenia—Change Version. New York, Biometrics Research, New York State Psychiatric Institute, 1978

Spitzer RL, Endicott J, Robins E: Research diagnostic criteria: rationale and reliability. Arch Gen Psychiatry 35:773–782, 1978

Sullivan MD, LaCroix AZ, Russo JE, et al: Depression and self-reported physical health in patients with coronary disease: mediating and moderating factors. Psychosom Med 63:248–256, 2001

Weissman A, Beck AT: Development and validation of the Dysfunctional Attitudes Scale: a preliminary investigation. Paper presented at the annual meeting of the Association for the Advancement of Behavior Therapy, Chicago, IL, November 1978

Yu DL, Seligman MEP: Preventing depression symptoms in Chinese children. Prev and Treat 5: Article 9, 2002. Available at: http://journals.apa.org/prevention/volume5/pre0050009a.html. Accessed September 26, 2006.

6

Vulnerability to Alcohol and Drug Use Disorders

Deborah Hasin, Ph.D.

Mark L. Hatzenbuehler, B.A.

Katherine Keyes-Wild, M.S.

Elizabeth Ogburn, M.S.

Substance use disorders have a complex etiology involving genetic and environmental factors. These occur along a continuum ranging from macro to micro, external to internal (Figure 6–1). In this chapter, we address these levels in turn. We begin with macro/external factors, including societal availability and desir-

This research was supported in part by grants from the National Institute on Alcoholism and Alcohol Abuse (K05 AA014223) and the National Institute on Drug Abuse (RO1 DA018652) and by the New York State Psychiatric Institute. The authors wish to thank Valerie Richmond, M.A., for editorial assistance and manuscript preparation.

ability of the substances, geographic and temporal differences, pricing, laws, and advertising. We next consider externally imposed stress. Intermediate-level factors include religiosity, parental, and peer social influences. Moving increasingly toward the micro and internal levels, we consider cognitive and personality variables, subjective responses to substances, and genetics. We conclude by discussing gene–environment interaction, addressing the idea that since etiological influences work at various levels, a factor at any level may emerge more clearly if other levels are considered conjointly.

THE MAIN PHENOTYPE OF INTEREST: DEPENDENCE

The main outcome of interest in this chapter is dependence; we present information on substance *use* as a necessary but not sufficient condition for dependence to develop. The substance dependence criteria in DSM-IV (American Psychiatric Association 1994) are based on the Alcohol Dependence Syndrome (ADS; Edwards and Gross 1976), which was generalized to drugs in 1981 (World Health Organization 1981). Dependence was considered a combination of physiological and psychological processes leading to increasingly impaired control over substance use in the face of negative consequences. Dependence was one "axis" of substance problems, and the consequences of heavy use (social, legal, medical problems, hazardous use) a different axis of substance problems. This biaxial concept (Edwards 1986) led to the distinction between abuse criteria (social, role, legal problems or hazardous use, most commonly driving while intoxicated) and dependence criteria (tolerance, withdrawal, numerous indicators of impaired control over use).

The focus on *dependence* is based on its centrality in research and on its psychometric properties. DSM-IV and ICD-10 (World Health Organization 1992) dependence have good to excellent reliability across samples and instruments (Bucholz et al. 1995; Canino et al. 1999; Grant et al. 1995; Hasin et al. 1996a, 1997a; Ustun et al. 1997), with few exceptions (rare substances; hallucinogens). Dependence validity has also been shown to be good via several study designs. These include multimethod comparisons (Cottler et al. 1997; Grant 1996; Hasin et al. 1996b, 1997a; Pull et al. 1997; Rounsaville et al. 1993; Schuckit et al. 1994); longitudinal studies (Hasin et al. 1990, 1997b, 1997c; Grant et al. 2001; Schuckit et al. 2000, 2001); latent variable analysis (C. Blanco, T.C. Harford, E. Nunes, et al.: "The Latent Structure of Substance Use Disorders: Results

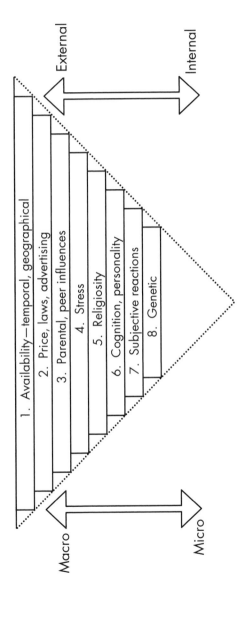

FIGURE 6–1.   External and internal vulnerability factors for substance use disorders.

From the National Longitudinal Alcohol Epidemiologic Survey (NLAES)," un-published work; Harford and Muthen 2001; Muthen et al. 1993); and construct validation (Hasin and Paykin 1999a; Hasin et al. 2003). Recently, animal models of a syndrome of cocaine dependence symptoms (as distinct from use patterns; Deroche-Gamonet et al. 2004; Robinson 2004; Vanderschuren and Everitt 2004) lend credence to the dependence syndrome not only as a cross-cultural phenomenon, as suggested by a World Health Organization study (Cottler et al. 1997; Hasin et al. 1997a; Pull et al. 1997), but a cross-species phenomenon as well.

Substance *abuse* is a different case. Contrary to clinical assumptions, abuse does not necessarily lead to dependence (Grant et al. 2001; Hasin et al. 1990, 1997b, 1997c; Schuckit et al. 2000, 2001). Furthermore, not all cases of alcohol or drug dependence involve abuse symptoms (Hasin and Grant 2004; Hasin et al. 2005). Latent variable analyses of DSM-IV alcohol abuse and dependence criteria (Harford and Muthen 2001; Muthen et al. 1993) show two distinct, correlated factors corresponding to alcohol dependence and abuse. Findings for cannabis and cocaine (C. Blanco, T.C. Harford, E. Nunes, et al: "The Latent Structure of Substance Use Disorders: Results From the National Longitudinal Alcohol Epidemiologic Survey (NLAES)" [unpublished work]) are similar. Dependence is more familial than abuse (Hasin and Paykin 1999a; Hasin et al. 1997c). DSM-IV alcohol abuse is most often diagnosed in the general population based on one symptom, driving while intoxicated (Hasin and Paykin 1999b; Hasin et al. 1999); preliminary analyses of national data (see below) show this is also the case for drug abuse. DSM-IV abuse may thus depend on the availability of a car, while dependence is a heritable, complex condition.

EPIDEMIOLOGY OF ALCOHOL AND DRUG USE, ABUSE, AND DEPENDENCE

Alcohol Consumption

Worldwide, alcohol consumption patterns vary. In eastern Mediterranean countries, yearly per capita consumption is 0.60 liters, in contrast to Western Europe, where it is 12.9 liters (Rehm et al. 2003). Alcohol consumption is also heterogeneous within countries. For example, about one-third of U.S. adults do not drink, although per capita consumption is 9.3 liters (Rehm et al. 2003; Room et al. 2003). Abstainers are rare in Eastern Europe (including Russia and Ukraine), where per capita consumption, 13.9 liters, is the highest in the world (Rehm et al.

2003). After immigration, immigrants tend to retain the drinking levels of their country of origin rather changing to the patterns of their new country, for example, Mexican immigrants in the U.S. (Grant et al. 2004b) and Russian immigrants in Israel (Hasin et al. 1998; Rahav et al. 1999).

Drug Use

In Western countries prior to the 1960s, drug use was rare and the few studies that addressed prevalence focused on heroin, with widely varying results (Du-Pont and Greene 1973; Greene et al. 1975; Singer 1971). More systematic surveys of U.S. drug use began in the 1960s. A series of national household surveys on drug use conducted by the National Institute on Drug Abuse and later by the Substance Abuse and Mental Health Services Administration showed that illicit drug use, especially marijuana, increased greatly after the late 1960s (Figure 6–2; Substance Abuse and Mental Health Services Administration 2002). Heroin use also increased in the late 1960s, when the profile of users changed from "bohemians" to inner-city, unemployed males. Yearly surveys of U.S. youth (Monitoring the Future; Johnston et al. 2003) since 1975 indicate that approximately 50% of twelfth-grade students have used an illicit drug, with a high of 66% in 1982, a low of 41% in 1992, and 51% in 2004. Since 1975, over 80% of students (ranging from 82.7% in 1992 to 90.4% in 1998) opined that marijuana was easily available.

Substance Use Disorders

The most comprehensive epidemiological information for the U.S. comes from the National Epidemiologic Survey on Alcohol and Related Conditions (NESARC), a survey of 43,093 respondents ages 18 years and older conducted in 2001–2002 (Grant et al. 2003, 2004c). The sample included noninstitutionalized individuals, with African Americans, Hispanics, and young adults oversampled; the response rate was 81%. The diagnostic interview was the Alcohol Use Disorder and Associated Disabilities Interview Schedule—DSM-IV Version (AUDADIS-IV; Grant et al. 2003), a structured interview for nonclinicians with high reliability and validity for substance use disorders (Canino et al. 1999; Grant et al. 1995; Hasin et al. 1996a; Ustun et al. 1997).

In the NESARC, the prevalence of current (past 12 months) alcohol abuse and dependence was 4.7% and 3.8%, respectively, for a total prevalence of 8.5% for any current alcohol use disorder. The prevalence of current drug abuse and dependence is 1.4%, and 0.6%, respectively, for a total prevalence of 2.0% (Grant et al. 2004a). Current alcohol and drug use disorders are more prevalent in men

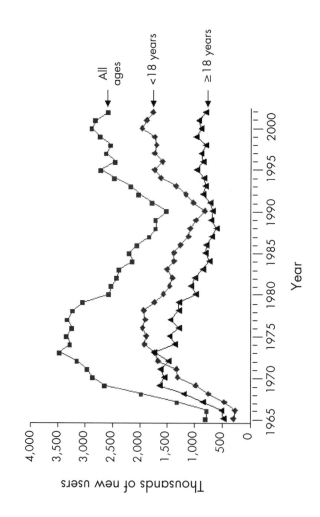

FIGURE 6–2.   New users of marijuana in the United States: 1965–2002.

Source.   Substance Abuse and Mental Health Services Administration 2002.

than in women, a consistent but unexplained finding, and prevalence declines steadily with age. There is no consistent trend by race for drug disorders, whereas for alcohol use disorders, whites generally have higher rates (Figure 6–3). Compared with a similar survey conducted 10 years earlier, the NESARC indicated that the prevalence of alcohol and drug disorders increased between 1992 and 2002 (Compton et al. 2004; Grant et al. 2004c), although this increase largely arose due to increases in abuse rather than dependence.

MACRO/EXTERNAL FACTORS IN THE ETIOLOGY OF SUBSTANCE USE DISORDERS

Substances must be available in the environment for individuals to use them. In Western societies, competing forces influence availability, and via availability, consumption of alcohol and drugs. Public health, moral/religious, "grassroots" and some governmental organizations attempt to reduce availability and consumption, while sellers of alcohol and drugs attempt to increase consumption. Widespread social attitudes toward substance use, as well as political events, can also influence availability and consumption.

Efforts to Reduce Availability and Consumption

Pricing

Alcohol taxation is the major determinant of state variation in the price of alcohol, and is thus a government intervention. An inverse relationship exists between state-level price of alcohol and per capita consumption or adverse consequences of drinking (Chaloupka et al. 2002). Furthermore, higher state-level beer tax is associated with lower prevalence of DSM-IV alcohol dependence (Henderson et al. 2004). Outside the United States, cutting the tax on spirits has been followed by increased per capita alcohol consumption (Heeb et al. 2003; Room 2004).

State Distribution Policies

In the United States, states differ in the ways they control availability of alcohol. Some states exert more control through operation of state alcoholic beverage sales, while others exert less control through the licensing of alcohol outlets. This difference impacts sales and consumption patterns (Wagenaar and Holder 1991). Compared with "wet" counties, "dry" counties, where alcohol is not sold,

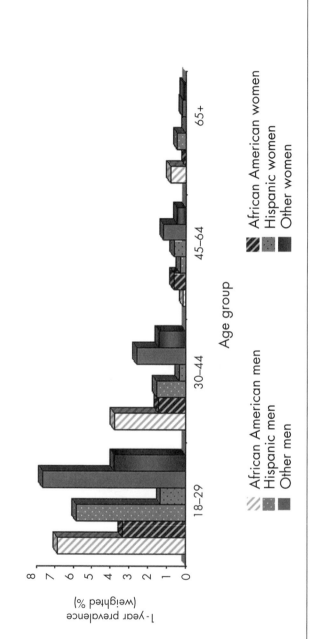

FIGURE 6–3. Trends in drug disorders by race/ethnicity: evidence from the National Epidemiologic Survey on Alcohol and Related Conditions.

have lower rates of alcohol-related accidents, "driving under the influence" (DUI) arrests, and cirrhosis mortality (Wilson et al. 1993). International studies corroborate these findings; in Norway, stringent alcohol regulations, such as mandatory closing on Saturdays, led to lower detoxification admissions (Room 2004).

Laws and Law Enforcement

Alcohol.   Laws and their enforcement also affect consumption patterns. In the United States between 1920 and 1933, the 18th Amendment to the Constitution outlawed the manufacture, transport, and sale of alcohol. Figure 6–4 illustrates that in 1935, per capita ethanol consumption was very low, but increased steadily afterward, consistent with cirrhosis mortality rates from the same period (Herd 1992; Lender and Martin 1982; Saadatmand et al. 1999; Yoon et al. 2003). Thus, the 18th Amendment achieved its purpose but was repealed because it was unacceptable to the public. Similar events occurred in the former Soviet Union, an area of very high per capita alcohol consumption (World Health Organization 1999). In the mid-1980s, the government attempted to restrict consumption. The policies were successful in reducing consumption but were so unpopular that they contributed to the downfall of the government (Shkolnikov and Nemtsov 1997).

In addition, stricter DUI laws and their enforcement are consistently related to decreased hazardous use (Maghsoodloo et al. 1988) and alcohol-related traffic fatalities (Asbridge et al. 2004; Hingson et al. 1998; Rogers and Schoenig 1994; Shults et al. 2002; Voas et al. 2003).

Drugs.   A literature on government efforts to reduce drug use by reducing availability is inconsistent. Some studies suggest the strategies are ineffective (Blumenthal et al. 1999; Oscapella 1995; Rydell et al. 1996; Weatherburn and Lind 1997; Wood et al. 2003), whereas others find supply reductions efficacious (Day et al. 2003; Weatherburn et al. 2003). Reducing the supply of specific drugs can have unintended consequences, including increases in other substances (Topp et al. 2003). Thus, the evidence is inconsistent on the efficacy of government attempts to limit drug use by reducing supply.

Outlet Density

Counties, cities, or states with higher alcohol outlet density have higher alcohol consumption and higher rates of alcohol-related problems, including hospital admissions, pedestrian injury collisions, and crashes and crash fatalities (Cohen

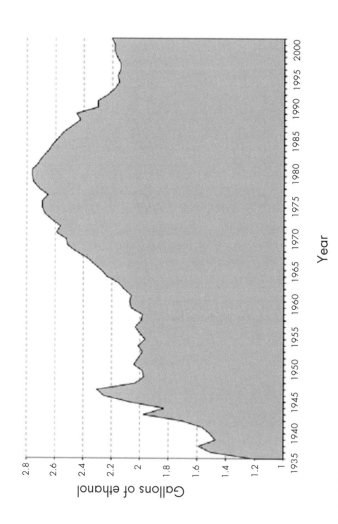

FIGURE 6–4.   Gallons of ethanol consumed in the United States, by year: 1935–2002.

Source.   Reprinted from Lakins NE, Williams GD, Yi H, et al.: *Surveillance Report #66: Apparent Per Capita Alcohol Consumption: National, State, and Regional Trends, 1977–2002.* Bethesda, MD, National Institute on Alcohol Abuse and Alcoholism, 2004.

et al. 2002; Escobedo and Ortiz 2002; Gruenewald et al. 1993; LaScala et al. 2001; Scribner et al. 2000; Tatlow et al. 2000; Weitzman et al. 2003). Multilevel analysis controlling for individual-level factors indicates that outlet density is related to higher mean group rates of consumption and drinking norms scores and to driving after drinking (Gruenewald et al. 2002; Scribner et al. 2000). The relationship of alcohol outlet density to individual risk for alcohol disorders is currently under investigation (R.C. Henderson, personal communication, 2005). Although information regarding outlet ("dealer") density is unavailable for drugs, the vigorous efforts of parents, schools, and law enforcement agencies to keep drug dealers away from schools are consistent with the same idea.

Grassroots Efforts

Mothers Against Drunk Driving (MADD) was started in 1980 by a group of women after a teenage girl was killed by a repeat-offense drunk driver. MADD, a very active organization, national since the early 1980s, has been highly effective in influencing state legislation pertaining to intoxicated driving, such as increasing the minimum drinking age from 18 to 21 years, and enforcement of maximum blood alcohol content (BAC) laws among drivers (Hamilton 2000; Russell et al. 1995). In particular, a highly publicized media campaign called "Rate the State," in which states were graded A through D on DUI countermeasures, put pressure on legislators to increase the stringency of these laws, shown as an effective strategy in reducing alcohol-impaired driving (e.g., Shults et al. 2002; Voas et al. 2000).

Countervailing Forces: Efforts to Increase Consumption

Alcohol Marketing and Advertising

Product development and marketing aim to increase sales and consumption (Centers for Disease Control and Prevention 2003). Alcohol companies allocate substantial resources to researching consumer preferences, developing new products, and promoting them (Jackson et al. 2000). For example, the alcohol beverage industry spent 696 million dollars on magazine advertising alone between 1997 and 2001, largely targeted to adolescents (Garfield et al. 2003). The alcohol industry does not publish the results of its marketing research, and resources necessary for definitive public health studies of advertising and other marketing effects are limited by comparison.

Public health concerns often focus on marketing that targets adolescents (Casswell 2004; Cooke et al. 2004). Existing data from longitudinal studies show associations between late childhood–early adolescent exposure to advertising and subsequent drinking initiation and frequency (Connolly et al. 1994; Ellickson et al. 2005; Stacy et al. 2004). Cross-sectional studies also show associations of various marketing and advertising strategies with positive attitudes about drinking and drinking frequency (Fleming et al. 2004; Grube and Wallack 1994; Kuo et al. 2003; Wyllie et al. 1998a, 1998b). Further, an imaging study of adolescent response to alcohol advertising indicated greater brain activation in areas linked to reward and desire among adolescents with alcohol use disorders than infrequent drinkers (Tapert et al. 2003), suggesting that advertisements are especially salient to vulnerable adolescents.

Political Events

Political events can also change availability. For example, in 2004, religiously motivated attacks occurred on alcohol retailers in Iraq (Hawley 2004). Also, after the Taliban government fell in Afghanistan in 2001, heroin production in Afghanistan increased greatly (Kulsudjarit 2004), coinciding with increased heroin use among U.S. teenagers (Tarabar and Nelson 2003). While the increase in use among adolescents cannot be definitively attributed to the increased availability of heroin from Afghanistan, the possibility of political events at a great distance geographically to influence local substance use patterns should not be ignored entirely when considering factors affecting vulnerability to substance use disorders.

Parental and Peer Influences

Parental Modeling of Substance Use

Twin studies indicate that up to half the liability to alcohol dependence is environmental (Rose et al. 2001). Parental modeling has been proposed as one such environmental factor affecting subsequent alcohol use in their children (Ellis et al. 1997). Adoption studies do not support this, however, since rates of alcoholism in adoptive children of alcoholic individuals are not elevated (Hopfer et al. 2003b).

Parenting Practices

Poor parental monitoring increases association with substance-abusing peers (Hawkins et al. 1992), a risk factor for alcohol misuse (see Peer Influence, below). Warm yet authoritative parenting styles protect adolescents from alcohol problems (Patock-Peckham et al. 2001). Harsh, inconsistent parenting predicts earlier initiation of alcohol use, conduct problems, and poor regulatory competencies (Kumpfer and Bluth 2004; Repetti et al. 2002).

Peer Influence

Peer influence is a strong predictor of adolescent drug and alcohol use and problems (Fergusson et al. 1995; Kandel 1973; Steinberg et al. 1994; Walden et al. 2004). Twin studies show that shared environmental influences such as peers have a significant effect on initiation of alcohol and any drug use (Rhee et al. 2003). Two models have been proposed to explain peer influence on adolescent substance use, social selection and socialization (Kandel 1985). The social selection theory proposes that young adolescents assortatively "mate" with friends; those children who display deviant behavior as children will be prone to choose deviant friendships in adolescence (Fergusson et al. 1999). This can lead to initiation of drug use (especially marijuana use) and may be a factor in the transition to "heavier" drugs. It has been further proposed that an underlying trait such as sensation seeking (see below) influences both the selection of peers and substance use (Donohew et al. 1999). In contrast, the socialization theory proposes that adolescents can be influenced to use substances by peers in their environment (Deater-Deckard 2001) via modeling, offers, development of expectancies, and social norms (Beyers et al. 2003; Borsari and Carey 2001; Clapper et al. 1994; Fergusson et al. 2002; Schulenberg et al. 1996). Substance use by older siblings is also associated with individual substance use (Brook et al. 1991; Bullock et al. 2002; Gfroerer 1987). Studies that could examine these various environmental effects while controlling for genetic influences are needed to resolve the social selection/ causation debate.

Peers may also be protective. Some U.S. ethnic/immigrant groups use substances less than the norm (e.g., Grant et al. 2004b). Adolescents from these groups with ethnically homogeneous peers encounter less pressure to use substances (J.S. Brook et al. 1998a, 1998b; D.W. Brook et al. 2002).

Stress

Drug disorders are often preceded and accompanied by disruptive behavior and conduct problems (Kuperman et al. 2001) that have a shared genetic vulnerability with drug disorders (Kendler et al. 2003). These behaviors evoke negative reactions from the environment, resulting in stressful life events that are not always independent of the individuals, making a causal direction between stress and disease onset difficult to discern. In animal studies where stress can be experimentally applied, cause and effect are clearer, as is also the case in studies of early stressful experiences in humans that antedate the onset of substance use disorders.

Animal Models

In animal studies, the timing of stress relative to normal development can be experimentally manipulated. In adult animals, substance use increases after physical stressors (Goeders and Guerin 1994; Piazza et al. 1990; Shaham and Stewart 1994) and social stressors (Covington and Miczek 2001; Haney et al. 1995; Kabbaj et al. 2001; Maccari et al. 1991a, 1991b; Miczek and Mutschler 1996; Tidey and Miczek 1997).

Early life stressors also contribute to drug using behaviors in animals. Neonatally isolated rats are more likely to acquire stimulant self-administration behaviors (Carroll et al. 2002; Hu et al. 2004; Kosten et al. 2000; Lynch and Carroll 1999; Lynch et al. 2005) and show higher dopamine levels in response to cocaine than handled rats, suggesting that early stress leads to greater cocaine reward (Brake et al. 2004; Kosten et al. 2003). Early-life rearing stressors predict ethanol seeking in primates (Barr et al. 2004). Isolated rearing led to increased drinking of morphine solution under various conditions (B.K. Alexander et al. 1981; Marks-Kaufman and Lewis 1984). Recently developed animal models of delta-9-tetrahydrocannabinol (Δ9-THC) self-administration (Braida et al. 2004) should allow similar studies for cannabis.

Early Stressors and Drug Use in Humans

Childhood stressors, including parental separation, neglect, and abuse (physical and sexual), are associated with later substance use, problems, and dependence (Dube et al. 2003; Hope et al. 1998; Kendler et al. 1996; Kessler et al. 1997). However, most studies failed to control for parental history of substance abuse, a potential confounder given that substance abuse is associated with poor parenting (Locke and Newcomb 2004). One informative study showed that among adolescents with a substance-abusing parent, strong family cohesion (the opposite of neglect) protected against drug problems (Hopfer et al. 2003a). Twin studies allow the study of environmental stressors while controlling for genetic influences, and have shown that childhood sexual abuse is an environmental risk factor for substance use disorders (Kendler et al. 2000; Nelson et al. 2002). Effects of other childhood adversities (e.g., neglect, physical and emotional abuse) have not been examined.

Religiosity

Religiosity has been called "one of the more important familial environmental factors that affect the risk for substance use and dependence" (Kendler et al. 1997, p. 322). An inverse relationship between religiosity and drinking is cross-cultural (e.g., Aharonovich et al. 2001; Perkins 1987). Longitudinal studies of adolescents, college and professional students show that religiosity protects against later heavy drinking (Barnes et al. 1994; Igra and Moos 1979; Margulies et al. 1977; Moore et al. 1990; Webb et al. 1991). Religiosity is strongly correlated within twin pairs due to shared environmental effects (Kendler et al. 1997; Kirk et al. 1999; Rose 1988; Truett et al. 1994). Heritability of drinking differs between religious and nonreligious twins, an example of gene–environment interaction (Koopmans et al. 1999). In twins studied longitudinally (Kendler et al. 1997), religiosity predicted later drinking more than drinking predicted later religiosity, suggesting that religiosity is more likely to influence drinking than the reverse. These studies indicate that religiosity is largely environmental and protects against alcohol use disorders. Religiosity also protects against drug disorders (e.g., C. Y. Chen et al. 2004; Miller et al. 2000), although this literature is less extensive.

MICRO/INTERNAL FACTORS IN THE ETIOLOGY OF SUBSTANCE USE DISORDERS

Psychological Factors

Alcohol Expectancies

Positive alcohol expectancies constitute an important risk factor for the development of alcohol dependence (e.g., Goldman et al. 1991; Shen et al. 2001). These expectancies can be derived from parents and peers, and a twin study found that such expectancies were environmental rather than genetic (Slutske et al. 2002).

Personality Traits

No single personality trait predicts alcoholism (Sher et al. 2005), but traits associated with the development of alcohol use disorders include novelty seeking (Cloninger et al. 1995) and sensation seeking (Martin et al. 2002, 2004; Zuckerman and Kuhlman 2000), traits that are often associated (Earleywine et al. 1992; Wills et al. 1994). The amount of heritability in sensation seeking is unclear, with some twin studies suggesting that approximately half of the variance can be attributed to genetic factors (Heath et al. 1994; Heiman et al. 2003, 2004; Hur and Bouchard 1997; Plomin and Daniels 1987; Stallings et al. 1996), and another suggesting it is largely due to the influence of similar environmental factors rather than genetic factors (Miles et al. 2001). Additional personality traits related to alcohol use disorders, albeit less consistently, are neuroticism/negative emotionality (e.g., Zimmerman et al. 2003), impulsivity/disinhibition (e.g., McGue et al. 1997), and extraversion/sociability (Hill et al. 2000).

Similar traits have been examined in relation to drug use disorders. For example, research has shown that impulsivity/inhibition is reliably lower among individuals with drug abuse/dependence (Conway et al. 2002; McGue et al. 1999), whereas negative emotionality tends to be higher (Conway et al. 2002; Swendsen et al. 2002).

Subjective Reactions

Level of response to alcohol indicates the quantity needed to obtain an effect. Those with a low level of response need to drink more to obtain an effect. This is a genetically influenced characteristic associated with enhanced risk for alcohol use disorders (Schuckit et al. 2004). Level of response varies by ethnicity. Several groups at high risk for alcohol use disorders show low response, including children of alcoholics, Native Americans, and Koreans (Ehlers et al. 1999; Monteiro et al. 1990; Wall et al. 1999), while high response is found among Jews (Schuckit et al. 2004), a group with relatively low levels of alcohol disorders (Hasin et al. 2002b; Levav et al. 1997). A low level of alcohol response predicts later onset of alcohol dependence in young adult males (Schuckit and Smith 1996) and may contribute to transition from lighter to heavier drinking in individuals in a heavy-drinking environment (Schuckit 1998). Several chromosomal regions have shown suggestive linkage results to level of response to alcohol (Wilhelmsen et al. 2003), but replication is needed.

Subjective reactions can also be characterized by whether they are positive or negative. A stimulating (reinforcing), rather than sedating, effect of alcohol has been identified in moderate/heavy drinkers (Holdstock et al. 2000), as well as untreated alcoholics (Thomas et al. 2004). In contrast, a flushing reaction to alcohol, found among Asians, includes unpleasant physical sensations (W.J. Chen et al. 1998; Higuchi et al. 1995; Tanaka et al. 1997). A strong flushing reaction precludes drinking, while moderate flushing protects against alcohol dependence. Individuals also vary in their subjective responses to marijuana, and positive and/or negative responses are moderately heritable (Lyons et al. 1997).

Genetics

Family and Twin Studies of Alcohol and Drug Dependence

Alcoholism (Bierut et al. 1998; Cotton 1979; Nurnberger et al. 2004) and drug disorders (Luthar et al. 1992; Merikangas et al. 1998) are familial. Twin studies of alcohol dependence show heritabilities of 50%–60% (Heath 1995; Kendler et al. 2000; Rhee et al. 2003). Heritability estimates for illicit drugs are more variable, perhaps due to more varied phenotypes (use, heavy use, abuse, and dependence); for drug dependence, heritability estimates are similar to alcohol dependence (Fu et al. 2002; Kendler et al. 2000; Rhee et al. 2003). Environmental factors appear to influence initiation and continuation of use past an experimental level, while genetic factors move individuals from use to dependence. Some twin studies investigating shared genetic variance of dependence on different substances have shown a high level of shared genetic variance between substances (Karkowski et al. 2000; Kendler et al. 2003; Tsuang et al. 2001), while other studies suggest that dependence on different classes of drugs is not genetically interchangeable (Bierut et al. 1998; Tsuang et al. 1998). Molecular genetics studies may be able to clarify these issues.

Genetic Linkage and Association Studies of Alcohol and Drug Dependence

Linkage studies attempt to identify chromosomal regions containing genes causing disorders via studies of families or sibling pairs. Fine gene mapping is then used to identify specific genes or single nucleotide polymorphisms associated with the disease or trait. Association studies compare genotypes between unrelated individuals with and without the trait of interest. The Collaborative Study on the Genetics of Alcoholism (COGA; Reich et al. 1998) has produced linkage results on several alcohol-related phenotypes, including dependence, drinking, comorbidity, and brain electrophysiological measures (Bierut et al. 2002; Porjesz et al. 2002). Alcohol dependence and related phenotypes (including comorbidity of alcohol dependence and major depression or alcohol dependence and habitual smoking) have shown linkage to regions on chromosomes 1, 2, 4, 7, 8, 15, and 16 (Corbett et al. 2005; Dick et al. 2004; Foroud et al. 1998, 2000; Wang et al. 2004). Linkage studies for drug use disorders began later than the COGA study and are currently under way in several locations in the U.S. A number of these are coordinated by the National Institute on Drug Abuse Genetics Consortium.

Genes Affecting the Metabolism of Substances

Alcohol is largely metabolized in the liver through a two-step process involving the enzymes alcohol dehydrogenase (ADH) and aldehyde dehydrogenase (ALDH; Edenberg 2000; Li 2000). ADH converts alcohol to acetaldehyde, a highly toxic substance. Acetaldehyde is quickly converted to acetate by ALDH and transported out of the liver. Excess acetaldehyde causes flushing and other unpleasant effects. Polymorphisms in ADH and ALDH genes encode isozymes with different activity levels that affect the efficiency of the alcohol-metabolizing process. The efficiency affects risk for heavy drinking and alcohol dependence, since individuals with an efficient process can drink more without subjectively unpleasant experiences, as is characteristic of most individuals with European background. Allele types contributing to an "inefficient" process of alcohol metabolism (e.g., *ALDH2*2*, *ADH1B*2*) are protective and are largely found in Asian groups (C.C. Chen et al. 1999; Goedde et al. 1992). The protective form of *ADH1B* is also found in U.S. and Israeli Jews, in whom it predicts less drinking (Carr et al. 2002; Hasin et al. 2002b; Neumark et al. 1998) and fewer alcohol dependence symptoms (Hasin et al. 2002a).

Cytochrome P450 is a family of enzymes crucial in drug metabolism, and genetically determined forms of these enzymes are associated with drug use disorders (Daly 2004; Ma et al. 2002). These enzymes affect the oxidation of drugs, which is the beginning of the metabolic process of making the drugs water-soluble so that they can be flushed more easily from the body and bloodstream (Ma et al. 2002). Genetic variants of these enzymes are hypothesized to affect ability to metabolize a wide range of drugs, including amphetamines and opiates, and this has been shown to affect the risk of dependence on these addictive drugs (Ingelman-Sundberg 2004; Sellers and Tyndale 2000).

Genes Involved in Neurotransmitter Systems

Considerable research has focused on the genes involved in neural pathways likely to affect substance-related behaviors. Genetic polymorphisms affecting neurotransmitters, including dopamine, serotonin, and γ-aminobutyric acid (GABA), have received attention because of their roles in processes related to substance abuse.

GABA receptor genes. GABA is the brain's chief inhibitory neurotransmitter, and alcohol enhances GABA activity. GABA type A ($GABA_A$) receptors mediate important effects of alcohol, including anxiolysis, sedation, disruption of motor coordination, tolerance, and also electroencephalograph activity in the beta band (Davies 2003). Early studies in humans and animals suggested that GABA receptor genes might affect risk for alcohol dependence (Grobin et al. 1998; Korpi and Lurz 1989; Loh et al. 1999; Valenzuela et al. 1998). A strong relationship was found between $GABA_A$ receptor alpha$_2$ subunit (*GABRA2*) genes on chromosome 4 and both alcohol dependence and brain oscillations in the beta frequency range (Edenberg et al. 2004), an endophenotype linked to alcohol dependence (Costa and Bauer 1997; Porjesz et al. 2002; Rangaswamy et al. 2002). The *GABRA2* results have since been replicated for alcohol dependence in U.S. (Covault et al. 2004) and Russian (Lappalainen et al. 2005) case–control studies, suggesting that polymorphisms in *GABRA2* play a role in the vulnerability to alcohol dependence. Other GABA receptor genes have also shown an association with alcohol dependence, including *GABRB2* (Loh et al. 2000; Radel et al. 2005), *GABRA6* (Loh et al. 1999; Radel et al. 2005), *GABRG2* (Loh et al. 2000) on chromosome 5q, and *GABRG3* (Dick et al. 2004) on chromosome 15q.

Dopamine receptors. Alcohol, opiates, and psychostimulants such as amphetamines all enhance the activity of dopaminergic neurons in humans and animals. Many genetic association studies of substance abuse or dependence have examined polymorphisms in dopamine receptor genes, especially *DRD2–DRD4* (Duaux et al. 2000), with inconsistent results (Blomqvist et al. 2000; Comings et al. 1999; Franke et al. 2000; Freimer et al. 1996; Gelernter et al. 1999; Li et al. 1997; Noble 1998; Young et al. 2004). Increased activity of the dopaminergic system has been considered to contribute to the reward and reinforcement properties of addictive drugs, but the mechanisms are more complex than originally thought and therefore not well understood. These complexities may have contributed to the inconsistencies in the genetic studies.

Serotonin-related genes. A low rate of serotonin turnover has been detected in alcoholism (Olsson et al. 2005). Serotonin levels are related to impulsive behavior (Reist et al. 2004), including suicide (Nielson et al. 1998), and also to major depressive disorder (Fehr et al. 2000), both common in substance abusers. Knockout mice for the serotonin 5-HT_{1B} receptor gene (*5HT1B*) have increased vulnerability to alcohol consumption and cocaine consumption (reviewed by Scearce-Levie et al. 1999). Among humans, a *5HT1B* polymorphism was associated with nonalcohol substance abuse although not alcohol dependence (Huang et al. 2003) and associated with antisocial alcohol dependence (Lappalainen et al. 1998; Soyka et al. 2004). However, a linkage disequilibrium study (Kranzler et al. 2002) did not find such an association in European American and African American samples, while a study designed to replicate Lappalainen et al. (1998) found an association but with a different allele (Fehr et al. 2000). Sander et al. (1998) found an association between antisocial alcoholism and the *SLC6A4* polymorphism of the serotonin transporter gene in a German sample. Because serotonin transporter sites serve as binding sites for cocaine (Jacobsen et al. 2000), polymorphism in the serotonin transporter gene was studied in relation to cocaine abuse in African Americans (Patkar et al. 2001). An association that was found initially when African American case patients were compared with racially mixed control subjects was no longer significant when control subjects were limited to African Americans. Thus, studies have been inconclusive regarding associations between serotonin-related genes and substance abuse and dependence.

Cannabinoid receptor genes.   Cannabinoid receptors are part of the drug reward pathway: they bind to Δ9-THC, the active ingredient in cannabis, creating alterations in memory and cognition as well as pain reduction. Variation in the gene protein encoded by the cannabinoid CN_1 receptor gene (*CNR1*) has been hypothesized to contribute to individual differences in drug vulnerabilities by modulating the reward pathway (Zhang et al. 2004). Results from association studies have been mixed. A preliminary study found genetic associations between alleles of an $(AAT)_n$ repeat section of *CNR1* and cocaine, amphetamine, and cannabis dependence in whites (Comings et al. 1997). However, this finding failed to replicate in case–control association studies with white and African American samples (Covault et al. 2001), as well as Chinese heroin and opiate users (Li et al. 2000). In the most complete study of the sequence and expression of the *CNR1* gene to date, Zhang et al. (2004) found an association between 6 different polymorphisms (including the $(AAT)_n$ repeat) and one haplotype ("TAG") and substance abuse in white, African American, and Japanese samples. This study provided evidence for a high level of functionality and conservation in the *CNR1* gene, pointing the way for promising future research. Animal studies of this gene have proven more consistent than human studies. In several studies, genetic variation resulting in downregulation in the endogenous cannabinoid receptor sites is associated with decrease in the craving and reward pathways induced by alcohol, cocaine, amphetamine, and cannabis (for a review, see Hungund and Basavarajappa 2004).

Mu-opioid receptor gene.   The mu-opioid receptor gene (*OPRM1*) on chromosome 6 is the primary action site for opioids, mediating their reinforcing effects, and also indirectly moderating the effects of other psychoactive substances, including cocaine and alcohol. Variability in the action of the mu-opioid receptor is at least partly under genetic control. In mice, the mu-opioid receptor gene has been shown to affect opioid dependence (R.C. Alexander et al. 1996; Berrettini et al. 1994) and sensitivity to the effects of cocaine (Hummel et al. 2004). Human genetics studies have been inconsistent, with some positive findings (Hoehe et al. 2000; Luo et al. 2003; Oslin et al. 2003) and some negative findings (Crowley et al. 2003; Franke et al. 2001).

In summary, results on alcohol metabolizing genes and $GABA_A$ receptors now appear fairly consistent. However, for other linkage and candidate gene studies, results have been less consistent. This might be due to several factors, including 1) inadequate phenotypes, 2) complexities of brain functioning not yet well enough understood to generate correct hypotheses, 3) comorbidity not addressed or controlled, 4) gene–gene interaction not taken into account, and 5) gene–environment interaction not taken into account.

Concerning phenotypes, as reviewed earlier, the reliability and validity of dependence is good to excellent regardless of study design. Further, transforming dependence into a quantitative trait based on the number of criteria met (0–7) yields a more informative phenotype (Hasin et al. 2002b; Heath et al. 2002). Thus, alcohol or drug dependence appears adequate as a clinical phenotype, although more specific clinical phenotypes are under investigation for use in future studies. As understanding of dependence progresses, biological endophenotypes should emerge. Such developments would reflect better understanding of brain functioning, which will assist not only in tests of single-gene hypotheses (the main type of study to date) but also in joint tests of multiple genes (e.g., C.C. Chen et al. 1999). Concerning comorbidity, some work has already been done on phenotypes involving dependence and psychiatric comorbidity (Nurnberger et al. 2001; Wang et al. 2004), and more are currently under way. More regular control for comorbidity, or at least examination of results with comorbid subjects included or removed from the sample (e.g., Covault et al. 2004), should begin to provide more information about the degree to which comorbidity has contributed to inconsistencies in groups of studies.

Gene–Environment Interaction

Twin studies have made a major contribution to our understanding of alcohol and drug dependence by showing that both genetic and environmental factors are important. However, surprisingly few studies have directly addressed whether specific genotype–phenotype relationships are modified by environmental circumstances. Recently, such studies have started to emerge in other areas of psychiatry. For example, a functional length polymorphism, the short allele of the 5-HTT (serotonin) promoter polymorphism has not shown main effects on the risk for major depression among individuals unexposed to environmental stressors. However, the short allele increased the risk for major depression among individuals exposed to recent stressful life events in four studies (Caspi et al. 2003; Eley et al. 2004; Kaufman et al. 2004; Kendler et al. 2005), with only one study failing to replicate this relationship (Gillespie et al. 2005). Because of the difficulty in detecting interactions and of obtaining consistency in genetics studies generally in psychiatry, these studies have generated considerable excitement about the new possibilities in understanding the vulnerability to major psychiatric disorders (Moffitt et al. 2005).

For substance use disorders, a few studies have addressed environmental modification of gene–phenotype relationships. A twin study showed that heritability of drinking differed between religious and nonreligious twins (Koopmans et al. 1999). During several years of increasing alcohol consumption in Japan, the prevalence of heterozygous ALDH2*2 increased significantly among Japanese alcoholics, suggesting that protection afforded by ALDH2*2 was increasingly counteracted over time by environmental factors (Higuchi et al. 1994). Examining small samples of contrasting Jewish Israeli groups, ADH1B*2 was protective against heavy drinking and alcohol dependence symptoms (Hasin et al. 2002a, 2002b). However, in recent Russian Jewish immigrants, exposed to an environment of heavy drinking before immigration (Hasin et al. 1998; Rahav et al. 1999), ADH1B*2 effects appeared much weaker, suggesting that earlier exposure to a heavy-drinking culture overrode the protective genetic effect (Hasin et al. 2002a, 2002b). This is now under further investigation in a larger study in Israel in conjunction with additional genetic and environmental risk factors and drug as well as alcohol phenotypes (D. Hasin, Principal Investigator). At least one other gene–environment interaction study is currently under way with a substance dependence phenotype, and results should emerge over the next few years.

Other environmental factors reviewed in this chapter have not yet been addressed in genetic studies of alcohol and drug dependence, but could affect the results. For example, relatives of substance-dependent probands may harbor genetic vulnerability to dependence, but may not express the disorder due to religiosity. If the proportion of relatives with high religiosity varies between family or sib-pair genetics studies, this could cause inconsistent results. Such factors could be assessed with little extra expense, although analytic procedures might require adjustment to take them into account.

CLINICAL IMPLICATIONS

Studying the interaction between certain genes and environments has important implications for the prevention of alcohol and drug use disorders. First, better knowledge in this area may help early identification of individuals unlikely to be able to use drugs or alcohol in moderation for early education, additional support or supervision. Second, the knowledge may help identify individuals exposed to particular stressors with specific genetic vulnerability to substance disorders that would benefit from early intervention. Third, clearer knowledge of the interaction of environmental with genetic effects may suggest new lines of investigation to determine the biological mechanisms of protective or risk-enhancing environmental events or conditions.

Finally, and in summary, a number of factors influencing the risk for substance dependence have been identified. However, investigators from different levels of factors (see Figure 6–1) rarely work together to address multilevel factors conjointly, although the need to do so is growing.

REFERENCES

Aharonovich E, Hasin D, Rahav G, et al: Differences in drinking patterns among Ashkenazic and Sephardic Israeli adults. J Stud Alcohol 62:301–305, 2001

Alexander BK, Beyerstein BL, Hadaway PF, et al: Effect of early and later colony housing on oral ingestion of morphine in rats. Pharmacol Biochem Behav 15:571–576, 1981

Alexander RC, Heydt D, Ferraro TN, et al: Further evidence for a quantitative trait locus on murine chromosome 10 controlling for morphine preference in inbred mice. Psychiatr Genet 6:29–31, 1996

American Psychiatric Association: Diagnostic and Statistical Manual of Mental Disorders, 4th Edition. Washington, DC, American Psychiatric Association, 1994

Asbridge M, Mann RE, Flam-Zalcman R, et al: The criminalization of impaired driving in Canada: assessing the deterrent impact of Canada's first per se law. J Stud Alcohol 65:450–459, 2004

Barnes GM, Farrell MP, Banerjee S: Family influences on alcohol abuse and other problem behaviors among black and white adolescents in a general population sample. J Res Adolesc 4:183–201, 1994

Barr CS, Schwandt ML, Newman TK, et al: The use of adolescent nonhuman primates to model human alcohol intake: neurobiological, genetic, and psychological variables. Ann N Y Acad Sci 1021:221–233, 2004

Berrettini WH, Ferraro TN, Alexander RC, et al: Quantitative trait loci mapping of three loci controlling morphine preference using inbred mouse strains. Nat Genet 7:54–58, 1994

Beyers JM, Bates JE, Pettit GS, et al: Neighborhood structure, parenting processes, and the development of youths' externalizing behaviors: a multilevel analysis. Am J Community Psychol 31:35–53, 2003

Bierut LJ, Dinwiddie SH, Begleiter H, et al: Familial transmission of substance dependence: alcohol, marijuana, cocaine, and habitual smoking: a report from the Collaborative Study on the Genetics of Alcoholism. Arch Gen Psychiatry 55:982–988, 1998

Bierut LJ, Saccone NL, Rice JP, et al: Defining alcohol-related phenotypes in humans. The Collaborative Study on the Genetics of Alcoholism. Alcohol Res Health 26:208–213, 2002

Blomqvist O, Gelernter J, Kranzler HR: Family-based study of DRD2 alleles in alcohol and drug dependence. Am J Med Genet 96:659–664, 2000

Blumenthal RN, Lorvick J, Kral AH, et al: Collateral damage in the war on drugs: HIV risk behaviors among injection drug users. International Journal of Drug Policy 10:25–38, 1999

Borsari B, Carey KB: Peer influences on college drinking: a review of the research. J Subst Abuse 13:391–424, 2001

Braida D, Iosue S, Pegorini S, et al: Delta9-tetrahydrocannabinol-induced conditioned place preference and intracerebroventricular self-administration in rats. Eur J Pharmacol 506:63–69, 2004

Brake WG, Zhang TY, Diorio J, et al: Influence of early postnatal rearing conditions on mesocorticolimbic dopamine and behavioral responses to psychostimulants and stressors in adult rats. Eur J Neurosci 19:1863–1874, 2004

Brook JS, Whiteman M, Brook DW, et al: Sibling influences on adolescent drug use: older brothers on younger brothers. J Am Acad Child Adolesc Psychiatry 30:958–966, 1991

Brook DW, Brook JS, Rosen Z, et al: Correlates of marijuana use in Colombian adolescents: a focus on the impact of the ecological/cultural domain. J Adolesc Health 31:286–298, 2002

Brook JS, Brook DW, De La Rosa M, et al: Pathways to marijuana use among adolescents: cultural/ecological, family, peer, and personality influences. J Am Acad Child Adolesc Psychiatry 37:759–766, 1998a

Brook JS, Balka EB, Brook DW, et al: Drug use among African Americans: ethnic identity as a protective factor. Psychol Rep 83:1427–1446, 1998b

Bucholz KK, Hesselbrock VM, Shayka JJ, et al: Reliability of individual diagnostic criterion items for psychoactive substance dependence and the impact on diagnosis. J Stud Alcohol 56:500–505, 1995

Bullock BM, Bank L, Burraston B: Adult sibling expressed emotion and fellow sibling deviance: a new piece of the family process puzzle. J Fam Psychol 16:307–317, 2002

Canino G, Bravo M, Ramirez R, et al: The Spanish Alcohol Use Disorder and Associated Disabilities Interview Schedule (AUDADIS): reliability and concordance with clinical diagnoses in a Hispanic population. J Stud Alcohol 60:790–799, 1999

Carr LG, Foroud T, Stewart T, et al: Influence of ADH1B polymorphism on alcohol use and its subjective effects in a Jewish population. Am J Med Genet 112:138–143, 2002

Carroll ME, Morgan AD, Lynch WJ, et al: Intravenous cocaine and heroin self-administration in rats selectively bred for differential saccharin intake: phenotype and sex differences. Psychopharmacol 161:304–313, 2002

Caspi A, Sugden K, Moffitt TE, et al: Influence of life stress on depression: moderation by a polymorphism in the 5-HTT gene. Science 301:386–389, 2003

Casswell S: Alcohol brands in young peoples' everyday lives: new developments in marketing. Alcohol Alcohol 39:471–476, 2004

Centers for Disease Control and Prevention: Point-of-purchase alcohol marketing and promotion by store type—United States, 2000–2001. MMWR 52:310–313, 2003

Chaloupka FJ, Grossman M, Saffer H: The effects of price on alcohol consumption and alcohol-related problems. Alcohol Res Health 26:22–34, 2002

Chen CC, Lu RB, Chen YC, et al: Interaction between the functional polymorphisms of the alcohol-metabolism genes in protection against alcoholism. Am J Hum Genet 65:795–807, 1999

Chen CY, Dormitzer CM, Bejarano J, et al: Religiosity and the earliest stages of adolescent drug involvement in seven countries of Latin America. Am J Epidemiol 159: 1180–1188, 2004

Chen WJ, Chen C-C, Yu J-M, et al: Self-reported flushing genotypes of ALDH2, ADH2, and ADH3 among Taiwanese Han. Alcohol Clin Exp Res 22:1048–1052, 1998

Clapper RL, Martin CS, Clifford PR: Personality, social environment, and past behavior as predictors of late adolescent alcohol use. J Subst Abuse 6:305–313, 1994

Cloninger CR, Sigvardsson S, Przybeck TR, et al: Personality antecedents of alcoholism in a national area probability sample. Eur Arch Psychiatry Clin Neurosci 245:239–244, 1995

Cohen DA, Mason K, Scribner R: The population consumption model, alcohol control practices, and alcohol-related traffic fatalities. Prev Med 34:187–197, 2002

Comings DE, Muhleman D, Gade R, et al: Cannabinoid receptor gene (CNR1): association with i.v. drug use. Mol Psychiatry 2:161–168, 1997

Comings DE, Gonzalez N, Wu S, et al: Homozygosity at the dopamine DRD3 receptor gene in cocaine dependence. Mol Psychiatry 4:484–487, 1999

Compton WM, Grant BF, Colliver JD, et al: Prevalence of marijuana use disorders in the United States: 1991–1992 and 2001–2002. JAMA 291:2114–2121, 2004

Connolly GM, Casswell S, Zhang JF, et al: Alcohol in the mass media and drinking by adolescents: a longitudinal study. Addiction 89:1255–1263, 1994

Conway KP, Swendsen JD, Rounsaville BJ, et al: Personality, drug of choice, and comorbid psychopathology among substance abusers. Drug Alcohol Depend 65:225–234, 2002

Cooke E, Hastings G, Wheeler C, et al: Marketing of alcohol to young people: a comparison of the UK and Poland. Eur Addict Res 10:1–7, 2004

Corbett J, Saccone NL, Foroud T, et al: A sex-adjusted and age-adjusted genome screen for nested alcohol dependence diagnoses. Psychiatr Genet 15:25–30, 2005

Costa L, Bauer L: Quantitative electroencephalographic differences associated with alcohol, cocaine, heroin and dual-substance dependence. Drug Alcohol Depend 46:87–93, 1997

Cottler LB, Grant BF, Blaine J, et al: Concordance of DSM-IV alcohol and drug use disorder criteria and diagnoses as measured by AUDADIS-ADR, CIDI and SCAN. Drug Alcohol Depend 47:195–205, 1997

Cotton NS: The familial incidence of alcoholism: a review. J Stud Alcohol 40:89–116, 1979

Covault J, Gelernter J, Kranzler H: Association study of cannabinoid receptor gene (CNR1) alleles and drug dependence. Mol Psychiatry 6:501–502, 2001

Covault J, Gelernter J, Hesselbrock V, et al: Allelic and haplotypic association of GABRA2 with alcohol dependence. Am J Med Genet 129B:104–109, 2004

Covington HE, Miczek KA: Repeated social-defeat stress, cocaine or morphine. Effects on behavioral sensitization and intravenous cocaine self-administration "binges." Psychopharmacol 158:388–398, 2001

Crowley JJ, Oslin DW, Patkar AA, et al: A genetic association study of the mu opioid receptor and severe opioid dependence. Psychiatr Genet 13:169–173, 2003

Daly AK: Pharmacogenetics of the cytochromes P450. Curr Top Med Chem 4:1733–1744, 2004

Davies M: The role of GABAA receptors in mediating the effects of alcohol in the central nervous system. J Psychiatry Neurosci 28:263–274, 2003

Day C, Topp L, Rouen D, et al: Decreased heroin availability in Sydney Australia in early 2001. Addiction 98:93–95, 2003

Deater-Deckard K: Annotation: recent research examining the role of peer relationships in the development of psychopathology. J Child Psychol Psychiatry 42:565–579, 2001

Deroche-Gamonet V, Belin D, Piazza PV: Evidence for addiction-like behavior in the rat. Science 305:1014–1017, 2004

Dick DM, Edenberg HJ, Xuei X, et al: Association of GABRG3 with alcohol dependence. Alcohol Clin Exp Res 28:4–9, 2004

Donohew RL, Hoyle RH, Clayton RR, et al: Sensation seeking and drug use by adolescents and their friends: models for marijuana and alcohol. J Stud Alcohol 60:622–631, 1999

Duaux E, Krebs MO, Loo H, et al: Genetic vulnerability to drug abuse. Eur Psychiatry 15:109–114, 2000

Dube SR, Felitti VJ, Dong M, et al: Childhood abuse, neglect, and household dysfunction and the risk of illicit drug use: the adverse childhood experiences study. Pediatrics 111:564–572, 2003

DuPont R, Greene M: The dynamics of a heroin addiction epidemic. Science 181:716–722, 1973

Earleywine M, Finn PR, Peterson JB, et al: Factor structure and correlates of the Tridimensional Personality Questionnaire. J Stud Alcohol 53:233–238, 1992

Edenberg HJ: Regulation of the mammalian alcohol dehydrogenase genes. Prog Nucleic Acid Res Mol Biol 64:295–341, 2000

Edenberg HJ, Dick DM, Xuei X, et al: Variations in GABRA2, encoding the a2 subunit of the GABAA receptor, are associated with alcohol dependence and with brain oscillations. Am J Hum Genet 74:705–714, 2004

Edwards G: The alcohol dependence syndrome: a concept as stimulus to enquiry. Br J Addict 81:171–183, 1986

Edwards G, Gross MM: Alcohol dependence: provisional description of a clinical syndrome. Br Med J 1:1058–1061, 1976

Ehlers CL, Garcia-Andrade C, Wall TL, et al: Electroencephalographic responses to alcohol challenge in Native American Mission Indians. Biol Psychiatry 45:776–787, 1999

Eley TC, Sugden K, Corsico A, et al: Gene-environment interaction analysis of serotonin system markers with adolescent depression. Mol Psychiatry 9:908–915, 2004

Ellickson PL, Collins RL, Hambarsoomians K, et al: Does alcohol advertising promote adolescent drinking? Results from a longitudinal assessment. Addiction 100:235–246, 2005

Ellis DA, Zucker RA, Fitzgerald HE: The role of family influences in development and risk. Alcohol Res Health 21:218–226, 1997

Escobedo, LG, Ortiz L: The relationship between liquor outlet density and injury and violence in New Mexico. Accid Anal Prev 34:689–694, 2002

Fehr C, Grintschuk N, Szegedi A, et al: The HTR1B 861G>C receptor polymorphism among patients suffering from alcoholism, major depression, anxiety disorders and narcolepsy. Psychiatry Res 97:1–10, 2000

Fergusson DM, Lynskey MT, Horwood LJ: The role of peer affiliations, social, family and individual factors in continuities in cigarette smoking between childhood and adolescence. Addiction 90:647–659, 1995

Fergusson DM, Woodward LJ, Horwood LJ: Childhood peer relationship problems and young people's involvement with deviant peers in adolescence. J Abnorm Child Psychol 27:357–369, 1999

Fergusson DM, Swain-Campbell NR, Horwood L: Deviant peer affiliations, crime and substance abuse: a fixed effects regression analysis. J Abnorm Clin Psychol 30:419–430, 2002

Fleming K, Thorson E, Atkin CK: Alcohol advertising exposure and perceptions: links with alcohol expectancies and intentions to drink or drinking in underaged youth and young adults. J Health Commun 9:3–29, 2004

Foroud T, Bucholz KK, Edenberg HJ, et al: Linkage of an alcoholism-related severity phenotype to chromosome 16. Alcohol Clin Exp Res 22:2035–2042, 1998

Foroud T, Edenberg HJ, Goate A, et al: Alcoholism susceptibility loci: confirmation studies in a replicate sample and further mapping. Alcohol Clin Exp Res 24:933–945, 2000

Franke P, Nothen MM, Wang T, et al: DRD4 exon III VNTR polymorphism-susceptibility factor for heroin dependence? Results of a case-control and a family based association approach. Mol Psychiatry 5:101–104, 2000

Franke P, Wang T, Nothem MM, et al: Nonreplication of association between mu-opioid-receptor gene (OPRM1) A118G polymorphism and substance dependence. Am J Med Genet 105:114–119, 2001

Freimer M, Kranzler H, Satel S, et al: No association between D3 dopamine receptor (DRD3) alleles and cocaine dependence. Addict Biol 1:281–287, 1996

Fu Q, Heath AC, Bucholz KK, et al: Shared genetic risk of major depression, alcohol dependence, and marijuana dependence: contribution of antisocial personality disorder in men. Arch Gen Psychiatry 59:1125–1132, 2002

Garfield CF, Chung PJ, Rathouz PJ: Alcohol advertising in magazines and adolescent readership. JAMA 289:2424–2429, 2003

Gelernter J, Kranzler H, Satel SL: No association between D2 dopamine receptor (DRD2) alleles or haplotypes and cocaine dependence or severity of cocaine dependence in European- and African-Americans. Biol Psychiatry 45:340–345, 1999

Gillespie NA, Whitfield JB, Williams B, et al: The relationship between stressful life events, the serotonin transporter (5-HTTLPR) genotype and major depression. Psychol Med 35:101–111, 2005

Gfroerer J: Correlation between drug use by teenagers and drug use by older family members. Am J Drug Alcohol Abuse 13:95–108, 1987

Goedde HW, Agarwal DP, Fritze G, et al: Distribution of ADH2 and ALDH2 genotypes in different populations. Hum Genet 88:344–346, 1992

Goeders NE, Guerin GF: Non-contingent electric footshock facilitates the acquisition of intravenous cocaine self-administration in rats. Psychopharmacol 114:63–70, 1994

Goldman MS, Brown SA, Christiansen BA, et al: Alcoholism and memory: broadening the scope of alcohol-expectancy research. Psychol Bull 110:137–146, 1991

Grant BF: DSM-IV, DSM-III-R, and ICD-10 alcohol and drug abuse/harmful use and dependence, United States, 1992: a nosological comparison. Alcohol Clin Exp Res 20:1481–1488, 1996

Grant BF, Harford TC, Dawson DA, et al: The Alcohol Use Disorder and Associated Disabilities Interview Schedule (AUDADIS): reliability of alcohol and drug modules in a general population sample. Drug Alcohol Depend 39: 37–44, 1995

Grant BF, Stinson FS, Harford TC: The 5-year course of alcohol abuse among young adults. J Subst Abuse 13:229–238, 2001

Grant BF, Dawson DA, Stinson FS, et al: The Alcohol Use Disorder and Associated Disabilities Interview Schedule-IV (AUDADIS-IV): reliability of alcohol consumption, tobacco use, family history of depression and psychiatric diagnostic modules in a general population sample. Drug Alcohol Depend 71:7–16, 2003

Grant BF, Stinson FS, Dawson DA, et al: Co-occurrence of 12-month alcohol and drug use disorders and personality disorders in the United States. Arch Gen Psychiatry 61:361–368, 2004a

Grant BF, Stinson FS, Hasin DS, et al: Immigration and lifetime prevalence of DSM-IV psychiatric disorders among Mexican Americans and non-Hispanic whites in the United States: results from the National Epidemiologic Survey on Alcohol and Related Conditions. Arch Gen Psychiatry 61:1226–1233, 2004b

Grant BF, Dawson DA, Stinson FS, et al: The 12-month prevalence and trends in DSM-IV alcohol abuse and dependence: United States, 1991–1992 and 2001–2002. Drug Alcohol Depend 74:223–234, 2004c

Greene M, Nightingale S, DuPont R: Evolving patterns of drug abuse. Ann Intern Med 83:402–411, 1975

Grobin AC, Matthews DB, Devaud LL, et al: The role of GABAA receptors in the acute and chronic effects of ethanol. Psychopharmacology (Berl) 139:2–19, 1998

Grube JW, Wallack L: Television beer advertising and drinking knowledge, beliefs, and intentions among schoolchildren. Am J Publ Health 84:254–259, 1994

Gruenewald PJ, Ponicki WR, Holder HD: The relationship of outlet densities to alcohol consumption: a time series cross-sectional analysis. Alcohol Clin Exp Res 17:38–47, 1993

Gruenewald PJ, Treno AJ, Johnson F: Outlets, drinking and driving: A multilevel analysis of availability. J Stud Alcohol 63:460–468, 2002

Hamilton W: Mothers Against Drunk Driving—MADD in the USA. Inj Prev 6:90–91, 2000

Haney M, Maccari S, Le Moal M, et al: Social stress increases the acquisition of cocaine self-administration in male and female rats. Brain Res 698:46–52, 1995

Harford TC, Muthen BO: The dimensionality of alcohol abuse and dependence: a multivariate analysis of DSM-IV symptom items in the National Longitudinal Survey of Youth. J Stud Alcohol 62:150–157, 2001

Hasin DS, Grant BF: The co-occurrence of DSM-IV alcohol abuse in DSM-IV alcohol dependence: results of the National Epidemiologic Survey on Alcohol and Related Conditions on heterogeneity that differ by population subgroup. Arch Gen Psychiatry 61:891–896, 2004

Hasin D, Paykin A: Alcohol dependence and abuse diagnoses: concurrent validity in a nationally representative sample. Alcohol Clin Exp Res 23:144–150, 1999a

Hasin D, Paykin A: DSM-IV alcohol abuse: investigation in a sample of at-risk drinkers in the community. J Stud Alcohol 60:181–187, 1999b

Hasin DS, Grant B, Endicott J: The natural history of alcohol abuse: implications for definitions of alcohol use disorders. Am J Psychiatry 147:1537–1541, 1990

Hasin D, Li Q, McCloud S, et al: Agreement between DSM-III, DSM-III-R, DSM-IV and ICD-10 alcohol diagnoses in US community-sample heavy drinkers. Addiction 91:1517–1527, 1996a

Hasin DS, Trautman K, Miele G, et al: Psychiatric Research Interview for Substance and Mental Disorders: reliability for substance abusers. Am J Psychiatry 153: 1195–1201, 1996b

Hasin D, Grant BF, Cottler L, et al: Nosological comparisons of alcohol and drug diagnoses: a multisite, multi-instrument international study. Drug Alcohol Depend 47: 217–26, 1997a

Hasin D, Van Rossem R, McCloud S, et al: Alcohol dependence and abuse diagnoses: validity in community sample heavy drinkers. Alcohol Clin Exp Res 21:213–219, 1997b

Hasin DS, Van Rossem R, McCloud S, et al: Differentiating DSM-IV alcohol dependence and abuse by course: community heavy drinkers. J Subst Abuse 9:127–135, 1997c

Hasin D, Rahav G, Meydan J, et al: The drinking of earlier and more recent Russian immigrants to Israel: comparison to other Israelis. J Subst Abuse 10:341–353, 1998

Hasin D, Paykin A, Endicott J, et al: The validity of DSM-IV alcohol abuse: drunk drivers versus all others. J Stud Alcohol 60:746–755, 1999

Hasin D, Aharonovich E, Liu X, et al: Alcohol and ADH2 in Israel: Ashkenazi, Sephardics, and recent Russian immigrants. Am J Psychiatry 159:1432–1434, 2002a

Hasin D, Aharonovich E, Liu X, et al: Alcohol dependence symptoms and alcohol dehydrogenase 2 polymorphism: Israeli Ashkenazis, Sephardics, and recent Russian immigrants. Alcohol Clin Exp Res 26:1315–1321, 2002b

Hasin DS, Schuckit MA, Martin CS, et al: The validity of DSM-IV alcohol dependence: what do we know and what do we need to know? Alcohol Clin Exp Res 27:244–252, 2003

Hasin DS, Hatzenbuehler M, Smith S, et al: Co-occurring DSM-IV Drug Abuse in DSM-IV Drug Dependence: results from the National Epidemiologic Survey on Alcohol and Related Conditions. Drug Alcohol Depend 80:117–123, 2005

Hawkins J, Catalano RF, Miller JY: Risk and protective factors for alcohol and other drug problems in adolescence and early adulthood: implications for substance abuse prevention. Psychol Bull 112:64–105, 1992

Hawley C: Wave of attacks on Iraqi alcohol sellers. BBC World News, July 22, 2004

Heath AC: Genetic influences on alcoholism risk: a review of adoption and twin studies. Alcohol Health Res World 19:166–171, 1995

Heath AC, Cloninger CR, Martin NG: Testing a model for the genetic structure of personality: a comparison of the personality systems of Cloninger and Eysenck. J Pers Soc Psychol 66:762–775, 1994

Heath AC, Martin NG, Lynskey MT, et al: Estimating two-stage models for genetic influences on alcohol, tobacco or drug use initiation and dependence vulnerability in twin and family data. Twin Res 5:113–124, 2002

Heeb J, Gmel G, Zurbrugg C, et al: Changes in alcohol consumption following a reduction in the price of spirits. Addiction 98:1433–1446, 2003

Heiman N, Stallings MC, Hofer SM, et al: Investigating age differences in the genetic and environmental structure of the Tridimensional Personality Questionnaire in later adulthood. Behav Genet 33:171–180, 2003

Heiman N, Stallings MC, Young SE, et al: Investigating the genetic and environmental structure of Cloninger's personality dimensions in adolescence. Twin Res 7:462–470, 2004

Henderson C, Liu X, Diez Roux AV, et al: The effects of US state income inequality and alcohol policies on symptoms of depression and alcohol dependence. Soc Sci Med 58:565–575, 2004

Herd D: Ideology, history and changing models of liver cirrhosis epidemiology. Br J Addict 87:1113–1126, 1992

Higuchi S, Matsushita S, Imazeki H, et al: Aldehyde dehydrogenase genotypes in Japanese alcoholics. Lancet 343:741–742, 1994

Higuchi S, Matsushita S, Murayama M, et al: Alcohol and aldehyde dehydrogenase polymorphisms and the risk for alcoholism. Am J Psychiatry 152:1219–1221, 1995

Hill SY, Shen S, Lowers L, et al: Factors predicting the onset of adolescent drinking in families at high risk for developing alcoholism. Biol Psychiatry 45:265–275, 2000

Hingson R, Heeren T, Winter M: Effects of Maine's 0.05% legal blood alcohol level for drivers with DWI convictions. Public Health Rep 113:440–446, 1998

Hoehe MR, Kopke K, Wendel B, et al: Sequence variability and candidate gene analysis in complex disease: association of mu opioid receptor gene variation with substance dependence. Hum Mol Genet 9:2895–2908, 2000

Holdstock L, King AC, DeWit H: Subjective and objective responses to ethanol in moderate/heavy and light social drinkers. Alcohol Clin Exp Res 24:789–794, 2000

Hope S, Power C, Rodgers B: The relationship between parental separation in childhood and problem drinking in adulthood. Addiction 93:505–514, 1998

Hopfer CJ, Stallings MC, Hewitt JK, et al: Family transmission of marijuana use, abuse, and dependence. J Am Acad Child Adolesc Psychiatry 42:834–841, 2003a

Hopfer CJ, Crowley TJ, Hewitt JK: Review of twin and adoption studies of adolescent substance abuse. J Am Acad Child Adolesc Psychiatry 42:710–719, 2003b

Hu M, Crombag HS, Robinson TE, et al: Biological basis of sex differences in the propensity to self-administer cocaine, Neuropsychopharmacol 29:81–85, 2004

Huang YY, Oquendo MA, Friedman JM, et al: Substance abuse disorder and major depression are associated with the human 5-HT1B receptor gene (HTR1B) G861C polymorphism. Neuropsychopharmacol 28:163–169, 2003

Hummel M, Ansonoff MA, Pintar JE, et al: Genetic and pharmacological manipulation of mu opioid receptors in mice reveals a differential effect on behavioral sensitization to cocaine. Neuroscience 125:211–220, 2004

Hungund BL, Basavarajappa BS: Role of endocannabinoids and cannabinoid CB1 receptors in alcohol-related behaviors. Ann N Y Acad Sci 1025:515–527, 2004

Hur YM, Bouchard TJ: The genetic correlation between impulsivity and sensation seeking traits. Behav Genet 27:455–463, 1997

Igra A, Moos RH: Alcohol use among college students: some competing hypotheses. J Youth Adolesc 8:393–405, 1979

Ingelman-Sundberg, M: Human drug metabolizing cytochrome P450 enzymes: properties and polymorphisms. Arch Pharmacol 369:89–104, 2004

Jackson MC, Hastings G, Wheeler C, et al: Marketing alcohol to young people: implications for industry regulation and research policy. Addiction 95 (suppl 4):S597–S608, 2000

Jacobsen LK, Staley JK, Malison RT, et al: Elevated central serotonin transporter binding availability in acutely abstinent cocaine-dependent patients. Am J Psychiatry 157:1134–1140, 2000

Johnston LD, O'Malley PM, Bachman JG, et al: Monitoring the Future: national survey results on drug use, 1975–2003, Vol 1: Secondary school students (NIH Publication No. 04-5507). Bethesda, MD, National Institute on Drug Abuse, 2003

Kabbaj M, Norton CS, Kollack-Walker S, et al: Social defeat alters the acquisition of cocaine self-administration in rats: role of individual differences in cocaine-taking behavior. Psychopharmacol 158:382–387, 2001

Kandel D: Adolescent marijuana use: the role of parents and peers. Science 181:1067–1070, 1973

Kandel DB: On processes of peer influences in adolescent drug use: a developmental perspective. Adv Alcohol Subst Abuse 4:139–163, 1985

Karkowski LM, Prescott CA, Kendler KS: Multivariate assessment of factors influencing illicit substance use in twins from female-female pairs. Am J Med Genet 96:665–670, 2000

Kaufman J, Yang BZ, Douglas-Palumberi H, et al: Social supports and serotonin transporter gene moderate depression in maltreated children. Proc Natl Acad Sci USA 101:17316–17321, 2004

Kendler KS, Neale MC, Prescott CA, et al: Childhood parental loss and alcoholism in women: a causal analysis using a twin-family design. Psychol Med 26:79–95, 1996

Kendler KS, Gardner CO, Prescott CA: Religion, psychopathology, and substance use and abuse; a multimeasure, genetic-epidemiologic study. Am J Psychiatry 154:322–329, 1997

Kendler KS, Bulik CM, Silberg J, et al: Childhood sexual abuse and adult psychiatric and substance use disorders in women: an epidemiological and co-twin control analysis. Arch Gen Psychiatry 57:953–959, 2000

Kendler KS, Jacobson KC, Prescott CA, et al: Specificity of genetic and environmental risk factors for use and abuse/dependence of cannabis, cocaine, hallucinogens, sedatives, stimulants, and opiates in male twins. Am J Psychiatry 160:687–695, 2003

Kendler KS, Kuhn JW, Vittum J, et al: The interaction of stressful life events and a serotonin transporter polymorphism in the prediction of episodes of major depression: a replication. Arch Gen Psychiatry 62:529–535, 2005

Kessler RC, Davis CG, Kendler KS: Childhood adversity and adult psychiatric disorder in the US National Comorbidity Survey. Psychol Med 27:1101–1119, 1997

Kirk KM, Maes HH, Neale MC, et al: Frequency of church attendance in Australia and the United States: models of family resemblance. Twin Res 2:99–107, 1999

Koopmans JR, Slutske WS, van Baal GC, et al: The influence of religion on alcohol use initiation: evidence for genotype X environment interaction. Behav Genet 29:445–453, 1999

Korpi ER, Lurz FW: GABAA receptor-mediated chloride flux in brain homogenates from rat lines with differing innate alcohol sensitivities. Neuroscience 32:387–392, 1989

Kosten TA, Miserebdino MJD, Kehoe P: Enhanced acquisition of cocaine self-administration in adult rats with neonatal isolation stress experience. Brain Res 875:44–50, 2000

Kosten TA, Zhang XY, Kehoe P: Chronic neonatal isolation stress enhances cocaine-induced increases in ventral striatal dopamine levels in rat pups. Brain Res Dev Brain Res 141:109–116, 2003

Kranzler HR, Hernandez-Avila CA, Gelernter J: Polymorphism of the 5-HT1B receptor gene (HTR1B): strong within-locus linkage disequilibrium without association to antisocial substance dependence. Neuropsychopharmacology 26:115–122, 2002

Kulsudjarit K: Drug problem in southeast and southwest Asia. Ann N Y Acad Sci 1025: 446–457, 2004

Kumpfer KL, Bluth B: Parent/child transactional processes predictive of resilience or vulnerability to "substance use disorders." Subst Use Misuse 39:671–698, 2004

Kuo M, Wechsler H, Greenberg P, et al: The marketing of alcohol to college students: the role of low prices and special promotions. Am J Prev Med 25:204–211, 2003

Kuperman S, Schlosser SS, Kramer JR, et al: Developmental sequence from disruptive behavior diagnosis to adolescent alcohol dependence. Am J Psychiatry 158:2022–2026, 2001

Lappalainen J, Long JC, Eggert M, et al: Linkage of antisocial alcoholism to the serotonin 5-HT$_{1B}$ receptor gene in 2 populations. Arch Gen Psychiatry 55: 989–994, 1998

Lappalainen J, Krupitsky E, Remizov M, et al: Association between alcoholism and gamma-aminobutyric acid alpha$_2$ receptor subtype in a Russian population. Alcohol Clin Exp Res 29:493–498, 2005

LaScala EA, Johnson FW, Gruenewald PJ: Neighborhood characteristics of alcohol-related pedestrian injury collisions: a geostatistical analysis. Prev Sci 2:123–134, 2001

Lender ME, Martin JK: Drinking in America: A History. New York, Free Press, 1982

Levav I, Kohn R, Golding JM, et al: Vulnerability of Jews to affective disorders. Am J Psychiatry 154:941–947, 1997

Li T, Xu K, Deng H, et al: Association analysis of the dopamine D4 gene exon III VNTR and heroin abuse in Chinese subjects. Mol Psychiatry 2:413–416, 1997

Li T, Liu X, Zhu ZH et al: No association between (AAT)n repeats in the cannabinoid receptor gene (CNR1) and heroin abuse in a Chinese population. Mol Psychiatry 5:128–130, 2000

Li TK: Pharmacogenetics of responses to alcohol and genes that influence alcohol drinking. J Stud Alcohol 61:5–12, 2000

Locke TF, Newcomb M: Child maltreatment, parent alcohol and drug-related problems, polydrug problems, and parenting practices: a test of gender differences and four theoretical perspectives. J Fam Psychol 18:120–134, 2004

Loh EW, Smith I, Murray R, et al: Association between variants at the GABAAb2, GABAAa6 and GABAAg2 gene cluster and alcohol dependence in a Scottish population. Mol Psychiatry 4:539–544, 1999

Loh EW, Higuchi S, Matsushita S, et al: Association analysis of the GABAA receptor subunit genes cluster on 5q33–34 and alcohol dependence in a Japanese population. Mol Psychiatry 5:301–307, 2000

Luo X, Kranzler HR, Zhao H, et al: Haplotypes at the OPRM1 locus are associated with susceptibility to substance dependence in European-Americans. Am J Genet B Neuropsychiatr Genet 120:97–108, 2003

Luthar SS, Anton SF, Merikangas KR, et al: Vulnerability to substance abuse and psychopathology among siblings of opioid abusers. J Nerv Ment Dis 180:153–161, 1992

Lynch WJ, Carroll ME: Sex differences in the acquisition of intravenously self-administered cocaine and heroin in rats. Psychopharmacology 144: 77–82, 1999

Lynch WJ, Mangigi LD, Taylor JR: Neonatal isolation stress potentiates cocaine seeking behavior in adult male and female rats. Neuropsychopharmacology 30:322–329, 2005

Lyons MJ, Toomey R, Meyer JM, et al: How do genes influence marijuana use? The role of subjective effects. Addiction 92:409–417, 1997

Ma MK, Woo MH, McLeod HL: Genetic basis of drug metabolism. Am J Health-Syst Pharm 59:2061–2069, 2002

Maccari S, Piazza PV, Deminiere JM, et al: Hippocampal type I and type II corticosteroid receptor affinities are reduced in rats predisposed to develop amphetamine self-administration. Brain Res 548:305–309, 1991a

Maccari S, Piazza PV, Deminiere JM, et al: Life events-induced decrease of corticosteroid type I receptors is associated with reduced corticosterone feedback and enhanced vulnerability to amphetamine self-administration. Brain Res 547:7–12, 1991b

Maghsoodloo S, Brown DB, Greathouse PA: Impact of the revision of DUI legislation in Alabama. Am J Drug Alcohol Abuse 14:97–108, 1988

Margulies RZ, Kessler RC, Kandel DB: A longitudinal study of onset of drinking among high-school students. J Stud Alcohol 38:897–912, 1977

Marks-Kaufman R, Lewis JL: Early housing experience modifies morphine self-administration and physical dependence in adult rats. Addict Behav 9:235–243, 1984

Martin CA, Kelly TH, Rayens MK, et al: Sensation seeking, puberty, and nicotine, alcohol, and marijuana use in adolescence. J Am Acad Child Adolesc Psychiatry 41:1495–1502, 2002

Martin CA, Kelly TH, Rayens MK, et al: Sensation seeking and symptoms of disruptive disorder: association with nicotine, alcohol, and marijuana use in early and mid-adolescence. Psychol Rep 94:1075–1082, 2004

McGue M, Slutske W, Taylor J, et al: Personality and substance use disorders: effects of gender and alcoholism subtype. Alcohol Clin Exp Res 21:513–520, 1997

McGue M, Slutske W, Iacono WG: Personality and substance use disorders, II: alcoholism versus drug use disorders. J Consult Clin Psychol 67:394–404, 1999

Merikangas KR, Stolar M, Stevens DE, et al: Familial transmission of substance use disorders. Arch Gen Psychiatry 55:973–979, 1998

Miczek KA, Mutschler NH: Activational effects of social stress on IV cocaine self administration in rats. Psychopharmacology 128:256–264, 1996

Miles DR, van den Bree MB, Gupman AE, et al: A twin study on sensation seeking, risk taking behavior and marijuana use. Drug Alcohol Depend 62:57–68, 2001

Miller L, Davies M, Greenwald S: Religiosity and substance use and abuse among adolescents in the National Comorbidity Survey. J Am Acad Child Adolesc Psychiatry 39:1190–1197, 2000

Moffitt TE, Caspi A, Rutter M: Strategy for investigating interactions between measured genes and measured environments. Arch Gen Psychiatry 62:473–481, 2005

Monteiro MG, Irwin M, Hauger RL, et al: TSH response to TRH and family history of alcoholism. Biol Psychiatry 27:905–910, 1990

Moore RD, Mead L, Pearson TA: Youthful precursors of alcohol abuse in physicians. Am J Med 88:332–336, 1990

Muthen BO, Grant B, Hasin D: The dimensionality of alcohol abuse and dependence: factor analysis of DSM-III-R and proposed DSM-IV criteria in the 1988 National Health Interview Survey. Addiction 88:1079–1090, 1993

Nelson EC, Heath AC, Madden PA, et al: Association between self-reported childhood sexual abuse and adverse psychosocial outcomes: results from a twin study. Arch Gen Psychiatry 59:139–145, 2002

Neumark YD, Friedlander Y, Thomasson HR, et al: Association of the ADH2*2 allele with reduced ethanol consumption in Jewish men in Israel: a pilot study. J Stud Alcohol 59:133–139, 1998

Nielson DA, Virkkunen M, Lappalainen J, et al: A tryptophan hydroxylase gene marker for suicidality and alcoholism. Arch Gen Psychiatry 55:593–602, 1998

Noble EP: The D2 dopamine receptor gene: a review of association studies in alcoholism and phenotypes. Alcohol 16:33–45, 1998

Nurnberger JI, Foroud T, Flury L, et al: Evidence for a locus on chromosome 1 that influences vulnerability to alcoholism and affective disorder. Am J Psychiatry 158:718–724, 2001

Nurnberger JI, Wiegand R, Bucholz K, et al: A family study of alcohol dependence: co-aggregation of multiple disorders in relatives of alcohol-dependent probands. Arch Gen Psychiatry 61:1246–1256, 2004

Olsson CA, Byrnes GB, Lotfi-Miri M, et al: Association between 5-HTTLPR genotypes and persisting patterns of anxiety and alcohol use: results from a 10-year longitudinal study of adolescent mental health. Mol Psychiatry 26, 2005 [Epub ahead of print]

Oscapella E: How Canadian laws and policies on "illegal" drugs contribute to the spread of HIV infection and hepatitis B and C. Ottawa: Canadian Foundation for Drug Policy, 1995

Oslin DW, Berrettini W, Kranzler HR, et al: A functional polymorphism of the mu-opioid receptor gene is associated with naltrexone response in alcohol-dependent patients. Neuropsychopharmacology 28:1546–1552, 2003

Patkar AA, Berrettini WH, Hoehe M, et al: Serotonin transporter (5-HTT) gene polymorphisms and susceptibility to cocaine dependence among African-American individuals. Addict Biol 6:337–345, 2001

Patock-Peckham JA, Cheong J, Balhorn ME, et al: A social learning perspective: a model of parenting styles, self-regulation, perceived drinking control, and alcohol use and problems. Alcohol Clin Exp Res 25:1284–1292, 2001

Perkins HW: Parental religion and alcohol use problems as intergenerational predictors of problem drinking among college youth. J Sci Study Relig 26:340–357, 1987

Piazza PV, Deminiere JM, le Moal M, et al: Stress- and pharmacologically induced behavioral sensitization increases vulnerability to acquisition of amphetamine self-administration. Brain Res 514:22–26, 1990

Plomin R, Daniels D: Why are children in the same family so different from each other? Behavioral Brain Sci 10:1–16, 1987

Porjesz B, Begleiter H, Wang K, et al: Linkage and linkage disequilibrium mapping of ERP and EEG phenotypes. Biol Psychol 61:229–248, 2002

Pull CB, Saunders JB, Mavreas V, et al: Concordance between ICD-10 alcohol and drug use disorder criteria and diagnoses as measured by the AUDADIS-ADR, CIDI and SCAN: results of a cross-national study. Drug Alcohol Depend 47:207–216, 1997

Radel M, Vallejo RL, Iwata N, et al: Haplotype-based localization of an alcohol dependence gene to the 4q34 gamma-aminobutyric acid type A gene cluster. Arch Gen Psychiatry 62:47–55, 2005

Rahav G, Hasin D, Paykin A: Drinking patterns of recent Russian immigrants and other Israelis: 1995 national survey results. Am J Public Health 89:1212–1216, 1999

Rangaswamy M, Porjesz B, Chorlian DB, et al: Beta power in the EEG of alcoholics. Biol Psychiatry 52:831–842, 2002

Rehm J, Rehn N, Room R, et al: The global distribution of average volume of alcohol consumption and patterns of drinking. Eur Addict Res 9:147–156, 2003

Reich T, Edenberg HJ, Goate A, et al: Genome-wide search for genes affecting the risk for alcohol dependence. Am J Med Genet 81:207–215, 1998

Reist C, Mazzanti C, Vu R, et al: Inter-relationships of intermediate phenotypes for serotonin function, impulsivity, and a 5-HT2A candidate allele: His452Tyr. Mol Psychiatry 9:871–878, 2004

Repetti RL, Taylor SE, Seeman TE: Risky families: family social environments and the mental and physical health of offspring. Psychol Bull 128:330–366, 2002

Rhee SH, Hewitt JK, Young SE, et al: Genetic and environmental influences on substance initiation, use, and problem use in adolescents. Arch Gen Psychiatry 60:1256–1264, 2003

Robinson TE: Neuroscience. Addicted rats. Science 305:951–953, 2004

Rogers PN, Schoenig SE: A time series evaluation of California's 1982 driving-under-the-influence legislative reforms. Accid Anal Prev 26:63–78, 1994

Room R: Effects of alcohol controls: Nordic research traditions. Drug Alcohol Rev 23:43–53, 2004

Room R, Graham K, Rehm J, et al: Drinking and its burden in a global perspective: policy considerations and options. Eur Addict Res 9:165–175, 2003

Rose RJ: Genetic and environmental variance in content dimensions of the MMPI. J Pers Soc Psychol 55:302–311, 1988

Rose RJ, Dick DM, Viken RJ, et al: Drinking or abstaining at age 14?: a genetic epidemiological study. Alcohol Clin Exp Res 25:1594–1604, 2001

Rounsaville BJ, Bryant K, Babor TF, et al: Cross system agreement for substance use disorders: DSM-III-R, DSM-IV, and ICD-10. Addiction 88:337–348, 1993

Russell A, Voas RB, Dejong W, et al: MADD rates the states: a media advocacy event to advance the agenda against alcohol-impaired driving. Public Health Rep 110: 240–245, 1995

Rydell CP, Caulkins JP, Everingham SE: Enforcement or treatment? modeling the relative efficacy of alternatives for controlling cocaine. Operations Research 44:687–695, 1996

Saadatmand F, Stinson FS, Grant BF, et al: Liver cirrhosis mortality in the United States, 1970–96. NIAAA Surveillance Report #52, 1999

Sander T, Harms H, Dufeu P, et al: Serotonin transporter gene variants in alcohol-dependent subjects with dissocial personality disorder. Biol Psychiatry 43:908–912, 1998

Scearce-Levie K, Chen JP, Gardner E, et al: 5-HT receptor knockout mice: pharmacological tools or models of psychiatric disorders. Ann N Y Acad Sci 868:701–715, 1999

Schuckit MA: Biological, psychological and environmental predictors of the alcoholism risk: a longitudinal study. J Stud Alcohol 59:485–494, 1998

Schuckit MA, Smith TL: An 8-year follow-up of 450 sons of alcoholic and control subjects. Arch Gen Psychiatry 53:202–210, 1996

Schuckit MA, Hesselbrock V, Tipp J, et al: Comparison of DSM-III-R, DSM-IV and ICD-10 substance use disorders diagnoses in 1922 men and women subjects in the COGA study. Addiction 89:1629–1638, 1994

Schuckit MA, Smith TL, Landi NA: The 5-year clinical course of high-functioning men with DSM-IV alcohol abuse or dependence. Am J Psychiatry 157:2028–2035, 2000

Schuckit MA, Smith TL, Danko GP, et al: Five-year clinical course associated with DSM-IV alcohol abuse or dependence in a large group of men and women. Am J Psychiatry 158:1084–1090, 2001

Schuckit MA, Smith TL, Kalmijn J: The search for genes contributing to the low level of response to alcohol: patterns of findings across studies. Alcohol Clin Exp Res 28:1449–1458, 2004

Schulenberg J, O'Malley PM, Bachman JG, et al: Getting drunk and growing up: trajectories of frequent binge drinking during the transition to young adulthood. J Stud Alcohol 57:289–304, 1996

Scribner RH, Cohen DA, Fisher W: Evidence of a structural effect for outlet density: a multilevel analysis. Alcohol Clin Exp Res 24:188–195, 2000

Sellers EM, Tyndale RF: Mimicking gene defects to treat drug dependence. Ann N Y Acad Sci 909:233–246, 2000

Shaham Y, Stewart J: Exposure to mild stress enhances the reinforcing efficacy of intravenous heroin self-administration in rats. Psychopharmacology 114:523–527, 1994

Shen S, Locke-Wellman J, Hill SY: Adolescent alcohol expectancies in offspring from families at high risk for developing alcoholism. J Stud Alcohol 62:763–772, 2001

Sher KJ, Grekin ER, Williams NA: The development of alcohol use disorders. Annu Rev Clin Psychol 1:493–523, 2005

Shkolnikov V, Nemtsov A: The anti-alcohol campaign and variations in Russian mortality, in Premature Death in the New Independent States. Edited by Bobadilla J, Costello C, Mitchell F. Washington, DC, National Academy Press, 1997, pp 239–261

Shults RA, Sleet DA, Elder RW, et al: Association between state level drinking and driving countermeasures and self reported alcohol impaired driving. Inj Prev 8:106–110, 2002

Singer M: The vitality of mythical numbers. Public Interest 4:3–9, 1971

Slutske WS, Cronk NJ, Sher KJ, et al: Genes, environment, and individual differences in alcohol expectancies among female adolescents and young adults. Psychol Addict Behav 16:308–317, 2002

Soyka M, Preuss UW, Koller G, et al: Association of 5-HT1B receptor gene and antisocial behavior in alcoholism. J Neural Transm 111:101–109, 2004

Stacy AW, Zogg JB, Unger JB, et al: Exposure to televised alcohol ads and subsequent adolescent alcohol use. Am J Health Behav 28:498–509, 2004

Stallings MC, Hewitt JK, Cloninger CR: Genetic and environmental structure of the Tridimensional Personality Questionnaire: three or four temperament dimensions? J Pers Soc Psychol 70:127–140, 1996

Steinberg L, Fletcher A, Darling N: Parental monitoring and peer influences on adolescent substance use. Pediatrics 93:1060–1064, 1994

Substance Abuse and Mental Health Services Administration: Results From the 2001 National Household Survey of Drug Abuse, Vol 1: Summary of National Findings (NHSDA Series H-17, DHHS Publication No. SMA 02-3758). Rockville, MD, SAMHSA Office of Applied Studies, 2002

Swendsen JD, Conway KP, Rounsaville BJ, et al: Are personality traits familial risk factors for substance use disorders? Results of a controlled family study. Am J Psychiatry 159:1760–1766, 2002

Tapert SF, Cheung EH, Brown GG, et al: Neural response to alcohol stimuli in adolescents with alcohol use disorder. Arch Gen Psychiatry 60:727–735, 2003

Tanaka F, Shiratori Y, Yokosuka O, et al: Polymorphism of alcohol-metabolizing genes affects drinking behavior and alcoholic liver disease in Japanese men. Alcohol Clin Exp Res 21:596–601, 1997

Tarabar AF, Nelson LS: The resurgence and abuse of heroin by children in the United States. Curr Opin Pediatr 15:210–215, 2003

Tatlow JR, Clapp JD, Hohman MM: The relationship between the geographic density of alcohol outlets and alcohol-related admissions in San Diego County. J Community Health 25:79–88, 2000

Thomas SE, Drobes DJ, Voronin K, et al: Following alcohol consumption, nontreatment-seeking alcoholics report greater stimulation but similar sedation compared with social drinkers. J Stud Alcohol 65:330–335, 2004

Tidey JW, Miczek KA: Acquisition of cocaine self-administration after social stress: role of accumbens dopamine. Psychopharmacology 130:203–212, 1997

Topp L, Day C, Degenhardt L: Changes in patterns of drug injection concurrent with a sustained reduction in the availability of heroin in Australia. Drug Alcohol Depend 70:275–286, 2003

Truett KR, Eaves LJ, Walters EE, et al: A model system for analysis of family resemblance in extended kinships of twins. Behav Genet 24:35–49, 1994

Tsuang MT, Lyons MJ, Meyer JM: Co-occurrence of abuse of different drugs in men: the role of drug-specific and shared vulnerabilities. Arch Gen Psychiatry 55:967–972, 1998

Tsuang MT, Bar JL, Harley RM, et al: The Harvard Twin Study of Substance Abuse: what we have learned. Harv Rev Psychiatry 9:267–279, 2001

Ustun B, Compton W, Mager D, et al: WHO Study on the reliability and validity of the alcohol and drug use disorder instruments: overview of methods and results. Drug Alcohol Depend 47:161–169, 1997

Valenzuela CF, Cardoso RA, Wick MJ, et al: Effects of ethanol on recombinant glycine receptors expressed in mammalian cell lines. Alcohol Clin Exp Res 22:1132–1136, 1998

Vanderschuren LJ, Everitt BJ: Drug seeking becomes compulsive after prolonged cocaine self-administration. Science 305:1017–1019, 2004

Voas RB, Tippetts AS, Fell J: The relationship of alcohol safety laws to drinking drivers in fatal crashes. Accid Anal Prev 32: 483–492, 2000

Voas RB, Tippetts AS, Fell JC: Assessing the effectiveness of minimum legal drinking age and zero tolerance laws in the United States. Accid Anal Prev 35:579–587, 2003

Wagenaar AC, Holder HD: A change from public to private sale of wine: results from natural experiments in Iowa and West Virginia. J Stud Alcohol 52:162–173, 1991

Walden B, McGue M, Iacono WG, et al: Identifying shared environmental contributions to early substance use: the respective roles of peers and parents. J Abnorm Psychol 113:440–450, 2004

Wall TL, Johnson ML, Horn SM, et al: Evaluation of the Self-Rating of the Effects of Alcohol form in Asian Americans with aldehyde dehydrogenase polymorphisms. J Stud Alcohol 60:784–789, 1999

Wang JC, Hinrichs AL, Stock H, et al: Evidence of common and specific genetic effects: association of the muscarinic acetylcholine receptor M2 (CHRM2) gene with alcohol dependence and major depressive syndrome. Hum Mol Genet 13:1903–1911, 2004

Weatherburn D, Lind B: The impact of law enforcement activity on a heroin market. Addiction 92:557–569, 1997

Weatherburn D, Jones C, Freeman K, et al: Supply control and harm reduction: lessons from the Australian heroin "drought." Addiction 98:83–91, 2003

Webb JA, Baer PE, Mclaughlin RJ, et al: Risk factors and their relation to initiation of alcohol use among early adolescents. J Am Acad Child Adolesc Psychiatry 30:563–568, 1991

Weitzman ER, Nelson TF, Wechsler H: Taking up binge drinking in college: the influences of person, social group, and environment. J Adolesc Health 32:26–35, 2003

Wilhelmsen KC, Schuckit M, Smith TL, et al: The search for genes related to a low-level response to alcohol determined by alcohol challenges. Alcohol Clin Exp Res 27:1041–1047, 2003

Wills TA, Vaccaro D, McNamara G: Novelty seeking, risk taking, and related constructs as predictors of adolescent substance use: an application of Cloninger's theory. J Subst Abuse 6:1–20, 1994

Wilson RW, Niva G, Nicholson T: Prohibition revisited: county alcohol control consequences. J Ky Med Assoc 91:9–12, 1993

Wood E, Tyndall MW, Spittal PM, et al: Impact of supply side policies for control of illicit drugs in the face of the AIDS and overdose epidemics: investigation of a massive heroin seizure. CMAJ 168:165–169, 2003

World Health Organization: Nomenclature and classification of drug- and alcohol-related problems: WHO memorandum. Bulletin of the World Health Organization 99:225–242, 1981

World Health Organization: International Statistical Classification of Diseases and Related Health Problems, 10th Revision (ICD-10). Geneva, Switzerland, World Health Organization, 1992

World Health Organization: Global Status Report on Alcohol. Geneva, Switzerland, World Health Organization, 1999

Wyllie A, Zhang JF, Casswell S: Positive responses to televised beer advertisements associated with drinking and problems reported by 18- to 29-year-olds. Addiction 93:749–760, 1998a

Wyllie A, Zhang JF, Casswell S: Responses to televised alcohol advertisements associated with drinking behaviour of 10–17-year-olds. Addiction 93:361–371, 1998b

Yoon YH, Yi H, Grant BF, et al: Surveillance Report #63: Liver Cirrhosis Mortality in the United States, 1970–2000. Bethesda, MD, NIAAA, Division of Biometry and Epidemiology, Alcohol Epidemiologic Data System, August 2003

Young RM, Lawford BR, Nutting A, et al: Advances in molecular genetics and the prevention and treatment of substance misuse: implications of association studies of the A1 allele of the D2 dopamine receptor gene. Addict Behav 29:1275–1294, 2004

Zhang PW, Ishiguro H, Ohtsuki T, et al: Human cannabinoid receptor 1: 5′ exons, candidate regulatory regions, polymorphisms, haplotypes and association with polysubstance abuse. Mol Psychiatry 9:916–931, 2004

Zimmerman P, Wittchen H, Hofler M, et al: Primary anxiety disorders and the development of subsequent alcohol use disorders: a 4-year community study of adolescents and young adults. Psychol Med 33:1211–1222, 2003

Zuckerman M, Kuhlman D: Personality and risk-taking: common biosocial factors. J Pers 68:999–1029, 2000

Part III

Prevention:
Lessons From Schizophrenia

7

Treatment of the Schizophrenia Prodrome

Barbara A. Cornblatt, Ph.D.
Todd Lencz, Ph.D.
Christopher Smith, M.A.
Andrea Auther, Ph.D.

A series of rapidly emerging research events has generated both optimism and concern about the administration of antipsychotic medication prior to the onset of psychosis: hope that early intervention will lead to the prevention of full-blown schizophrenia, but concern that antipsychotic treatment alone may be insufficient to achieve this goal. Although the supporting research is encouraging, it is still in its early years. Current findings (Heinssen et al. 2001; McGlashan et al. 2001b, 2006; McGorry et al. 2001, 2002; Woods et al. 2003) are promising but are not yet conclusive, and the possibility of prevention remains open. In this chapter, we discuss both the promise and the problems characterizing this area of research. We begin by addressing two very preliminary questions: 1) Why is schizophrenia, arguably the most severe and difficult to treat of the mental illnesses, considered preventable? and 2) Why does pharmacological intervention during the prodromal phase of schizophrenia appear justified or even acceptable as a starting point in prevention programs? We discuss the evidence in support of the use of early pharmacotherapy as well as some of the controversies that have emerged in response to the early clinical interventions. We conclude by reporting early treatment findings emerging from the Hillside Recognition and Prevention Program, which has attempted to integrate a high-risk research methodology within a treatment framework and has, as a result, adopted a strategy somewhat different from that of many other prodromal studies now under way.

WHY WE THINK THAT SCHIZOPHRENIA IS PREVENTABLE

Prevention is suggested by the neurodevelopmental nature of schizophrenia. Over the past two decades or so, schizophrenia has become widely viewed as a brain disease with its roots in very early, probably prenatal, development. Yet florid psychosis, the end point of the illness, typically does not emerge until the late teens or early 20s, suggesting that an extensive period of time exists during which preventive intervention might take place. One major challenge is accurate identification of vulnerable individuals sufficiently early to enable initiation of effective interventions; such identification has traditionally been the task of genetic high-risk studies. A second critical challenge is determination of the most effective type of treatment. In the sections to follow, we argue that whereas intervention has, to date, been approached from the perspective of previous treatment trials, in the case of prodromal intervention (which involves treatment of an "at risk" population), elements of traditional high-risk studies should also be incorporated.

Neurodevelopmental Hypothesis

The neurodevelopmental hypothesis was originally proposed as a theoretical alternative to the traditional view of schizophrenia as a neurodegenerative illness. The notion that schizophrenia follows a degenerative course dates back to Kraepelin (1919/1971), who believed that schizophrenia was an early form of dementia (i.e., dementia praecox). Recent studies provide evidence countering the degenerative hypothesis. Several studies have indicated that structural anomalies such as enlarged ventricles are found in schizophrenia patients at their initial episode of illness and do not appear to increase as the illness progresses (e.g., Cannon 1991; Degreef et al. 1992; Hoff et al. 1992; Hoffman et al. 1991; but see DeLisi et al. 1995). Moreover, clinically, it appears that few patients show the progressive deterioration characteristic of the dementias, and, in fact, some patients improve over time. The alternative viewpoint—that at least some aspects of schizophrenia are neurodevelopmental—has evolved far more recently and is supported by indirect but consistent data. Developmental abnormalities on the cellular level, including abnormal synaptic pruning, defects in embryonic cell migration, and abnormal myelination of axons, have been reported that support the neurodevelopmental model (Cannon 1998; Falkai et al. 1988; Green 1998; Jakob and Beckmann 1986; Kovelman and Scheibel 1986).

A neurodevelopmental perspective suggests that preventive intervention should be quite possible, given that the unfolding of the clinical illness is a long-term process. As illustrated in Figure 7–1, according to most views, this process most likely begins with an early (prenatal) series of biological insults or errors that require the presence of a disease genotype and may also involve other factors (e.g., infection, environmental trauma). As a result, the brain develops abnormalities, which might be structural, functional, or biochemical, or some combination of the three. Whatever the exact nature of the brain disturbance, it is currently believed to be the source of the susceptibility or vulnerability to later schizophrenia.

Although schizophrenia is frequently described as being "clinically silent" throughout much of adolescence, it has been increasingly recognized that the biological substrate of illness is reflected in subtle premorbid neurocognitive deficits and nonspecific prodromal behavioral/clinical disturbances. This underlying susceptibility is likely to be essential for future illness to develop, though it may not be sufficient. For example, full disease expression may require some sort of "trigger," such as an independent environmental or biological stressor or a second genetic "hit." It therefore follows that if the underlying susceptibility is successfully treated, it may be possible to eliminate or reduce the impact of the trigger(s). The resulting questions are 1) Which of the markers or risk factors should be targeted? 2) Which are most amenable to treatment? 3) When should treatment be initiated? and 4) What types of medication should be used?

Causal Risk Factors

Neurocognitive Deficits

Kraemer et al. (2001) has suggested that only *causal* risk factors are reasonable targets for intervention. We propose that neurocognitive deficits are strong candidates, since they are among the most widely studied early risk factors and also appear to be causally involved in the development of schizophrenia. This is based on the following evidence:

1. Findings from traditional genetic high-risk studies have indicated that neurocognitive deficits (especially compromised attention and working memory) can be detected in early childhood and precede other types of symptoms by many years (Cannon and Mednick 1993; Cornblatt and Keilp 1994; Cornblatt and Obuchowski 1997; Cornblatt et al. 1999; Erlenmeyer-Kimling et al. 2000). These deficits have been referred to as "biobehavioral markers" because they are intermediate between basic biological functions and more complex clinical behaviors and are thought to be direct reflections (or markers) of the underlying brain abnormalities.

2. Data collected over 20 years in the New York High-Risk Project (NYHRP) have indicated that the attentional deficits detected in childhood (typically by age 9 years) are stable across development and appear to be causally related to subsequent social difficulties in adolescence and to increasing social isolation in adulthood (e.g., Cornblatt and Erlenmeyer-Kimling 1985; Cornblatt et al. 1992, 1998; Erlenmeyer-Kimling and Cornblatt 1978, 1987, 1992; Erlenmeyer-Kimling et al. 2000).

3. Impaired attention, in particular, and neurocognitive dysfunction, in general, do not appear to be related to positive (psychotic) symptoms (Cornblatt et al. 1997, 1998; Green et al. 2000). This set of findings indicates that neurocognition is a separate domain, most likely involved in the underlying vulnerability that precedes the emergence of positive symptoms.

4. In affected patients, cognitive disturbances have been reported to relate more directly to functional outcome than do either positive or negative symptoms (Green 1996; Green et al. 2000).

These findings suggest that treating pre-illness cognitive markers may substantially influence the extent to which subsequent "triggers" will result in the expression of the full psychotic illness. Moreover, it can be speculated that treating long-standing cognitive deficits may reduce the social difficulties and functional disability associated with the range of schizophrenia spectrum disorders.

Attenuated Negative Features

Although neurocognitive deficits have traditionally been the most widely studied pre-illness risk factors, a number of other clinical and functional abnormalities have also been identified. There is considerable evidence, especially from prospective and follow-back high-risk studies, to suggest that attenuated negative symptoms, such as deficits in social functioning, are important characteristics of the prodromal phase of illness (e.g., Davidson et al. 1999; Jones and Done 1997; Klostarkötter et al. 1997; Loffler and Hafner 1999; Tsuang et al. 2000b).

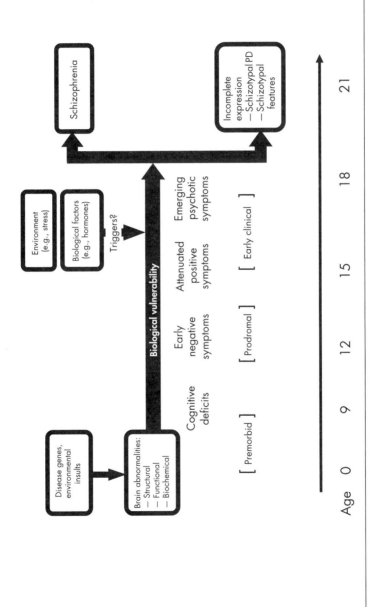

FIGURE 7–1. Simplified neurodevelopmental model of schizophrenia.

PD = personality disorder.

Incorporating these research findings as well as early data from the Hillside Recognition and Prevention Program, we have proposed (Cornblatt 2002, 2003) a specific profile in adolescence that appears to reflect risk for schizophrenia-related disorders. This profile is referred to as the CASIS cluster (consisting of Cognitive, Affective and Social Impairments as well as School decline and failure). School failure in this context primarily reflects withdrawal from school (and often increasing refusal to attend school) rather than "acting out" difficulties, and this withdrawal is typically accompanied by a decline in academic performance. This view is similar but not identical to the concept of schizotaxia proposed by Tsuang and colleagues (Tsuang 2000; Tsuang et al. 2000a). Consistent with Tsuang's view of schizotaxia, it is assumed that the CASIS cluster does not inevitably lead to full-blown schizophrenia but rather appears to be a risk factor for it. Therefore, treatment targeting these difficulties would be assumed to decrease that risk.

While each individual feature entering into this cluster is quite nonspecific and can signal any number of emerging difficulties, it may be that it is the particular combination of features that is predictive of later schizophrenia. Thus, it is proposed that this cluster of pre-illness features may serve two roles. First, as a combined profile, it may function as a way to accurately predict later illness. (Future research will determine whether predictive validity is improved by the addition of attenuated positive symptoms.) Second, it may inform prevention efforts by providing risk factors that represent optimal targets for early treatment.

This view has substantial implications for intervention. As we discuss in detail below, many of the prodromal intervention programs now in progress focus on positive symptoms, consistent with clinical trials involving already-psychotic patients. This focus, in turn, leads to the assumption that antipsychotic medication is the optimal starting point for psychopharmacology. However, an increased emphasis on treatment of cognitive deficits and attenuated negative symptoms prior to the emergence of positive symptoms suggests a broader choice of medication or, possibly, cognitive remediation or other types of psychosocial interventions. This broadened focus is further supported by the widely accepted understanding that in affected patients, antipsychotics are more effective in treating positive symptoms than in improving either negative symptoms or cognitive deficits.

Prodromal Indicators

Because interest in the schizophrenia prodrome is relatively new, the signs and symptoms defining this phase of the illness continue to evolve (McGlashan and

Johannessen 1996; McGlashan et al. 2001a; McGorry et al. 1999, 2000; Miller et al. 1999; Yung and McGorry 1996a, 1996b; Yung et al. 1996, 2006). Developmentally, the prodrome can be viewed as the transition between the premorbid and the psychotic stages of illness. Prodromal indicators therefore emerge at a later time point than do the premorbid neurocognitive risk factors discussed above. Because prodromal indicators are closer to the onset of illness, it is assumed that they will have considerably greater predictive accuracy than either the neurocognitive or the other CASIS cluster markers. However, the extent to which this is actually the case remains to be determined.

The schizophrenia prodrome is currently identified almost entirely by the presence of mild (i.e., attenuated) positive symptoms, which are psychotic-like but have not reached the intensity of true psychosis. Such attenuated symptoms are considered the forerunners of psychosis. These signs and symptoms are thus not causal risk factors for psychosis, but instead are its first manifestations—that is, are part of the disease process itself. As a result, interventions based on the identification of positive symptom indicators are, at best, early secondary prevention, since the illness has already begun. This is in contrast to primary or pre-illness intervention that can result from treatment of the CASIS predictors, once these are firmly established.

Even if prodromal intervention is started after the illness has actually begun, it can be seen as having considerable value in preventing further deterioration and disability. It is also possible to conduct such programs now, whereas pre-illness interventions are still many years away. However, a number of problems remain to be resolved. Despite assumptions that prodromal indicators accurately signal impending schizophrenia, more research is needed. To date, prediction is in the 40%–50% range (McGlashan et al. 2001a; Phillips et al. 1999; Yung et al. 1998). Therefore, when current criteria (consisting primarily of attenuated positive symptoms) are used, about 50% of the individuals targeted for treatment in prodromal programs will have been misidentified as requiring such an intervention. This false-positive rate is problematic, especially for the design of clinical intervention trials.

Selection criteria focusing on positive symptoms have been inherited from the treatment tradition. It is quite possible that predictive accuracy will be considerably improved by adding some of the risk factors identified by high-risk studies, especially those making up the CASIS cluster of risk factors, as discussed above. To do so, however, may change the way treatment is approached in the next generation of prodromal intervention programs.

Pharmaco-Intervention: Justification and Controversies

Benefits of Early Treatment

A number of studies have now suggested that the earlier medication is begun after the onset of psychosis, the better the outcome (Haas et al. 1998; Larsen et al. 1998; Lieberman and Koreen 1993; Loebel et al. 1992; McGlashan 1996; Wyatt 1991; Wyatt et al. 1997). This notion—that the longer psychosis remains untreated, the poorer the prognosis—is typically referred to as the *duration of untreated psychosis* (DUP) effect and is tied to the belief (as yet not well supported) that psychosis, in and of itself, may be toxic to the brain (Lieberman 1999; Wyatt 1991; Wyatt et al. 1997). This assumption led McGlashan (1996, 1998, 1999) to suggest that the DUP effect justifies prodromal intervention in spite of the possibility of false-positive identifications. However, the importance of DUP has been challenged by several recent studies (Ho et al. 2000; Robinson et al. 1999; Starostin et al. 2000) that report no association between DUP and outcome. Furthermore, several researchers have raised questions about the direction of causality, maintaining that a correlation between DUP and prognosis, even if one were to exist, may simply reflect other factors, such as severity of illness or level of premorbid functioning (Harvey and Davidson 2002; Verdoux et al. 2001). Nevertheless, regardless of whether the DUP does directly impact prognosis, as pointed out by McGorry and Edwards (2002), intervention during the prodromal stage can still result in many psychosocial, psychological, educational, and other advantages.

Introduction of Second-Generation Antipsychotic Medications

Up until recently, intervention could not be attempted, regardless of whether stable risk factors could be identified. This was because standard antipsychotics, the most effective pharmacological treatment previously available, were associated with quite severe side effects (e.g., tardive dyskinesia and other types of movement disorders). Given its likelihood of involving a relatively high rate of false-positive identifications, pre-illness intervention was not considered either feasible or ethical. However, the emergence of second-generation antipsychotics changed this situation and appeared, at least initially, to provide the tools for preventive intervention. Although the newer antipsychotic medications appeared to reduce many of the side effects associated with the earlier neuroleptics (Brown et al. 1999; Rajarethinam et al. 2001; Sharma et al. 1998), increasing evidence of new side effects (e.g., substantial weight gain) and other difficulties have raised questions about whether antipsychotics should be the first-line treatment for prodromal symptoms (Cornblatt et al. 2001).

Type of Medication

It was initially assumed by most treatment-oriented prodromal researchers that second-generation antipsychotics would be the most effective tools for achieving the prevention of psychosis. This is because administration of antipsychotic medication to prodromal individuals appears to be a logical extension of treatment for the fully expressed disorder. However, this strategy is justified only if attenuated positive symptoms are accepted as the first-line targets for intervention—an assumption which, from a high-risk research perspective, can be challenged.

By definition, individuals considered to be prodromal do not display florid psychotic symptoms, the symptoms most improved by antipsychotic medication. They do, however, typically display the range of features included in the CASIS cluster discussed above. Nevertheless, little attention has been directed toward designing treatments for these other risk features.

The need for an alternative treatment strategy is illustrated by Figure 7–2. Rather than viewing the unfolding of the illness as a single linear process (as shown earlier in Figure 7–1), there are two defined pathways, with the implication that many additional pathways to psychosis may, in reality, be involved. However, even from the simplified viewpoint in Figure 7–2, it is clear that the two pathways are likely to involve different types of intervention. To begin with, the vulnerability pathway *(bottom arrow)* consists of enduring traits that begin at a developmentally earlier time point. The clinical pathway involves emerging positive symptoms *(top arrow)*, which, beginning considerably later, most likely have their origins in a different part of the brain and may benefit from early treatment with antipsychotics. It may be that only by treating *both* pathways can the illness be fully eliminated.

Of particular interest here is what effect treating one pathway will have on the other. Intervention with antipsychotics in the clinical *(top)* pathway may reduce the likelihood of psychosis but may still result in an individual characterized by schizotypal personality disorder or other schizophrenia-spectrum features or personality disorders. If the vulnerability *(bottom)* process is reduced by early intervention, it may be possible to reduce or eliminate not only the later emerging psychotic symptoms but also the associated disability.

Heterogeneity of the Prodrome

Schizophrenia is considered to be a heterogeneous disorder by most researchers—heterogeneous in terms of clinical characteristics and in terms of etiology (e.g., Venables 1995). It is therefore logical that the prodromal stage that precedes the fully expressed illness will be equally heterogeneous. This heterogene-

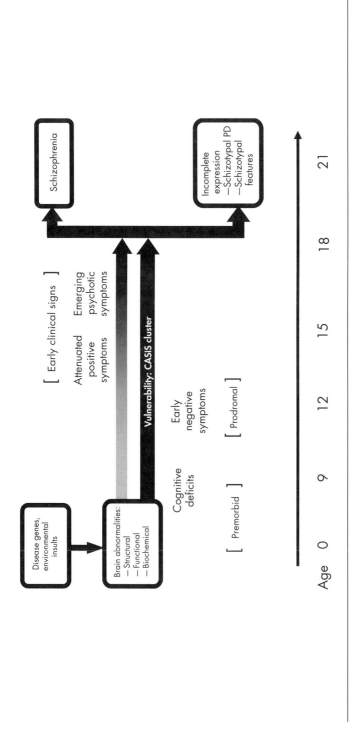

FIGURE 7–2.   Expanded neurodevelopmental model of schizophrenia, with at least two independent pathways required for the illness to be fully expressed.

CASIS = Cognitive, Affective, Social Impairment/Isolation, and School difficulties/failure; PD = personality disorder.

ity will pose still further complications when researchers attempt to evaluate treatment effectiveness, since different prodromal patterns may respond differently to a common intervention.

An illustration of this is the highly influential diagnostic system developed by McGorry, McGlashan, and their colleagues (Miller et al. 1999; Venables 1995; Yung and McGorry 1996a, 1996b; Yung et al. 1996, 1998), which consists of three separate categories of selection criteria. Category 1 requires at least one of the following attenuated positive symptoms: ideas of reference, odd beliefs or magical thinking, perceptual disturbance, odd thinking and speech, paranoid ideation, and odd behavior or appearance. Category 2 requires the experience of transient psychotic symptoms that have spontaneously resolved within 1 week. Category 3 combines genetic risk (i.e., being the first-degree relative of an individual with a diagnosis of schizophrenia) with state change in functioning (i.e., must have undergone a substantial decline in the previous year). An individual meeting any one of these three categories is considered to be prodromal for schizophrenia, with the prodrome itself viewed as a single clinical entity.

This type of approach incorporates several potential difficulties. First, there is no evidence to indicate that these three categories involve a common etiology. Second, if the categories are etiologically distinct, it is likely that each category involves a different conversion rate. Third (and related to points 1 and 2), different treatment approaches may be optimal for each of the three categories. When the categories are combined into a single broad group, treatment successes or failures may well be masked. However, separation into individual cells increases the problems associated with small sample sizes and further complicates clinical trials by requiring much broader recruitment.

Developmental Concerns

An additional concern involves the lack of solid information describing the developmental course of the prodromal phase. As now conceptualized, this period can last from weeks to years (Beiser et al. 1993; Yung and McGorry 1996a) and involves a complex developmental picture. The extent to which the prodrome consists of common stages (e.g., initial emergence of attenuated negative symptoms followed by attenuated positive symptoms; see discussion of the Hillside Recognition and Prevention Program below) is unknown. Such information would contribute to an understanding of when treatment would be most profitably initiated, what type of treatment is most appropriate for each prodromal phase, and which criteria are most useful for evaluating short-term treatment effects (i.e., in delaying or preventing the progression of illness). We propose that naturalistic research can help to clarify such unresolved descriptive issues. This approach provides the framework for the Hillside Recognition and Prevention Program, which will be the focus of the balance of this chapter.

THE HILLSIDE RECOGNITION AND PREVENTION PROGRAM

In contrast with most of the other prodromal studies now in progress, the Hillside Recognition and Prevention (RAP) Program integrates components of both genetic high-risk research and traditional clinical trials. This results from our notion that treatment programs developed for patients who already have schizophrenia may not be appropriate for prodromal adolescents who are "at risk" for developing psychosis. In particular, the way to measure outcome (i.e., the successfulness of the intervention) is unclear in a high-risk as opposed to an affected patient population. To a considerable extent, this difficulty results from the absence of well-established conversion rates. If the rate of conversion from the prodrome to schizophrenia without treatment has not yet been established, it cannot be determined whether an intervention is effective in reducing the number of new cases (incidence) of the disorder. Although some researchers have suggested that conversion rates in placebo controls can provide this information, that solution has been judged to be highly flawed, at least at this stage of prodromal research (Cornblatt et al. 2001).

To address the lack of base-rate information, the RAP program was designed to collect fundamental clinical data before moving on to clinical trials. We have incorporated a prospective research methodology borrowed from traditional genetic high-risk studies (Cornblatt and Obuchowski 1997; Erlenmeyer-Kimling and Cornblatt 1987), many of which involve long-term naturalistic follow-up of at-risk adolescents with no attempt to intervene (e.g., more than 30 years in the NYHRP). The RAP program is following this strategy by obtaining baseline data and then naturalistically following all research participants. However, unlike the earlier genetic high-risk (GHR) adolescents, who were typically symptom-free, all RAP adolescents are symptomatic. Ethically, they require treatment. We have therefore incorporated the clinic component into our naturalistic framework. There is no attempt to do any sort of systematic treatment intervention or to conduct prevention trials in the current RAP program. Instead, we are tracking the course the prodrome follows when treated as it would be in the community. We expect this approach—both the naturalistic follow-up and the naturalistic treatment program—to provide much of the basic information now missing from the field: for example, to establish the validity of the diagnostic criteria now in use, the heterogeneity of the prodrome, its developmental course, and the best type of medication for use at particular stages of the prodrome.

Description of Program

The Hillside RAP Program has been conducted at the Zucker Hillside Hospital of the North Shore–Long Island Jewish Health System in New York since 1998. The program consists of a clinic treating prodromal adolescents and a number of related high-risk and naturalistic treatment research projects. The RAP clinic provides treatment to all adolescents between the ages of 12 and 18 years (in some cases, however, participants may be as old as 22 years of age when admitted) who meet our entry criteria, regardless of whether they participate in any of the research protocols. Following admission into the clinic, patients and their families are asked if they are interested in enrolling in our research program. Approximately 80% of the patients undergoing treatment in the RAP clinic elect to participate in research (with full consent obtained from parents and assent from minors).

Our primary research project involves baseline neurocognitive, biobehavioral, and clinical assessments and then at least 3 years of prospective follow-up of all participants (regardless of whether they continue to receive treatment in the RAP clinic). For research purposes, we refer to this primary project as the Clinical High-Risk (CHR) Project, because the label "prodrome," widely used clinically, implies a greater likelihood of developing subsequent illness than can currently be definitively established. In fact, as we have discussed above, the validity of prodromal indicators has not yet been solidly established, and doing so is one of the major goals of the RAP research program. It is therefore not inevitable, or even highly likely, that youngsters displaying these symptoms will develop schizophrenia. At present, they are assumed, at most, to be at elevated risk for illness, but the extent of that elevation is another major issue to be resolved by the RAP Program. In the balance of this report, therefore, adolescents who display signs and symptoms considered as prodromal will be referred to as being at *clinical high risk* (CHR), to differentiate them from individuals at *genetic high risk* (GHR).

The RAP program recently completed a 2-year pilot phase (1998–2000) and the first two years of the funded 5-year prospective study (2000–2005, referred to as Phase I). In addition to establishing the baseline characteristics of prodromal adolescents, the pilot study included a treatment component that followed the naturalistic strategy described above. As a result, RAP clinic psychiatrists treated presenting symptoms as they would in their routine practice. It should be noted here that the RAP clinic is independent of the research program. Treating psychiatrists in the clinic do not attend research meetings and are not familiar with our hypotheses.

Initial Selection Strategy

In the absence of well-defined selection criteria matching our theoretical orientation, the initial recruitment strategy during the pilot phase was to circulate two lists of putative prodromal indicators to the intake staff at Schneider Children's Hospital. These lists were derived to a great extent from the early work of McGorry and collaborators (e.g., McGorry et al. 1995; Yung and McGorry 1996a, 1996b). The first list consisted of nonspecific, attenuated negative characteristics of schizophrenia considered to be early features of the prodrome and included depressed mood, social withdrawal, deterioration in functioning, impairment in personal hygiene, reduced concentration, reduced motivation, sleep disturbance, and anxiety. The second list, directed at the more-positive, schizophrenia-like symptoms, consisted of features assumed to appear later in the prodrome, included suspiciousness, peculiar behavior, inappropriate affect, vague or overelaborate speech, circumstantial speech, odd beliefs, magical thinking, and unusual perceptual experiences. Intake staff were asked to refer any adolescents displaying these symptoms; no specific combinations or minimum numbers were required. Each referral was considered by the RAP intake team on an individual basis. As mentioned, upon acceptance into the clinic, each individual and his or her family was fully informed about the research protocol and invited to participate.

Clinical Subgroups

A total of 81 patients (mean age, 15.7 years; age range, 11–22 years; 70% male) completed baseline testing at the close of the Phase I pilot study. Based on analyses of the structured and semistructured Axis I Schedule for Affective Disorders and Schizophrenia for School-Age Children—Epidemiologic Version, 5th Revision (K-SADS; Orvaschel and Puig-Antich 1994), Axis II Structured Interview for DSM-IV Personality (SIDP-IV; Pfohl et al. 1997), and prodromal symptoms (Structured Interview for Prodromal Symptoms [SIPS] and Schedule of Prodromal Symptoms [SOPS]; Miller et al. 1999) interviews, a rigorous algorithm was developed to divide the sample into three clinical subgroups (see Lencz et al. 2004 for more detail). We consider these subgroups to reflect prodromal symptoms as they naturally occur in the types of clinical populations commonly treated by health care professionals (especially psychiatrists and pediatricians).

As shown in Figure 7–3, going from left to right, the first subgroup consists of patients with the least-severe RAP profile, characterized by either attenuated negative symptoms (in particular, social withdrawal/isolation and school withdrawal/difficulties). We refer to this group as the *CHR-negative* (clinical high risk characterized by attenuated negative/disorganized symptoms) subgroup. We hypothesize that these subjects may represent the earliest stage at which true prodromal subjects can be identified.

The middle subgroup consists of patients considered to be in the prodrome according to criteria similar to those developed by McGlashan (Miller et al. 1999) and by McGorry and colleagues (McGorry et al. 1995). We refer to this group as the *CHR-positive* (attenuated positive symptoms) subgroup. We consider these patients to be in the later stages of the prodrome, because they display attenuated positive symptoms in addition to the attenuated negative features they share with the CHR-negative subgroup.

Somewhat to our surprise, when patients were assessed in depth, just over one-third of those accepted into the RAP clinic displayed symptoms that had already reached psychotic intensity. These individuals, represented by the third box, do not meet criteria for schizophrenia, because they lack the number or chronicity of psychotic symptoms or the level of functional deterioration required. This group is labeled as having *schizophrenia-like psychosis* (SLP). It should be noted that although subjects with SLP are no longer within the strictly defined prodromal phase of illness, they are nevertheless of considerable interest within the RAP program. From a clinical perspective, the primary goal for both the CHR-negative and CHR-positive subgroups is to prevent the onset of psychosis. Although it is too late to prevent psychosis in the SLP subgroup, it is still possible to prevent chronic schizophrenia, which is the major goal for SLP patients in the RAP intervention program.

From a research perspective, all three of these subgroups seem to formulate a coherent developmental model that is fully compatible with the neurodevelopmental hypothesis of schizophrenia. On the basis of this model, we hypothesize that schizophrenia typically involves a premorbid period (not included in the model), during which only subtle neurocognitive deficits are evident, followed by a phase of relatively mild, nonspecific, and attenuated negative symptoms. The early prodromal stage then flows into the middle to late prodromal phases, when positive symptoms begin to emerge in attenuated form. Untreated, these attenuated symptoms will gradually increase in intensity until they reach the level of psychosis, and, eventually, full-blown schizophrenia will take hold.

Of the 81 youngsters who completed the pilot study, 54 had complete medication data and at least 6 months of clinical follow-up. We refer to these 54 adolescents as our Pilot Phase I Treatment Sample. As shown in Figure 7–3, 14 of the 54 were in the CHR-negative group, 25 were in the CHR-positive group,

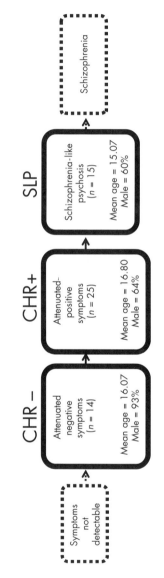

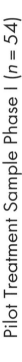

FIGURE 7–3.   Hillside Recognition and Prevention (RAP) Program developmental clinical model of schizophrenia.

CHR– = clinical high risk–negative; CHR+ = clinical high risk–positive; SLP = schizophrenia-like psychosis.

and 15 were in the SLP group. Across the three subgroups, the mean age ranged from 15 to 16 years. There were also more males than females in all three subgroups, but the difference was particularly marked in the CHR-negative subgroup, which was 93% male. Given the small sample size, continued recruitment into this subgroup will be necessary before we can determine whether the sex disparity reflects an ascertainment bias or is legitimate, and, if so, what the implications are for diagnosis and outcome.

Preliminary Clinical Outcome

Deterioration in the RAP program refers to a symptom exacerbation of sufficient magnitude to require a shift in clinical subgroup (e.g., from CHR-negative to CHR-positive or from CHR-positive to SLP; see Lencz et al. for more detail). *Conversion* indicates that criteria for DSM-IV (American Psychiatric Association 1994) schizophrenia or schizoaffective disorder were met. By the end of Phase I, 12 youngsters out of the 54 had deteriorated (22%), with 9 (17%) converting to schizophrenia. Broken down by subgroup, in the CHR-negative group, 2 subjects (14%) deteriorated, with 1 converting to schizophrenia (7%). Among CHR-positive subjects, there was a similar pattern, with 4 subjects deteriorating (16%) and 2 of these 4 converting (8%). For the SLP subgroup, however, as might be expected, the risk was far higher, with 6 of the 15 adolescents deteriorating (40%) and all 6 converting to schizophrenia.

These early findings are of interest from a number of perspectives. To begin with, the initial pattern of deterioration/conversion displayed by RAP adolescents was not fully consistent with our expectations or with the literature. We had predicted that the CHR-negative group, which was characterized by nonspecific symptoms and therefore likely to have the highest false-positive rate, would show the lowest number of deterioration/conversions. We further expected that the CHR-positive group would have conversion rates in the 40% range, consistent with the literature, and that the rates would be higher still for subjects in the SLP group.

Contrary to expectation, rates of both conversion and deterioration were equivalent for the two prodromal groups (i.e., CHR-negative *and* CHR-positive) and, for both, were considerably lower than those reported in the literature. About 15% of each of the two prodromal subgroups deteriorated during follow-up, which lasted, on average, just under a year. Approximately 7.5% of each group converted to schizophrenia. As expected, conversion rates within the SLP subgroup were much higher than those within the other two subgroups, but, to our surprise, they were very similar to the 40% rate reported by other prodromal research groups.

Several factors must be considered when evaluating these data. First, our subjects are considerably younger than those in prodromal samples in studies by both McGorry and McGlashan, which tended to focus on young adults (McGlashan et al. 2001b; McGorry et al. 2001). It may be that interventions begun in adolescence are particularly effective in delaying/eliminating symptoms. Alternatively, it may require several more years before the full symptom picture emerges, with symptom stability during adolescence not fully indicative of later outcome. These competing possibilities can only be resolved with long-term follow-up, which is currently under way.

Differences in diagnostic procedures must also be taken into account, in that in some cases it is possible that subjects considered as prodromal according to other diagnostic systems were classified within the SLP group according to our algorithm (see Lencz et al. 2004 for more detail). This possibility is supported by the similarity in conversion rates between the SLP subgroup and the more general prodromal populations reported by McGlashan, McGorry, and their colleagues (McGlashan et al. 2001b; McGorry et al. 2001). In the end, though, the possibility must also be recognized that our sample simply has a considerably lower conversion rate to schizophrenia than was initially expected.

These early outcome data also provide some very preliminary support for the developmental model. The 12 adolescents who deteriorated tended to follow a lawful progression, moving from box to box in the model. This suggests that for at least some schizophrenia patients, the developmental sequences proposed in the model may hold.

Early Treatment Findings

As noted earlier, throughout the RAP pilot study, treatment was delivered within a naturalistic framework. Treating clinicians were asked to provide medication as they would in standard practice and were given no guidelines or special instructions. The primary goals of our naturalistic treatment study were 1) to determine how prodromal symptoms are typically treated and 2) to evaluate the extent to which standard care is effective in reducing or eliminating prodromal signs and symptoms.

How Are Prodromal Symptoms Typically Treated?

The primary initial observation resulting from the pilot data addressing this question is that there is a very high level of polypharmacy. About 75% of the prodromal adolescents participating in the CHR study received some type of pharmacotherapy, with a considerable majority of these subjects treated with more than one class of medication. The categories most commonly used included second-generation antipsychotics, antidepressants (mainly selective serotonin reuptake inhibitors [SSRIs]), mood stabilizers, anxiolytics, and, in some cases, stimulants. A number of factors undoubtedly lead to this high level of polypharmacy in standard care—for example, pressure from parents and schools for immediate symptom reduction, lack of criteria for clear physician choice of medication, and, probably most importantly, the high rate of comorbidity.

Comorbidity. Many of the prodromal adolescents participating in the CHR project meet criteria for other Axis I disorders, in many cases more than one. The five most common comorbid illnesses are attention-deficit/hyperactivity disorder (ADHD), oppositional defiant disorder, major depression, social phobia, and obsessive-compulsive disorder (OCD). Aside from leading to considerable polypharmacy, this pattern of comorbidity raises a number of diagnostic issues. Of primary interest is the extent to which the additional diagnoses represent independent illnesses with distinct etiologies or, in fact, are actually risk factors for schizophrenia that, on the surface, appear to be other childhood disorders. For example, the attention deficits that are major determinants of the ADHD diagnosis are also well-established childhood precursors of schizophrenia. As a result, ADHD diagnoses in CHR subjects are always somewhat suspect. The high rate of comorbidity should also be evaluated in regard to the population rates of both illnesses. If the two are etiologically independent, ADHD would not be expected to be found in prodromal subjects to any greater extent than in the general population. Yet the rate is considerably higher (greater than 25%).

Similar concerns can be raised about the other comorbid disorders. For example, depression has been reported by Hafner and colleagues (e.g., Hafner and Nowotny 1995; Loffler and Hafner 1999) to be the earliest of the prodromal symptoms. Thus, are the depressive symptoms that are ever-present among prodromal adolescents risk factors, or is depression a frequent comorbid disorder? Similarly, obsessions during adolescence can either signal the presence of OCD or be forerunners of delusions. Whether these and other symptoms represent comorbid disorders or are risk factors for later schizophrenia (or early symptom presentations) is important from a treatment perspective. True comorbidity suggests that polypharmacy might be the preferred strategy.

How Effective Is Standard Care in Treating Prodromal Symptoms?

Again, some preliminary answers to this question were provided by the pilot data obtained from the Phase I treatment sample. Outcome for each of the three groups was assessed as a function of type of medication used. Medication was divided into antidepressants (with or without mood stabilizers and/or anxiolytics), second-generation antipsychotics (with or without any of the other medications), or no medication.

It should first be emphasized that across all three subgroups, the majority of patients treated in the RAP program (77%) have either stabilized or improved clinically, suggesting that early intervention may indeed be beneficial. It should also be noted that all individuals treated within the RAP clinic receive some form of psychosocial treatment: group, family, or individual therapy, and in most cases some combination of these three.

Outcome as a function of medication (or no medication) was quite different for each of the three groups, as described below.

CHR-negative subgroup.   As might be expected, the highest proportion of subjects not treated pharmacologically was in the CHR-negative group (close to 40%). In nearly all cases, this was because psychosocial treatment, frequently group therapy focusing on social skills, was considered to be the preferred treatment. Only in a handful of cases was medication prescribed but not taken. Approximately 40% of the remaining CHR-negative subjects were treated with antidepressants (primarily SSRIs). This finding was in no way surprising, given the nonspecific nature of the attenuated negative and disorganized symptoms characterizing this group. The balance of the CHR-negative group (around 20%) received second-generation antipsychotic treatment.

With respect to outcome after 1 year of treatment, most of the adolescents in the CHR-negative group remained clinically stable over the follow-up period. Neither psychosocial therapy nor pharmacological treatment with either antidepressants or second-generation antipsychotics resulted in major improvement in any notable number of CHR-negative subjects. There was also a minimum of deterioration, but in the few cases where this occurred, it was related to nonadherence to prescribed medication.

CHR-positive subgroup.   Because this subgroup most closely corresponds to the "prodromal" diagnosis as it is typically described in the literature, our expectation was that second-generation antipsychotics would be the optimal treatment. In fact, about half of the subjects in the CHR-positive subgroup were treated with second-generation antipsychotics (mainly olanzapine or risperidone). What was surprising in light of the presence of mild positive symptoms, however, was the high rate of antidepressant treatment: approximately 30% of CHR-positive adolescents received antidepressants, often in combination with anxiolytics or mood stabilizers, but not second-generation antipsychotics. Moreover, there was considerable clinical improvement among CHR-positive subjects over the follow-up period, but the rate of improvement was comparable regardless of whether these patients were treated with antidepressants or with second-generation antipsychotics. The other result of special note was that the balance of the CHR-positive group (about 25%) was off medication throughout the follow-up period. However, in contrast with CHR-negative subjects, in most cases this reflected nonadherence to prescribed treatment. Nearly all of the CHR-positive individuals who deteriorated/converted were considered nonadherent. Details about the final Phase I naturalistic treatment findings can be found in Cornblatt et al. (in press).

SLP subgroup.   All individuals in the SLP subgroup were prescribed a second-generation antipsychotic to treat the psychotic symptoms already in evidence. However, nearly one-third of the SLP subjects were largely nonadherent. This circumstance, as it turns out, had considerable implications for outcome. Of those individuals who were relatively adherent, 100% improved clinically. Of those adolescents in the SLP group who deteriorated (i.e., converted to schizophrenia), all were nonadherent to prescribed medication.

Treatment Conclusions

The preliminary data collected over the pilot phase of the RAP study suggest that early pharmacological intervention is very helpful in controlling prodromal symptoms. However, these findings challenge the assumption that antipsychotics are necessarily the best first-line treatment, given that antidepressants had a comparably beneficial effect in adolescents who were free of psychotic symptoms (i.e., CHR-negative and CHR-positive subjects). However, it must be kept in mind that these findings were generated from an open-label, naturalistic study without random assignment. Controlled research is necessary to conclusively establish the comparability of antipsychotics and antidepressants in prepsychosis intervention. Possibly the strongest finding, however, is the effect of adherence to medication regimens. Refusal to take prescribed medication—regardless of whether that medication consisted of antidepressants or antipsychotics—appears to be the strongest risk factor for subsequent conversion to schizophrenia. The reasons for this effect will be a subject of intense scrutiny throughout the newly initiated 5-year RAP research program.

CONCLUSION

Interest in pharmacological intervention prior to the onset of psychosis has dramatically increased over the past 5 years. This has largely resulted from three research developments: 1) widespread acceptance of the neurodevelopmental view of schizophrenia; 2) emerging evidence that the earlier treatment is initiated *after* onset of psychosis, the better the outcome—leading to the assumption that treatment initiated *before* onset will be better still; and 3) introduction of the second-generation antipsychotics. The convergence of these three developments has generated considerable enthusiasm for the possibility that schizophrenia can be prevented. However, a great deal of preliminary groundwork is needed to support full-scale prevention trials. Information about the predictive validity of the prodromal indicators currently in use is essential. In addition, considerable research is needed to address such questions as the developmental course and heterogeneity of the prodrome, the identity of the causal risk factors that should be targeted for early treatment, and precisely what the treatment should consist of. The Hillside RAP Program is a naturalistic, prospective clinical high-risk study that has been designed to answer many of these preliminary questions.

Preliminary findings from Phase I, the initial 3-year pilot phase of the RAP program, has highlighted three major areas of particular interest. First, a group of early features—the CASIS cluster (i.e., cognitive, affective, increasing social impairments, along with school difficulties/failure)—appears to precede positive symptoms and may represent a core risk profile for schizophrenia and related spectrum disorders. Second, medications other than antipsychotics may be effective for treating early prodromal symptoms and for treatments other than pharmacological (Cornblatt et al. 2001, [in press]). Third, the single most important risk factor for clinical deterioration identified during the early treatment phase was noncompliance with medication, whether antipsychotics or antidepressants. On the basis of these and other findings, it can be concluded that the prodrome is a developmentally complex phase of schizophrenia and that considerably more research is essential for optimizing intervention programs.

CLINICAL IMPLICATIONS

Our findings, and much of the available literature in the field, support the view that earlier clinical treatment for psychosis is associated with better outcomes than is later treatment. At present, this usually means that treatment initiated soon after psychosis is preferable to treatment initiated later. It is also becoming clearer, however, that initiating treatment during the prodromal phase, or in response to problems that are components of the CASIS cluster, may be essential to obtaining the most positive outcome possible. Given that some or many of these problems may not involve psychosis, effective treatment may not involve antipsychotic medication. As these clinical treatments or combinations of treatments receive experimental validation, earlier intervention and prevention strategies will become increasingly feasible.

REFERENCES

American Psychiatric Association: Diagnostic and Statistical Manual of Mental Disorders, 4th Edition. Washington, DC, American Psychiatric Association, 1994

Beiser M, Erickson D, Fleming JA, et al: Establishing the onset of psychotic illness. Am J Psychiatry 150:1349–1354, 1993

Brown CS, Markowitz JS, Moore TR, et al: Atypical antipsychotics, part II: adverse effects, drug interactions, and costs. Ann Pharmacother 33:210–217, 1999

Cannon TD: Genetic and perinatal sources of structural brain abnormalities in schizophrenia, in Fetal Neural Development and Adult Schizophrenia. Edited by Mednick SA, Cannon TD, Barr CE, et al. New York, Cambridge University Press, 1991, pp 174–198

Cannon TD: Genetic and perinatal influences in the etiology of schizophrenia: a neurodevelopmental model, in Origins and Development of Schizophrenia: Advances in Experimental Psychopathology. Edited by Lenzenweger M, Dworkin RH. Washington, DC, American Psychological Association, 1998, pp 67–92

Cannon TD, Mednick SA: The schizophrenia high-risk project in Copenhagen: three decades of progress. Acta Psychiatr Scand Suppl 370:33–47, 1993

Cornblatt BA: The New York High-Risk Project to the Hillside Recognition and Prevention (RAP) Program. Am J Med Genet 114:956–966, 2002

Cornblatt BA, Erlenmeyer-Kimling L: Global attentional deviance as a marker of risk for schizophrenia: specificity and predictive validity. J Abnorm Psychol 94:470–486, 1985

Cornblatt BA, Keilp JG: Impaired attention, genetics, and the pathophysiology of schizophrenia. Schizophr Bull 20:31–46, 1994

Cornblatt B, Obuchowski M: Update of high-risk research: 1987–1997. Int Rev Psychiatry 9:437–447, 1997

Cornblatt BA, Lenzenweger MF, Dworkin RH, et al: Childhood attentional dysfunctions predict social deficits in unaffected adults at risk for schizophrenia. Br J Psychiatry 161 (suppl 18):59–64, 1992

Cornblatt B, Obuchowski M, Schnur DB, et al: Attention and clinical symptoms in schizophrenia. Psychiatr Q 68:343–359, 1997

Cornblatt B, Obuchowski M, Schnur D, et al: Hillside study of risk and early detection in schizophrenia. Br J Psychiatry Suppl 172:26–32, 1998

Cornblatt B, Obuchowski M, Roberts S, et al: Cognitive and behavioral precursors of schizophrenia. Dev Psychopathol 11:487–508, 1999

Cornblatt BA, Lencz T, Kane JM, et al: Treatment of the schizophrenia prodrome: is it presently ethical? Schizophr Res 51:31–38, 2001

Davidson M, Reichenberg A, Rabinowitz J, et al: Behavioral and intellectual markers for schizophrenia in apparently healthy male adolescents. Am J Psychiatry 156:1328–1335, 1999

Degreef G, Ashtari M, Bogerts B, et al: Volumes of ventricular system subdivisions measured from magnetic resonance images in first-episode schizophrenic patients. Arch Gen Psychiatry 49:531–537, 1992

DeLisi LE, Tew W, Xie S, et al: A prospective follow-up study of brain morphology and cognition in first-episode schizophrenic patients: preliminary findings. Biol Psychiatry 38:349–360, 1995

Erlenmeyer-Kimling L, Cornblatt B: Attentional measures in a study of children at high-risk for schizophrenia. J Psychiatric Res 14:93–98, 1978

Erlenmeyer-Kimling L, Cornblatt B: High-risk research in schizophrenia: a summary of what has been learned. J Psychiatric Res 21:401–411, 1987

Erlenmeyer-Kimling L, Cornblatt BA: Summary of attentional findings in the New York High-Risk Project. J Psychiatric Res 26:405–426, 1992

Erlenmeyer-Kimling L, Rock D, Roberts SA, et al: Attention, memory, and motor skills as childhood predictors of schizophrenia-related psychoses: the New York High-Risk Project. Am J Psychiatry 157:1416–1422, 2000

Falkai P, Bogerts B, Rozumek M: Limbic pathology in schizophrenia: the entorhinal region—a morphometric study. Biol Psychiatry 24:515–521, 1988

Green MF: What are the functional consequences of neurocognitive deficits in schizophrenia. Am J Psychiatry 153:321–330, 1996

Green MF: Schizophrenia From a Neurocognitive Perspective: Probing the Impenetrable Darkness. Boston, MA, Allyn & Bacon, 1998

Green MF, Kern RS, Braff DL, et al: Neurocognitive deficits and functional outcome in schizophrenia: are we measuring the "right stuff"? Schizophr Bull 26:119–136, 2000

Haas GL, Garratt LS, Sweeney JA: Delay to first antipsychotic medication in schizophrenia: impact on symptomatology and clinical course of illness. J Psychiatr Res 32:151–159, 1998

Hafner H, Nowotny B: Epidemiology of early onset schizophrenia. Eur Arch Psychiatry Clin Neurosci 245:80–92, 1995

Harvey PD, Davidson M: Schizophrenia: course over the lifetime, in Neuropsychopharmacology: The Fifth Generation of Progress. Edited by Davis KL, Charney DS, Coyle JT, et al. Philadelphia, PA, Lippincott Williams & Wilkins, 2002, pp 47–64

Heinssen RK, Perkins DO, Appelbaum PS, et al: Informed Consent in Early Psychosis Research: National Institute of Mental Health Workshop, November 15, 2000. Schizophr Bull 27:571–583, 2001

Ho BC, Andreasen NC, Flaum M, et al: Untreated initial psychosis: its relation to quality of life and symptom remission in first-episode schizophrenia. Am J Psychiatry 157:808–815, 2000

Hoff AL, Riordan H, O'Donnell D, et al: Anomalous lateral sulcus asymmetry and cognitive function in first-episode schizophrenia. Schizophr Bull 18:257–270, 1992

Hoffman WF, Ballard L, Turner EH, et al: Three-year follow-up of older schizophrenics: extrapyramidal syndromes, psychiatric symptoms, and ventricular brain ratio. Biol Psychiatry 30:913–926, 1991

Jakob H, Beckmann H: Prenatal developmental disturbances in the limbic allocortex in schizophrenics. J Neural Transm 65:303–326, 1986

Jones PB, Done DJ: From birth to onset: a developmental perspective of schizophrenia in two national birth cohorts, in Neurodevelopment and Adult Psychopathology. Edited by Keshavan MS, Murray RM. New York, Cambridge University Press, 1997, pp 119–136

Klostarkötter J, Schultze-Lutter F, Gross G, et al: Early self-experienced neuropsychological deficits and subsequent schizophrenic diseases: an 8-year average follow-up prospective study. Acta Psychiatr Scand 95:396–404, 1997

Kovelman JA, Scheibel AB: A neurohistological correlate of schizophrenia. Biol Psychiatry 19:1601–1621, 1986

Kraemer HC, Stice E, Kazdin A, et al: How do risk factors work together? Mediators, moderators, and independent, overlapping, and proxy risk factors. Am J Psychiatry 158:848–856, 2001

Kraepelin E: Dementia Praecox and Paraphrenia (1919). Huntington, NY, Robert Krieger, 1971

Larsen TK, Johannessen JO, Opjordsmoen S: First-episode schizophrenia with long duration of untreated psychosis. Pathways to care. Br J Psychiatry Suppl 172:45–52, 1998

Lencz T, Smith CW, Auther A, et al: Nonspecific and attenuated negative symptoms in patients at clinical risk for schizophrenia. Schizophr Res 68:37–48, 2004

Lieberman JA: Is schizophrenia a neurodegenerative disorder? A clinical and neurobiological perspective. Biol Psychiatry 46:729–739, 1999

Lieberman JA, Koreen AR: Neurochemistry and neuroendocrinology of schizophrenia: a selective review. Schizophr Bull 19:371–429, 1993

Loebel AD, Lieberman JA, Alvir JM, et al: Duration of psychosis and outcome in first-episode schizophrenia. Am J Psychiatry 149:1183–1188, 1992

Loffler W, Hafner H: Ecological pattern of first admitted schizophrenics in two German cities over 25 years. Soc Sci Med 49:93–108, 1999

McGlashan TH: Early detection and intervention in schizophrenia: research. Schizophr Bull 22:327–345, 1996

McGlashan TH: The profiles of clinical deterioration in schizophrenia. J Psychiatric Res 32:133–141, 1998

McGlashan TH: Duration of untreated psychosis in first-episode schizophrenia: marker or determinant of course. Biol Psychiatry 46:899–907, 1999

McGlashan TH, Johannessen JO: Early detection and intervention with schizophrenia: rationale. Schizophr Bull 22:201–222, 1996

McGlashan TH, Miller TJ, Woods SW, et al: Instrument for the assessment of prodromal symptoms and states, in Early Intervention in Psychotic Disorders. Edited by Miller T, Mednick SA, McGlashan TH, et al. Dordrecht, The Netherlands, Kluwer Academic, 2001a, pp 135–149

McGlashan TH, Miller TJ, Woods SW: Pre-onset detection and intervention research in schizophrenia psychoses: current estimates of benefit and risk. Schizophr Bull 27:563–570, 2001b

McGlashan TH, Zipursky RB, Perkins D, et al: Randomized, double-blind trial of olanzapine versus placebo in patients prodromally symptomatic for psychosis. Am J Psychiatry 163:790–799, 2006

McGorry PD, Edwards J: Response to "The prevention of schizophrenia: what interventions are safe and effective?" (letter). Schizophr Bull 28:177–180, 2002

McGorry PD, McFarlane C, Patton GC, et al: The prevalence of prodromal features of schizophrenia in adolescence: a preliminary survey. Acta Psychiatr Scand 92:241–249, 1995

McGorry PD, McKenzie D, Jackson HJ, et al: Can we improve the diagnostic efficiency and predictive power of prodromal symptoms for schizophrenia? Schizophr Res 42:91–100, 2000

McGorry P, Yung A, Phillips L: People at risk of schizophrenia and other psychoses: comments on the Edinburgh High-Risk Study. Br J Psychiatry 175:586–587, 1999

McGorry PD, Yung A, Phillips L: Ethics and early intervention in psychosis: keeping up the pace and staying in step. Schizophr Res 51:17–29, 2001

McGorry PD, Yung A, Phillips L, et al: Randomized controlled trial of interventions designed to reduce the risk of progression to first-episode psychosis in a clinical sample with subthreshold symptoms. Arch Gen Psychiatry 59:921–928, 2002

Miller TJ, McGlashan TH, Woods SW, et al: Symptom assessment in schizophrenic prodromal states. Psychiatr Q 70:273–287, 1999

Orvaschel H, Puig-Antich J: Schedule for Affective Disorders and Schizophrenia for School-Age Children—Epidemiologic Version (K-SADS-E), 5th Revision. Philadelphia, PA, Western Psychiatric Institute and Clinic, 1994

Pfohl B, Blum N, Zimmerman M: Structured Interview for DSM-IV Personality (SIDP-IV). Washington, DC, American Psychiatric Press, 1997

Phillips L, Yung AR, Hearn N, et al: Preventative mental health care: accessing the target population. Austr N Z J Psychiatry 33:241–247, 1999

Rajarethinam R, DeQuardo JR, Miedler J, et al: Hippocampus and amygdala in schizophrenia: assessment of the relationship of neuroanatomy to psychopathology. Psychiatry Res 108:79–87, 2001

Robinson D, Woerner MG, Alvir JM, et al: Predictors of relapse following response from a first episode of schizophrenia or schizoaffective disorder. Arch Gen Psychiatry 56:241–247, 1999

Sharma T, Lancaster E, Lee D, et al: Brain changes in schizophrenia: volumetric MRI study of families multiply affected with schizophrenia—the Maudsley Family Study 5. Br J Psychiatry 173:132–138, 1998

Starostin A, Staudenmaier HM, Allgower CE, et al: Measurement of pi(0)pi(0) production in the nuclear medium by pi(−) interactions at 0.408 GeV/c. Phys Rev Lett 85(26 Pt 1):5539–5542, 2000

Tsuang MT: Genes, environment, and mental health wellness. Am J Psychiatry 157:489–491, 2000

Tsuang MT, Stone WS, Faraone SV: Toward reformulating the diagnosis of schizophrenia. Am J Psychiatry 147:1041–1050, 2000a

Tsuang MT, Stone WS, Faraone SV: Towards the prevention of schizophrenia. Biol Psychiatry 48:349–356, 2000b

Venables PH: Schizotypal status as a developmental stage in studies of risk for schizophrenia, in Schizotypal Personality. Edited by Raine A, Lencz T, Mednick SA. Cambridge, UK, Cambridge University Press, 1995, pp 107–131

Verdoux H, Liraud F, Bergey C, et al: Is the association between duration of untreated psychosis and outcome confounded? A 2-year follow-up study of first-admitted patients. Schizophr Res 49:2331–2410, 2001

Woods SW, Breier A, Zipursky RB, et al: Randomized trial of olanzapine versus placebo in the symptomatic and acute treatment of the schizophrenic prodrome. Biol Psychiatry 54:453–464, 2003

Wyatt RJ: Neuroleptics and the natural course of schizophrenia. Schizophr Bull 17:325–351, 1991

Wyatt RJ, Green MF, Tuma AH: Long-term morbidity associated with delayed treatment of first admission schizophrenic patients: a re-analysis of the Camarillo State Hospital data. Psychol Med 27:261–268, 1997

Yung AR, McGorry PD: The initial prodrome in psychosis: descriptive and qualitative aspects. Austr N Z J Psychiatry 30:587–599, 1996a

Yung AR, McGorry PD: The prodromal phase of first-episode psychosis: past and current conceptualizations. Schizophr Bull 22:363–370, 1996b

Yung AR, McGorry PD, McFarlane CA, et al: Monitoring and care of young people at incipient risk of psychosis. Schizophr Bull 22:283–304, 1996

Yung AR, Phillips LJ, McGorry PD, et al: Prediction of psychosis. A step towards indicated prevention of schizophrenia. Br J Psychiatry Suppl 172:14–20, 1998

Yung AR, Standford C, Cosgrave E, et al: Testing the ultra high risk (prodromal) criteria for the prediction of psychosis in a clinical sample of young people. Schizophr Res 84:57–66, 2006

8

Adolescent Neurodevelopment

A Critical Period for Preventive Intervention

Elaine F. Walker, Ph.D.
Amanda McMillan, B.A.
Kevin Tessner, M.A.
Vijay Mittal, M.A.
Hanan Trotman, B.A.

Advances in neuroimaging and molecular biology have provided researchers with highly sophisticated tools to explore the neurobiological basis of mental disorders. In the case of schizophrenia, arguably the most debilitating mental illness, we have seen a dramatic increase in published reports on the brain abnormalities and genetic factors associated with this illness. The techniques and findings are impressive, but when viewed as a whole, no simple road map is emerging. Rather, contemporary research is yielding a picture of diverse and seemingly complex neuropathological processes.

It appears that both structural and functional brain abnormalities are linked with schizophrenia and that multiple neural systems are affected. One or more of these neural abnormalities may be critical for the emergence of psychotic symptoms, while other neural systems play a modulating role in potentiating the expression of dysfunction in key systems. Furthermore, the nature of the brain abnormalities seems to change with development. There is strong evidence that maturational changes play a role in the expression of the basic neuropathology and, as a consequence, the clinical manifestations.

It has been suggested that the neural systems governing the response to stress may function to potentiate the expression of the core vulnerability to schizophrenia (Cunningham et al. 2002; Walker and Diforio 1997). Walker and Diforio (1997) pointed out four general lines of investigation yielding support for this hypothesis. First, behavioral studies have shown that clinical symptoms can be exacerbated by exposure to stress. Second, medical disorders (e g., Cushing's) that involve elevated levels of the "stress" hormone, cortisol, are associated with increased risk for psychosis. Third, research in psychotic patients has revealed abnormalities in several aspects of the neural system that governs cortisol release—namely, the hypothalamic-pituitary-adrenal (HPA) axis. For example, patients with schizophrenia and other psychotic disorders show an elevated rate of nonsuppression in response to dexamethasone challenge. Recent reports indicate that unmedicated patients also manifest heightened baseline cortisol (Muck-Seler et al. 2004), and even patients whose condition was stabilized while taking antipsychotics manifest elevated ratios of cortisol/dehydroepiandrosterone (DHEA) compared with healthy control subjects (Ritsner et al. 2004). Higher cortisol levels are associated with more severe schizophrenia symptoms (Shirayama et al. 2002; Walder et al. 2000). Furthermore, the fact that baseline cortisol level is elevated in never-medicated, first-episode patients indicates that elevated HPA axis activity precedes clinical onset (Ryan et al. 2003, 2004a, 2004b). Finally, perhaps the most compelling evidence that the HPA system is implicated in schizophrenia is the data showing significant hippocampal volume reduction and structural abnormalities (Harrison 2004). This finding is relevant to HPA function because, as described below, the hippocampus appears to play an important role in regulating the activity of the HPA axis (Altamura et al. 1999).

In this chapter we review research findings that bear on adolescent vulnerability to psychosis and neurodevelopment of the HPA–hippocampal system, with an emphasis on implications for preventive intervention. Our model posits that the HPA–hippocampal system can moderate the expression of constitutional vulnerability for psychosis. We assume that adolescence is a critical period for this moderating effect, because postpubertal neurodevelopment of the HPA axis and hippocampus increases susceptibility to the adverse effects of stress-induced glucocorticoid secretion, and because hormonal changes during this period can trigger latent genetic vulnerabilities. Finally, we present preliminary data from our recent research that suggest how psychopharmacological interventions might alter the transition to psychosis in adolescents with schizotypal and other personality disorders.

THE HPA AXIS

The HPA axis is a neural system that is pivotal in controlling the mammalian response to environmental challenges. The HPA axis is particularly sensitive to stress and is activated in response to physical and psychological factors that threaten homeostasis (Charmandari et al. 2003; Dorn and Chrousos 1997). The initial step in the neurohormonal cascade of the HPA axis is the release of the hypothalamic secretagogue, corticotropin-releasing hormone (CRH). This, in turn, triggers the release of adrenocorticotropic hormone (ACTH) from the anterior pituitary. ACTH then acts on the adrenal glands, leading to the release of glucocorticoids (cortisol in primates) from the adrenal cortex into circulation. An acute rise in cortisol levels can be adaptive, because it serves to increase the availability of energy substrates; however, persistent elevations can be maladaptive.

The actions of cortisol are mediated by two types of receptors: mineralocorticoid receptors and glucocorticoid receptors, also referred to as type I and type II receptors, respectively. Mineralocorticoid receptors and glucocorticoid receptors are two closely related members of the steroid nuclear receptor family of transcription factors that bind cortisol. These receptors are present on many cells throughout the body, including the brain, and they are pivotal in the self-modulation of the HPA axis. Thus, glucocorticoids act to suppress their own release through activation of mineralocorticoid receptors and glucocorticoid receptors, which initiates both fast- and slow-acting negative-feedback systems that inhibit ACTH release. These feedback systems act through the hypothalamus and pituitary, although other regions also play a role.

THE HIPPOCAMPUS AND HPA FUNCTION

The hippocampus is relevant to functioning of the HPA axis for two reasons. First, as noted, it plays a role in modulation of the HPA system, presumably because of the high concentration of steroid receptors on hippocampal neurons (Watzka et al.

2000). Second, the hippocampus may be uniquely sensitive to the adverse effects of sustained high levels of glucocorticoid secretion (Charmandari et al. 2003; Dorn and Chrousos 1997). Thus, heightened levels may have neurotoxic effects that structurally compromise the hippocampus. For both of these reasons, an inverse relation between glucocorticoid levels and hippocampal volume would be predicted.

Consistent with the hypothesized modulating role of the hippocampus, studies using rodent models have revealed an inverse relationship between glucocorticoid levels and hippocampal volume (Hibberd et al. 2000; Meaney et al. 1995, 1996). Similar findings have been reported in the rhesus monkey (Coe et al. 2003) and the tree shrew (Ohl et al. 2000). A recent study suggests that the relation can be measured at the cellular level; in pigs exposed to chronic stress, basal cortisol is negatively correlated with hippocampal neuron number as well as volume (van der Beek et al. 2004). These effects were most pronounced in the left dentate gyrus.

Subsequent neuroimaging studies of human subjects have also revealed a relation between glucocorticoid secretion and hippocampal volume. Consistent with the notion of hippocampal negative feedback, the findings show an inverse relation. In patients with dementia, higher serum cortisol concentrations are associated with reductions of cerebral volume in both the hippocampus and temporal lobes (Ferrari et al. 2000). Similarly, a longitudinal study revealed that in aged humans, a measure of hippocampal atrophy was positively correlated with both basal cortisol and the magnitude of cortisol elevation over time (Lupien et al. 1998). Furthermore, prolonged cortisol elevation was linked with hippocampus-dependent memory deficits. More recently, a study of both young (ages 19–30 years) and older (ages 59–76 years) healthy male subjects showed that hippocampal volume was inversely associated with 24-hour urinary cortisol and corticotropin (ACTH) levels, after age and cerebral vault size were controlled for (Wolf et al. 2002).

We recently conducted an investigation of the relation between salivary cortisol and hippocampal volume in a group of 14 healthy young (mean age 25 years) males. The study employed a double-blind crossover design. There were two experimental conditions: placebo and hydrocortisone (cortisol) administration. Each subject was assessed under both conditions, with half of the sample randomly assigned to each of the two conditions. The placebo or drug (100 mg) was administered approximately 2 hours prior to entry into the magnetic resonance imaging (MRI) scanner. Saliva was then sampled at regular 15-minute intervals, beginning at 60 minutes prior to entering the scanner, then immediately before entering the scanner. The average of all cortisol samples was computed for each subject within each condition. As expected, administration of hydrocortisone resulted in a dramatic increase in cortisol secretion above levels in the placebo condition. Controlling for whole-brain volume, there was a trend toward a significant inverse correlation between hippocampal volume and mean cortisol in the placebo condition ($r = -0.26$, $P = 0.06$). In the hydrocortisone condition, the correlation was higher and was statistically significant ($r = -0.59$, $P < 0.05$). These findings lend further support to the hypothesized link between hippocampal volume and cortisol secretion and suggest that the relation is more pronounced when cortisol secretion is elevated. Thus, the hippocampus may play a greater role in modulating HPA activity when it is elevated above baseline in response to challenge.

As noted, the relation between cortisol levels and hippocampal volume appears to be partially due to an effect of elevated cortisol on hippocampal morphology. When compared with age-matched controls, patients receiving chronic corticosteroid therapy have smaller hippocampal volumes, declarative memory deficits, and lower hippocampal levels of N-acetylaspartate (NAA) (E.S. Brown et al. 2004). Also, functional neuroimaging of human subjects has revealed that acute administration of cortisol selectively reduces hippocampal glucose utilization, suggesting that cortisol elevation has direct and acute effects on hippocampal function (de Leon et al. 1997).

But the adverse effects of elevated cortisol on hippocampal structure and function may be reversible, under some circumstances. Sapolsky (1994) found reversible morphological changes in animals exposed to moderate stress—a finding suggestive of hippocampal plasticity in animals—and recent findings indicate that this is also the case in humans. For example, after cortisol levels decline to normal concentrations in treated Cushing's patients, there is an increase in hippocampal volume that is accompanied by functional improvement in verbal learning (Starkman et al. 1999, 2003). At this point, there is no database for drawing inferences about the temporal course of plasticity; the hippocampal change may occur shortly after reductions in cortisol levels, or it may extend over long time periods.

In summary, it appears that there is a dynamic relation between circulating glucocorticoids and hippocampal morphology. The specific neural mechanisms have not been elucidated, nor do we know the time course for these events. But as described below, there may be critical developmental periods for these processes.

THE HIPPOCAMPUS AND SCHIZOPHRENIA

As noted, numerous studies of diagnosed patients with schizophrenia have revealed significantly smaller hippocampal volumes in patients compared with matched control subjects (Harrison 2004; Shenton et al. 2001). When effect sizes for differentiating diagnostic groups are compared across brain regions, hippocampal volume shows the largest diagnostic group difference. Other research suggests that reductions in hippocampal volume are present early in the illness and are at least partly a consequence of nongenetic factors. Studies of young first-onset schizophrenia patients reveal hippocampal volume reductions (Seidman et al. 2003).

Furthermore, twin studies indicate that both environmental and genetic factors contribute to hippocampal reductions in schizophrenia. In 1990, the National Institute of Mental Health studies of discordant monozygotic (MZ) twins revealed that the affected twins showed significantly smaller brain volumes compared with their healthy co-twins (Suddath et al. 1990). Of all brain regions examined, however, the hippocampal/amygdala complex was most markedly reduced in volume. Other studies of discordant MZ twins have yielded the same pattern of results. An investigation conducted in the Netherlands revealed that schizophrenic twins, whether from concordant or discordant pairs, had smaller whole-brain volumes than did control twins; however, the probands of discordant pairs showed more hippocampal volume reduction than their healthy co-twins or concordant twins (van Haren et al. 2004). The same pattern of findings has been reported in at least two other studies of discordant MZ twins (Baare et al. 2001; van Erp et al. 2004). These findings suggest that genetic risk for schizophrenia is associated with generalized reductions in brain volume, but that reductions in the hippocampus are most pronounced in association with the clinical syndrome of schizophrenia. These results are consistent with the notion that the HPA–hippocampal system moderates the expression of genetically determined constitutional vulnerability for schizophrenia.

Extending this further, it has been shown that the intraclass correlation for hippocampal volume in healthy MZ twin pairs is larger than that for discordant MZ twin pairs, and that the estimate for additive genetic effects on hippocampal volume is larger in healthy twins than in discordant twins (van Erp et al. 2004). Thus, hippocampal volume is largely affected by genetic factors in healthy individuals, but is subject to significantly greater modulation by environmental factors in schizophrenic patients and their relatives. Similar findings have been reported for cortisol levels in healthy versus discordant MZ twin pairs; intraclass correlations for cortisol are high and significant for healthy twin pairs, but not for discordant twins.

At the cellular level, there is evidence of reductions in hippocampal glucocorticoid receptors in schizophrenia patients. A study of postmortem brain specimens showed that glucocorticoid receptor mRNA levels were reduced in several regions of the hippocampus (dentate gyrus, CA4, CA3, and CA1) in schizophrenia patients but not in mood disorder patients (Webster et al. 2002). The dentate gyrus is a region that is especially sensitive to the affects of stress-induced corticosteroids (Sousa and Almeida 2002; van der Beek et al. 2004), as well as exposure to alcohol and nicotine (Jang et al. 2002). A reduction in gluco-corticoid receptors in the hippocampus would be expected to compromise negative feedback to the HPA axis, and thus contribute to HPA dysregulation (Heuser et al. 2000).

Additional evidence of functional abnormality in schizophrenia comes from a study of the effects of cortisol (hydrocortisone) administration on regional patterns of brain activity (Ganguli et al. 2002). These investigators found increased regional cerebral activity in response to elevated cortisol in the left hippocampal region in the schizophrenia group, while the control group showed evidence of decreased regional cerebral activity in the same anatomical location. The specific implications for neuronal function are not clear, but the findings do show that schizophrenia patients differ from healthy control subjects in the way hippocampal neurons respond to cortisol binding with mineralocorticoid receptors and glucocorticoid receptors.

In addition to the role of the hippocampus in the HPA system, it is well established that the hippocampus is critical for working memory. The presence of hippocampal abnormality in schizophrenia is consistent with the extensive evidence of memory deficits in patients with this illness (Antonova et al. 2004).

ADOLESCENCE AS A CRITICAL NEURODEVELOPMENTAL PERIOD

It is widely recognized that there are developmental changes in clinical expression of vulnerability to psychosis. Notable among these is the marked rise in risk of clinical onset that occurs in adolescence and early adulthood (Walker 2002). Numerous studies have documented that individuals who are diagnosed with schizophrenia during the modal risk period, early adulthood, manifest a gradual deterioration in function that begins in early adolescence. These findings support the notion that postpubertal neurodevelopmental processes interact with the expression of vulnerability.

Adolescent neurodevelopment is characterized by marked increases in neurohormone secretion. In addition to rising gonadal hormones, there is now mounting evidence of a pubertal increase in activity of the HPA axis. Most cross-sectional and longitudinal studies of salivary and urinary cortisol find an increase with age during the adolescent years. Cross-sectional studies of healthy children reveal a gradual rise in salivary and urinary cortisol during middle childhood, followed by a marked increase that begins around 13 years of age and continues through adolescence (Kenny et al. 1966a, 1966b; Kiess et al. 1995; Lupien et al. 2002; Wingo 2002). Recent longitudinal studies have also revealed increases in cortisol release during adolescence, with the most significant augmentation occurring at age 13 years (Wajs-Kuto et al. 1999; Walker 2002). Studies that have examined pubertal stage indicate that the changes are strongly linked with sexual maturation (Kenny et al. 1966a, 1966b; Kiess et al. 1995; Tornhage 2002).

It has been proposed that the HPA axis—in particular, pituitary release of ACTH and adrenal release of cortisol—may be involved in triggering sexual maturation (Weber et al. 1997). Consistent with this notion, Weber et al. (1997) found that individuals with glucocorticoid deficiency were more likely to have delayed or absent adrenarche. Conversely, children with an early onset of adrenarche, as measured by the early (before age 8 years) appearance of Tanner stages II–III, show signs of heightened HPA activity (Dorn et al. 1999). Compared with age-matched controls, girls with premature adrenarche show significantly higher concentrations of cortisol, as well as estradiol, thyroid-stimulating hormone, and adrenal androgens.

Changes in circulating steroid hormones are important for brain structure and function, because these hormones are transported through the bloodstream, triggering cellular activity and regulating a range of physiological functions (Beach 1975; Kawata 1995; Keenan and Soleymani 2001). Hormones affect the way neurons function, because they modulate the response parameters of neurons to neurotransmitters (Mesce 2002). Unlike neurotransmitters, however, they do not communicate through synapses; rather, hormones diffuse in the extracellular space and influence individual neurons, as well as the structure and activity of neuronal circuits.

Two general classes of hormonal effects on the brain have been described: *activational* and *organizational* (Arnold and Breedlove 1985; Charmandari et al. 2003). Activational effects are conceptualized as transient inductions of time-limited, functional changes in neural circuitry. Hormones can have activational influences on sensory processes, autonomic nervous system activity, and enzyme systems (and thus, cellular permeability to electrolytes, water, and nutrients). In contrast, organizational effects are those that result in changes in the way the brain is organized—its structural characteristics (Buchanan et al. 1992).

Until recently, it was generally assumed that activational effects occurred during adulthood, whereas organizational effects were restricted to fetal neurodevelopment. But it now appears that some organizational effects of hormones occur later in life, including adolescence (Arnold and Breedlove 1985; Charmandari et al. 2003). The magnitude of these effects is suggested by accumulating longitudinal studies of human adolescents, which demonstrate that the brain undergoes significant organizational changes during this period.

Rapidly accumulating data on the postnatal development of the human brain demonstrate that the maturational process extends through adolescence, and probably into early adulthood (Gogtay et al. 2004). Notable among these developments is an increase in the volume of the hippocampus. With MRI, strong age-related increases are observed in the combined area of subiculum and CA1–CA3 (CAS) of the hippocampus (Saitoh et al. 2001).

ADOLESCENT SENSITIVITY TO THE ADVERSE EFFECTS OF STRESS

Several recent reviews have documented that adolescence is a period of heightened stress-sensitivity and vulnerability to mental disorder (Compas et al. 2004; Cunningham et al. 2002; Spear 2000; Walker 2002). This has been shown repeatedly in animal models, and recent studies of human subjects also suggest this (Chambers et al. 2003). For example, rodents show hippocampal volume increases during the peri-/postpubertal period (28–77 days) (Isgor et al. 2004). But exposure to physical stress in early postpuberty reduces hippocampal growth, especially in the CA1 and CA3 pyramidal cell layers and in the dentate gyrus granular cell layer. Exposure to chronic stress induced hippocampal volume deficits that were first observable 3 weeks later, but not 24 hours after exposure. Moreover, these volume deficits were associated with cognitive impairments (i.e., Morris water-maze navigation), sustained downregulation in hippocampal glucocorticoid receptor gene expression, and greater acute stress-induced corticosterone secretion. Volume changes both due to normal maturation and following chronic stress exposure were independent of neuron number. Thus, exposure of adolescents to chronic stress may lead to significant alterations in the HPA axis and changes in hippocampal structure and cognitive function that persist into adulthood. At the receptor level, there is evidence that glucocorticoids have differential effects on the regional expression of mRNA N-methyl-D-aspartate (NMDA) receptor subunits in the hippocampus. Studies of rodents indicate that there may be a window during adolescence in which the receptor genes are especially responsive to glucocorticoids (Lee et al. 2003).

In human adolescents, there are also data indicating increased sensitivity of the hippocampus. In subjects with a history of alcohol abuse, earlier age at onset and longer duration of abuse was associated with reduced volume of the hippocampus (De Bellis et al. 2000). The volume of other brain regions was not associated with alcohol abuse. These findings were interpreted to suggest that during adolescence, the hippocampus may be particularly susceptible to the adverse effects of alcohol.

Briefly summarizing, it appears that postpubertal neuromaturation entails significant changes in the HPA axis and the hippocampus. These maturational changes may result in greater sensitivity of the HPA axis to external stress and increased sensitivity of the hippocampus to insult, including the damaging effects of glucocorticoid elevations. As described above, the HPA–hippocampal system also appears to play a role in the behavioral expression of vulnerability to psychiatric symptoms. Numerous studies indicate heightened cortisol secretion in schizophrenia and other psychiatric disorders. In MZ twins discordant for psychosis, the affected co-twin has a smaller hippocampus, and discordant twins do not manifest normal concordance for cortisol levels (Walker et al. 2002), consistent with the notion that the HPA–hippocampal system moderates the expression of constitutional vulnerability for schizophrenia. Specifically, vulnerable individuals who experience dysregulation of, or damage to, this system may be at increased risk for developing the clinical syndrome. The fact that these systems are hypersensitive during adolescence may account for the rise in prodromal symptoms that has been observed at this developmental stage.

IMPLICATIONS FOR PREVENTIVE INTERVENTION

Interest in the possibility of preventing the onset of psychotic disorders has burgeoned in the past decade. To date, studies have yielded evidence that such prevention may be feasible. At this point, we do not know the critical mechanisms of action of antipsychotics, although a reduction in dopaminergic activity figures prominently in theories about efficacy, and it has been demonstrated that the magnitude of reduction in symptoms is correlated with occupancy of striatal dopamine receptors by antipsychotics. But antipsychotics are known to have a myriad of other neurobiological effects, including a significant reduction in cortisol levels in adult patients (Walker and Diforio 1997).

Several studies have shown that typical antipsychotics, including haloperidol, reduce plasma cortisol (Wik 1995). Similarly, treatment with the atypical antipsychotics olanzapine or risperidone can decrease plasma cortisol in schizophrenia patients (Ryan et al. 2004a, 2004b). One study showed that clozapine did not affect plasma cortisol in schizophrenia patients (Breier et al. 1994); however, another investigation revealed that after withdrawing haloperidol, clozapine treatment of schizophrenia patients resulted in a reduction of plasma cortisol (Markianos et al. 1999). Clozapine was also found to reduce the cortisol response to D-fenfluramine challenge in schizophrenia (Curtis et al. 1995). The apparent dampening effects of antipsychotics on cortisol are consistent with dopamine antagonism. Given the evidence of more severe symptoms in patients with higher baseline and challenge-induced cortisol, it is possible that this effect also serves to reduce symptom severity. Moreover, cortisol reduction may also be implicated in the prophylactic effects of antipsychotic drugs. Several recent reports indicate that administration of antipsychotics to individuals with prodromal or schizotypal symptoms may delay the onset of clinical syndromes of psychosis (McGlashan et al. 2003; McGorry et al. 2002; Miller et al. 2003).

The effects of other psychotropics, especially antidepressants, on cortisol secretion have been of particular interest, because the HPA axis is assumed to play a role in the etiology of some mood disorders. In adults, some antidepressants have been shown to alter cortisol, although the direction of the effects varies (Pariante et al. 2004). Discrepant findings can be attributed, at least in part, to the differential effects of certain subtypes of antidepressants. For example, at least one antidepressant, citalopram, a selective serotonin reuptake inhibitor (SSRI), appears to heighten cortisol secretion in healthy control subjects and depressed patients (Bhagwagar et al. 2002; Harmer et al. 2003). In contrast, however, studies of other SSRIs reveal either no effect on cortisol (Deuschle et al. 2003; Inder et al. 2001; Muck-Seler et al. 2002) or a decrease in cortisol secretion (Thakore et al. 1997).

Findings from studies of tricyclic antidepressants also vary, with some showing no change in cortisol (Inder et al. 2001; Sonntag et al. 1996) and others showing declines (Deuschle et al. 2003; Kunzel et al. 2003; Rodenbeck et al. 2003; Sonntag et al. 1996). Finally, the antidepressant mirtazapine, which does not inhibit the reuptake of norepinephrine or serotonin but is an antagonist of presynaptic alpha$_2$ receptors and postsynaptic 5-hydroxytryptamine type 2 (5-HT$_2$) and type 3 (5-HT$_3$) receptors, has been shown to produce a reduction in salivary cortisol in both responding and nonresponding depressed patients (Laakmann et al. 2003), as well as in healthy controls (Laakmann et al. 1999). Taken together, the findings on antidepressants and cortisol suggest that the medication subtypes have varied effects. This, along with methodological factors, such as sampling method (plasma versus saliva) and subject characteristics, has probably contributed to the divergent findings.

The few studies examining stimulants and cortisol secretion, all conducted in adults, reveal either a drug-induced cortisol elevation in response to methylphenidate (Joyce et al. 1986) or no change (W.A. Brown and Williams 1976). A stimulant-induced cortisol increase would be predicted to result via the agonistic effect on dopamine. Grady et al. (1996) found that plasma cortisol levels increased after intravenous D-amphetamine administration to healthy adults. Along these same lines, Meltzer et al. (2001) administered apomorphine, a dopamine agonist, to healthy control subjects and drug-free schizophrenia patients; they found an increase in plasma cortisol in the controls, but a blunted response in the schizophrenia patients, possibly due to the residual effects of antipsychotics.

The apparent effects of psychotropics on HPA function in adults raises important questions about the effects of these drugs on hormone secretion in adolescents, who are presumably at a critical period for hormonal maturation. It is of interest to know how psychotropics alter cortisol secretion in youth at risk for mental disorders, because there may be implications for the clinical progression. We are examining this issue in our ongoing research on adolescents at risk for psychosis.

EMORY STUDY OF AT-RISK ADOLESCENTS

In our recent research, we have focused on adolescents who manifest personality disorder, including schizotypal personality disorder, and are presumed to be at heightened risk for psychotic disorders. In total, 114 adolescents (mean age 14 years, SD = 1.2 years) have been recruited for participation in the study. A battery of diagnostic measures was administered, including the Structured Interview for DSM-IV Personality Disorders (SIDP-IV; Pfohl et al. 1997), the Structured Clinical Interview for Axis I DSM-IV Disorders (SCID; First et al. 1995), an interview with the parent, and the Child Behavior Checklist, a parent-report measure. Of the total sample, 79 met diagnostic criteria for a DSM-IV (American Psychiatric Association 1994) Axis II disorder and 35 did not meet criteria for a DSM-IV disorder. About 30% were currently receiving one or more of three classes of medications: antidepressants, antipsychotics, or stimulants. All participants underwent a diagnostic assessment, and saliva samples for cortisol assay were obtained hourly, at least four times. Cortisol levels were examined as a function of current and past medication.

In the analyses described here, the relation between cortisol secretion and current and past psychotropic medication treatment is examined in a mixed sample of healthy adolescents and adolescents with Axis II disorders. We considered the three most common classes of medication: antidepressants, stimulants, and antipsychotics. It should be noted that this was a naturalistic study, in that medication status was predetermined by the child's physician, prior to enrollment in the research. On the basis of past findings, as well as the known actions of stimulants, it was predicted that those currently taking stimulants would show elevations in cortisol. For antipsychotic medications, based on both empirical findings and these agents' mechanisms of action, a reduction in cortisol secretion was predicted. Excluding citalopram, the extant empirical literature suggests a dampening effect of antidepressants on cortisol.

Mean cortisol levels (saliva samples 1–3) for the total sample ($n = 114$), by current medication status, are shown in Figures 8–1 through 8–3. As described above, previous research findings indicate that the three classes of psychotropics differ in the direction of their relation with cortisol in adult populations. The mean values listed in Figures 8–1 through 8–3 are generally consistent with earlier reports. The same pattern was found for the Axis II disorder group when examined separately. Given this pattern of results, as well as the high rate of coadministration, regression analyses were conducted so that the effect of each medication class was tested, with statistical controls for the other medications. Furthermore, the effects of age were controlled in the analyses.

Hierarchical regression analyses were conducted with mean cortisol as the dependent variable. Separate analyses were conducted to test the relation of cortisol with each of the three general classes of medication. For these regression equations, age and the "control" medication were entered in the first block. In the second block, the target medication was entered as a predictor variable, and the magnitude of R^2 change was used to test for significance.

As shown in Table 8–1, antipsychotic and stimulant medication accounted for a significant proportion of the variance in cortisol level. For both of these classes of medication, there was a significant increment in R^2 for Block II. Again, the same pattern of findings held when children who did not meet clinical criteria were excluded.

Because there is evidence that citalopram may be associated with an increase in cortisol, whereas other antidepressants decrease cortisol, data were also analyzed excluding subjects on citalopram. There was no significant relation between antidepressant use and cortisol, although the trend was toward lower cortisol in youth taking antidepressants. The same pattern held when data from the clinical subgroup (i.e., those with an Axis II diagnosis) were analyzed separately.

To examine the effects of past medication treatment, we employed the same analytic procedure described above. For these analyses, there was no significant relation between past use of any of the three drug classes and cortisol.

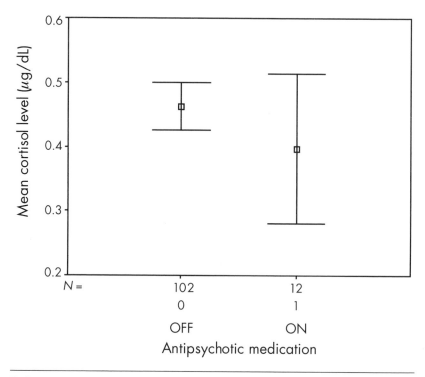

FIGURE 8–1. Mean cortisol levels, by current antipsychotic medication status (0 = off; 1 = on), in a mixed sample of healthy adolescents and adolescents with Axis II disorders (*n*=114) in the Emory Study of At-Risk Adolescents.

In summary, after age and other medications were controlled for, current stimulant medication was associated with significantly higher mean cortisol. Antipsychotic medication was associated with significantly lower cortisol. There was no relation between antidepressant medication and cortisol level, although there was a trend toward lower cortisol in youth on antidepressants.

Because this was not a controlled experimental study, we cannot conclude that the relation between cortisol and medication reflects a causal effect of the psychotropics. It is possible that the differences reflect characteristics of the adolescents that predated their use of medication. Nonetheless, there are several reasons for tentatively concluding that the relation reflects a medication effect. First, we found a relation only between the cortisol secretion and *current* medication use; *past* psychotropic exposure was not linked with cortisol. Second, the pattern of findings was generally consistent with those observed in controlled studies with adults. Finally, the pattern of findings was consistent with what

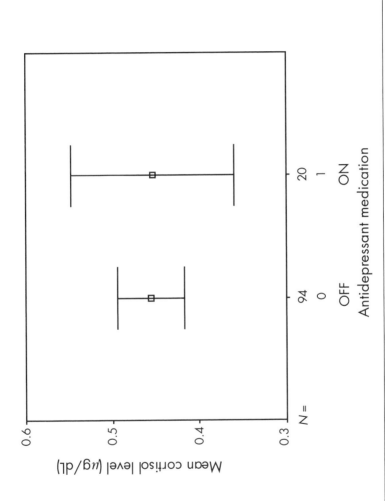

FIGURE 8–2. Mean cortisol levels, by current antidepressant medication status (0 = off; 1 = on), in a mixed sample of healthy adolescents and adolescents with Axis II disorders (*n*=114) in the Emory Study of At-Risk Adolescents.

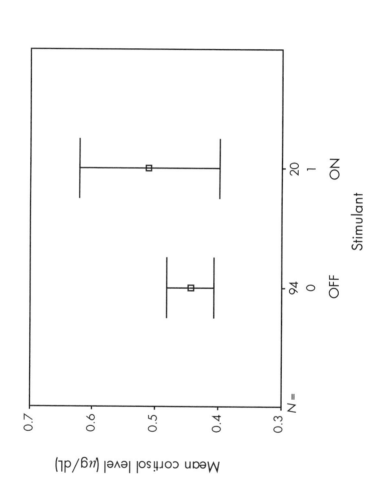

FIGURE 8–3.   Mean cortisol levels, by current stimulant medication status (0 = off; 1 = on), in a mixed sample of healthy adolescents and adolescents with Axis II disorders ($n=114$) in the Emory Study of At-Risk Adolescents.

Table 8–1. Results of regression analyses to test for the relationship between current medication and cortisol

Block II predictor	Block I predictors (age, control medications)				Block II			
	R	df	F	P	R	df	F change	P
Antipsychotic medication	.35	3, 110	5.04	0.003	.39	1, 109	4.19	0.040
Stimulant medication	.34	3, 110	4.92	0.003	.39	1, 109	4.51	0.040
Antidepressant medication	.39	3, 110	6.58	0.0001	.39	1, 109	.162	0.690

would be expected from the mechanisms of action of the drugs. Thus, it is most likely that the relations between cortisol and current medication use observed in this study reflect the effects of the drugs on glucocorticoid secretion.

CONCLUSION

Evidence is gradually accumulating that the HPA–hippocampal system is impaired in patients with schizophrenia and other psychotic disorders. Moreover, it appears that this impairment precedes the onset of the clinical disorder. Specifically, evidence of hippocampal volumetric reduction is observed in young first-episode patients who have never been treated with psychotropics. Furthermore, past research has shown that increases in cortisol secretion precede symptom exacerbations in diagnosed patients (for a review, see Walker and Diforio 1997). This pattern of findings mirrors evidence from studies of healthy control subjects, as well as some clinical samples, which show an inverse relation between hippocampal volume and cortisol levels, consistent with the notion that the hippocampus serves to modulate HPA activity. Although we are not aware of similar studies in psychotic patients, it is reasonable to assume that the same association would be found.

In this chapter we have also presented evidence that adolescence is a sensitive period for the development of the HPA–hippocampal system, and that psychotropic drugs can alter cortisol secretion. In light of the documented rise in psychotropic medication of youth, it is especially important to understand how these drugs affect steroid hormones. The findings reported here suggest one mechanism of action for both beneficial and detrimental effects. On the positive side, the suppression of cortisol by antipsychotics may be one component of these drugs' therapeutic action. It has been suggested that the augmentation of dopamine activity produced by cortisol release may account for the apparent exacerbation of psychotic symptoms following stress exposure (Walker and Diforio 1997). Recent studies of at-risk individuals have increased optimism that antipsychotics may have prophylactic effects with respect to the onset of psychosis (Miller et al. 2003). Assuming that such a prophylactic effect is confirmed in future research, it may be partially attributable to a dampening of cortisol release by antipsychotics. Thus, antipsychotics may exert a preventive effect via reductions in the biological response to stress. On the other hand, there may be unforeseen adverse consequences of dampening cortisol secretion in youth. Given the evidence that developmental increases in cortisol secretion serve to trigger key maturational processes, suppressing secretion may interfere with those processes. Conversely, augmentation of cortisol secretion by stimulants may also have both benefits and risks. The therapeutic effects of stimulant medication, with respect to both behavior and cognitive functioning, have been well documented in youth. But the present findings suggest that stimulants could alter maturational processes or enhance stress sensitivity by augmenting cortisol release.

CLINICAL IMPLICATIONS

Researchers are continuing to pursue studies of the prodromal phase of psychosis, and it is expected that the findings will shed further light on predictors of transition to psychotic symptoms. It is clear that psychotropic medications, as well as numerous other factors, have the potential to alter neurohormonal systems, thereby influencing the expression of vulnerability. Documenting the effects of psychotropic medications on at-risk youth may shed light on the role of the HPA–hippocampal system and also provide leads on approaches to preventive intervention. More generally, the importance of stress in the development of psychosis underscores the need to assess and treat maladaptive responses to stress as early as possible.

REFERENCES

Altamura AC, Boin F, Maes M: HPA axis and cytokine dysregulation in schizophrenia: potential implications for antipsychotic treatment. Eur Neuropsychopharmacol 10:1–4, 1999

American Psychiatric Association: Diagnostic and Statistical Manual of Mental Disorders, 4th Edition. Washington, DC, American Psychiatric Association, 1994

Antonova E, Sharma T, Morris R, et al: The relationship between brain structure and neurocognition in schizophrenia: a selective review. Schizophr Res 70:117–145, 2004

Arnold AP, Breedlove SM: Organizational and activational effects of sex steroids on brain and behavior: a reanalysis. Horm Behav 19:469–498, 1985

Baare WF, van Oel CJ, Hulshoff Pol HE, et al: Volumes of brain structures in twins discordant for schizophrenia. Arch Gen Psychiatry 58:33–40, 2001

Beach FA: Behavioral endocrinology: an emerging discipline. Am Sci 63:178–187, 1975

Bhagwagar Z, Hafizi S, Cowen PJ: Acute citalopram administration produces correlated increases in plasma and salivary cortisol. Psychopharmacology 163:118–120, 2002

Breier A, Buchanan RW, Waltrip RW, et al: The effect of clozapine on plasma norepinephrine: relationship to clinical efficacy. Neuropsychopharmacology 10:1–7, 1994

Brown ES, Woolston D, Frol A, et al: Hippocampal volume, spectroscopy, cognition, and mood in patients receiving corticosteroid therapy. Biol Psychiatry 55:538–545, 2004

Brown WA, Williams BW: Methylphenidate increases serum growth hormone concentrations. J Clin Endocrinol Metab 43:937–939, 1976

Buchanan CM, Eccles JS, Becker JB: Are adolescents the victims of raging hormones? Evidence for activational effects of hormones on moods and behavior at adolescence. Psychol Bull 111:62–107, 1992

Chambers RA, Taylor JR, Potenza MN: Developmental neurocircuitry of motivation in adolescence: a critical period of addiction vulnerability. Am J Psychiatry 160:1041–1052, 2003

Charmandari E, Kino T, Souvatzoglou E, et al: Pediatric stress: hormonal mediators and human development. Horm Res 59:161–179, 2003

Coe CL, Kramer M, Czeh B, et al: Prenatal stress diminishes neurogenesis in the dentate gyrus of juvenile rhesus monkeys. Biol Psychiatry 54:1025–1034, 2003

Compas BE, Connor-Smith J, Jaser SS: Temperament, stress reactivity, and coping: implications for depression in childhood and adolescence. J Clin Child Adolesc Psychol 33:21–31, 2004

Cunningham MG, Bhattacharyya S, Benes FM: Amygdalo-cortical sprouting continues into early adulthood: implications for the development of normal and abnormal function during adolescence. J Comp Neurol 453:116–130, 2002

Curtis VA, Wright P, Reveley A, et al: Effect of clozapine on d-fenfluramine-evoked neuroendocrine responses in schizophrenia and its relationship to clinical improvement. Br J Psychiatry 166:642–646, 1995

De Bellis MD, Clark DB, Beers SR, et al: Hippocampal volume in adolescent-onset alcohol use disorders. Am J Psychiatry 157:737–744, 2000

de Leon MJ, McRae T, Rusinek H, et al: Cortisol reduces hippocampal glucose metabolism in normal elderly, but not in Alzheimer's disease. J Clin Endocrinol Metab 82:3251–3259, 1997

Deuschle M, Hamann B, Meichel C, et al: Antidepressive treatment with amitriptyline and paroxetine: effects on saliva cortisol concentrations. J Clin Psychopharmacol 23:201–205, 2003

Dorn LD, Chrousos GP: The neurobiology of stress: understanding regulation of affect during female biological transitions. Semin Reprod Endocrinol 15:19–35, 1997

Dorn LD, Hitt SF, Rotenstein D: Biopsychological and cognitive differences in children with premature vs. on-time adrenarche. Arch Pediatr Adolesc Med 153:137–146, 1999

Ferrari E, Fioravanti M, Magri F, et al: Variability of interactions between neuroendocrine and immunological functions in physiological aging and dementia of the Alzheimer's type. Ann N Y Acad Sci 917:582–596, 2000

First M, Spitzer RL, Gibbon M, et al: Structured Clinical Interview for the DSM-IV Axis I Disorders (SCID-I), Patient Edition. Washington, DC, American Psychiatric Press, 1995

Ganguli R, Singh A, Brar J, et al: Hydrocortisone induced regional cerebral activity changes in schizophrenia: a PET scan study. Schizophr Res 56:241–247, 2002

Gogtay N, Giedd JN, Lusk L, et al: Dynamic mapping of human cortical development during childhood through early adulthood. Proc Natl Acad Sci U S A 101:8174–8179, 2004

Grady TA, Broocks A, Canter SK, et al: Biological and behavioral responses to D-amphetamine, alone and in combination with serotonin3 receptor antagonist ondasterone, in healthy volunteers. Psychiatry Res 64:1–10, 1996

Harmer CJ, Bhagwagar Z, Shelley N, et al: Contrasting effects of citalopram and reboxetine on waking salivary cortisol. Psychopharmacology 167:112–114, 2003

Harrison PJ: The hippocampus in schizophrenia: a review of the neuropathological evidence and its pathophysiological implications. Psychopharmacology 174:151–162, 2004

Heuser I, Deuschle M, Weber B, et al: Increased activity of the hypothalamus-pituitary-adrenal system after treatment with mineralocorticoid receptor antagonist spironolactone. Psychoneuroendocrinology 25:513–518, 2000

Hibberd C, Yau JL, Seckl JR: Glucocorticoids and the aging hippocampus. J Anat 197:553–562, 2000

Inder WJ, Prickett TCR, Mulder RT, et al: Reduction in basal afternoon plasma ACTH during early treatment of depression with fluoxetine. Psychopharmacology (Berl) 156:73–78, 2001

Isgor C, Kabbaj M, Akil H, et al: Delayed effects of chronic variable stress during peripubertal-juvenile period on hippocampal morphology and on cognitive and stress axis functions in rats. Hippocampus 14:636–648, 2004

Jang MH, Shin MC, Jung SB, et al: Alcohol and nicotine reduce cell proliferation and enhance apoptosis in dentate gyrus. Neuroreport 13:1509–1513, 2002

Joyce PR, Donald RA, Nicholls MG, et al: Endocrine and behavioral responses to methylphenidate in normal subjects. Biol Psychiatry 21:1015–1023, 1986

Kawata M: Roles of steroid hormones and their receptors in structural organization in the nervous system. Neurosci Res 24:1–46, 1995

Keenan PA, Soleymani RM: Gonadal steroids and cognition, in Medical Neuropsychology (Critical Issues in Neuropsychology), 2nd Edition. Edited by Tarter RE, Butters M, Beers SR. Dordrecht, Netherlands, Kluwer Academic, 2001, pp 181–197

Kenny FM, Gancayo GP, Heald FP, et al: Cortisol production rate in adolescent males in different stages of sexual maturation. J Clin Endocrinol 26:1232–1236, 1966a

Kenny FM, Preeyasombat C, Migeon CJ: Cortisol production rate, II: normal infants, children and adults. Pediatrics 37:34–42, 1966b

Kiess W, Meidert A, Dressendorfer RA, et al: Salivary cortisol levels throughout childhood and adolescence: relation with age, pubertal stage and weight. Pediatr Res 37:502–506, 1995

Kunzel HE, Binder EB, Nickel T, et al: Pharmacological and nonpharmacological factors influencing hypothalamic-pituitary-adrenocortical axis reactivity in acutely depressed psychiatric in-patients, measured by the Dex-CRH test. Neuropsychopharmacology 28:2169–2178, 2003

Laakmann G, Hennig J, Baghai T, et al: Influence of mirtazapine on salivary cortisol in depressed patients. Neuropsychobiology 47:31–36, 2003

Laakmann G, Schule C, Baghai T, et al: Effects of mirtazapine on growth hormone, prolactin, and cortisol secretion in healthy male subjects. Psychoneuroendocrinology 24:769–784, 1999

Lee PR, Brady D, Koenig JI: Corticosterone alters N-methyl-D-aspartate receptor subunit mRNA expression before puberty. Mol Brain Res 115:55–62, 2003

Lupien SJ, de Leon M, de Santi S, et al: Cortisol levels during human aging predict hippocampal atrophy and memory deficits. Nat Neurosci 1:69–73, 1998

Lupien SJ, Wilkinson CW, Briere S, et al: The modulatory effects of corticosteroids on cognition: studies in young human populations. Psychoneuroendocrinology 27:401–416, 2002

Markianos M, Hatzimanolis J, Lykouras L: Switch from neuroleptics to clozapine does not influence pituitary-gonadal axis hormone levels in male schizophrenic patients. Eur Neuropsychopharmacology 9:533–536, 1999

McGlashan TH, Zipursky RB, Perkins D, et al: The PRIME North America randomized double-blind clinical trial of olanzapine versus placebo in patients at risk of being prodromally symptomatic for psychosis, I: study rationale and design. Schizophr Res 61:7–18, 2003

McGorry PD, Yung AR, Phillips LJ, et al: Randomized controlled trial of interventions designed to reduce the risk of progression to first-episode psychosis in a clinical sample with subthreshold symptoms. Arch Gen Psychiatry 59:921–928, 2002

Meaney MJ, O'Donnell D, Rowe W, et al: Individual differences in hypothalamic-pituitary-adrenal activity in later life and hippocampal aging. Exp Gerontology 30:229–251, 1995

Meaney MJ, Diorio J, Francis D, et al: Early environmental regulation of forebrain glucocorticoid receptor gene expression: implications for adrenocortical responses to stress. Dev Neurosci 18:49–72, 1996

Meltzer HY, Myung LA, Jayathilake K: The blunted plasma cortisol response to apomorphine and its relationship to treatment response in patients with schizophrenia. Neuropsychopharmacology 24:278–290, 2001

Mesce KA: Metamodulation of the biogenic amines: second-order modulation by steroid hormones and amine cocktails. Brain Behav Evol 60:339–349, 2002

Miller TJ, Zipursky RB, Perkins D, et al: The PRIME North America randomized double-blind clinical trial of olanzapine versus placebo in patients at risk of being prodromally symptomatic for psychosis, II: baseline characteristics of the "prodromal" sample. Schizophr Res 61:19–30, 2003

Muck-Seler D, Pivac N, Sagud M, et al: The effects of paroxetine and tianeptine on peripheral biochemical markers in major depression. Prog Neuropsychopharmacol Biol Psychiatry 26:1235–1243, 2002

Muck-Seler D, Pivac N, Mustapic M, et al: Platelet serotonin and plasma prolactin and cortisol in healthy, depressed and schizophrenic women. Psychiatry Res 127:217–226, 2004

Ohl F, Michaelis T, Vollmann-Honsdorf GK, et al: Effect of chronic psychosocial stress and long-term cortisol treatment on hippocampus-mediated memory and hippocampal volume: a pilot study in tree shrews. Psychoneuroendocrinology 25:357–363, 2000

Pariante CM, Thomas SA, Lovestone S, et al: Do antidepressants regulate how cortisol affects the brain? Psychoneuroendocrinology 29:423–447, 2004

Pfohl B, Blum N, Zimmerman M: Structured Interview for DSM-IV Personality (SIDP-IV). Washington, DC, American Psychiatric Press, 1997

Ritsner M, Maayan R, Gibel A, et al: Elevation of the cortisol/dehydroepiandrosterone ratio in schizophrenia patients. Eur Neuropsychopharmacol 14:267–273, 2004

Rodenbeck A, Cohrs S, Jordan W, et al: The sleep-improving effects of doxepin are paralleled by a normalized plasma cortisol secretion in primary insomnia: a placebo-controlled, double-blind, randomized, cross-over study followed by an open treatment over 3 weeks. Psychopharmacology 170:423–428, 2003

Ryan MC, Collins P, Thakore JH: Impaired fasting glucose tolerance in first-episode, drug-naive patients with schizophrenia. Am J Psychiatry 160:284–289, 2003

Ryan MC, Flanagan S, Kinsella U, et al: The effects of atypical antipsychotics on visceral fat distribution in first episode, drug-naive patients with schizophrenia. Life Sci 74: 1999–2008, 2004a

Ryan MC, Sharifi N, Condren R, et al: Evidence of basal pituitary-adrenal overactivity in first episode, drug naive patients with schizophrenia. Psychoneuroendocrinology 29:1065–1070, 2004b

Saitoh O, Karns CM, Courchesne E: Development of the hippocampal formation from 2 to 42 years: MRI evidence of smaller area dentata in autism. Brain 124:1317–1324, 2001

Sapolsky RM: Why Zebras Don't Get Ulcers. New York, Friedman, 1994

Seidman LJ, Pantelis C, Keshavan MS, et al: A review and new report of medial temporal lobe dysfunction as a vulnerability indicator for schizophrenia: a magnetic resonance imaging morphometric family study of the parahippocampal gyrus. Schizophr Bull 29:803–830, 2003

Shenton ME, Dickey CC, Frumin M, et al: A review of MRI findings in schizophrenia. Schizophr Res 49:1–52, 2001

Shirayama Y, Hashimoto K, Suzuki Y, et al: Correlation of plasma neurosteroid levels to the severity of negative symptoms in male patients with schizophrenia. Schizophr Res 58:69–74, 2002

Sonntag A, Rothe B, Guldner J, et al: Trimipramine and imipramine exert different effects on the sleep EEG and on nocturnal hormone secretion during treatment of major depression. Depression 4:1–13, 1996

Sousa N, Almeida OF: Corticosteroids: sculptors of the hippocampal formation. Rev Neurosci 13:59–84, 2002

Spear LP: The adolescent brain and age-related behavioral manifestations. Neurosci Biobehav Rev 24:417–463, 2000

Starkman MN, Giordani B, Gebarski SS, et al: Decrease in cortisol reverses human hippocampal atrophy following treatment of Cushing's disease. Biol Psychiatry 46:1595–1602, 1999

Starkman MN, Giordani B, Gebarski SS, et al: Improvement in learning associated with increase in hippocampal formation volume. Biol Psychiatry 53:233–238, 2003

Suddath RL, Christison GW, Torrey EF, et al: Anatomical abnormalities in the brains of monozygotic twins discordant for schizophrenia. N Engl J Med 322:789–794, 1990

Thakore JH, Barnes C, Joyce J, et al: Effects of antidepressant treatment on corticotropin-induced cortisol responses in patients with melancholic depression. Psychiatry Res 73:27–32, 1997

Tornhage CJ: Reference values for morning salivary cortisol concentrations in healthy school-aged children. J Pediatr Endocrinol Metab 15:197–204, 2002

van der Beek EM, Wiegant VM, Schouten WG, et al: Neuronal number, volume, and apoptosis of the left dentate gyrus of chronically stressed pigs correlate negatively with basal saliva cortisol levels. Hippocampus 14:688–700, 2004

van Erp TG, Saleh PA, Huttunen M, et al: Hippocampal volumes in schizophrenic twins. Arch Gen Psychiatry 61:346–353, 2004

van Haren NE, Picchioni MM, McDonald C, et al: A controlled study of brain structure in monozygotic twins concordant and discordant for schizophrenia. Biol Psychiatry 56:454–461, 2004

Wajs-Kuto E, De Beeck LO, Rooman RP, et al: Hormonal changes during the first year of oestrogen treatment in constitutionally tall girls. Eur J Endocrinol 141:579–584, 1999

Walder DJ, Walker EF, Lewine RJ: Cognitive functioning, cortisol release, and symptom severity in patients with schizophrenia. Biol Psychiatry 48:1121–1132, 2000

Walker EF: Adolescent neurodevelopment and psychopathology. Current Directions in Psychological Science 11:24–28, 2002

Walker E, Diforio D: Schizophrenia: a neural diathesis-stress model. Psychol Rev 104:1–19, 1997

Walker EF, Bonsall R, Walder DJ: Plasma hormones and catecholamine metabolites in monozygotic twins discordant for psychosis. Neuropsychiatry Neuropsychol Behav Neurol 15:10–17, 2002

Watzka M, Beyenburg S, Blumcke I, et al: Expression of mineralocorticoid and gluco-corticoid receptor mRNA in the human hippocampus. Neurosci Lett 290:121–124, 2000

Weber A, Clark AJ, Perry LA, et al: Diminished adrenal androgen secretion in familial glucocorticoid deficiency implicates a significant role for ACTH in the induction of adrenarche. Clin Endocrinol 46:431–437, 1997

Webster MJ, Knable MB, O'Grady J, et al: Regional specificity of brain glucocorticoid receptor mRNA alterations in subjects with schizophrenia and mood disorders. Mol Psychiatry 7:985–994, 2002

Wik G: Effects of neuroleptic treatment on cortisol and 3-methoxy-4-hydroxyphenyl-ethyl glycol levels in blood. J Endocrinol 144:425–429, 1995

Wingo MK: The adolescent stress response to a naturalistic driving stressor. Diss Abstr Int: Sec B: The Sciences and Engineering 63:1082, 2002

Wolf OT, Convit A, de Leon MJ, et al: Basal hypothalamo-pituitary-adrenal axis activity and corticotropin feedback in young and older men: relationships to magnetic resonance imaging-derived hippocampus and cingulate gyrus volumes. Neuroendocrinology 75:241–249, 2002

9

Toward Prevention of Schizophrenia

Early Detection and Intervention

Ming T. Tsuang, M.D., Ph.D., D.Sc.

William S. Stone, Ph.D.

Michael J. Lyons, Ph.D.

Family studies have indicated that the biological relatives of schizophrenia patients are at increased risk for schizophrenia, other nonaffective psychoses, schizoaffective disorder, and schizotypal personality disorder (Tsuang et al. 1999a). Twin studies have demonstrated genetic influence through a greater concordance of monozygotic (MZ) compared with dizygotic (DZ) twins. Environmental influences are suggested by the 50% concordance rate in MZ twin pairs. The results of twin studies suggest that approximately 70% of the vulnerability to schizophrenia is attributable to genetic factors (Tsuang et al. 1999a). Adoption studies indicate that biological, but not adoptive, relatives of individuals with schizophrenia are at increased risk for the illness (Tsuang et al. 1999a). Biological children of nonschizophrenic parents are not at greater risk for schizophrenia when raised by schizophrenic adoptive parents. Although family, twin, and adoption studies show that genetic factors play a substantial role in the etiology of schizophrenia, molecular genetic studies have been slow in identifying susceptibility genes that contribute a large proportion of vulnerability (Tsuang et al. 1999a).

In their review of the relationship between the neuropathology and genetics of schizophrenia, Harrison and Weinberger (2005) identify seven putative susceptibility genes with positive findings in at least three published independent samples: catechol-O-methyl transferase (COMT), neuregulin (NRG1), dysbindin (DTNBP1), disrupted-in-schizophrenia 1 (DISC1), regulator of G-protein signaling (RGS4), metabotropic glutamate receptor 3 (GRM3; mGluR3), and G72 (and D-amino acid oxidase [DAAO]). The authors speculate that these genes may converge on schizophrenia risk via influence on synaptic plasticity, given that three of the above genes affect plasticity and synaptogenesis (NRG1, DTNBP1, DISC1), two affect receptors (GRM3, G72), and one affects signal transduction (RGS4). The glutamatergic system is most often implicated in association with these genes, although they are also strongly linked to the dopaminergic (viz. COMT) and GABAergic (gamma-aminobutyric acid [GABA]) systems. In addition, alteration of gene expression rather than of protein structure appears to be the rule.

GENETIC AND PHENOTYPIC HETEROGENEITY MODEL

Figure 9–1 presents a model that takes into account the complexity of the phenotypes that we wish to study and the determinants of those phenotypes. The figure indicates that individuals who are influenced by the relevant genetic and environmental risk factors may have one of three outcomes: 1) they may be free of symptoms of the disorder; 2) they may have an attenuated version of the disorder that does not reach the full diagnostic criteria, in which case they are considered to have a "spectrum" disorder; and 3) they may manifest the clinical phenotype (i.e., they meet full diagnostic criteria for the relevant disorder). The figure also indicates that there may be individuals who meet the diagnostic criteria but do not manifest the disorder from an etiological perspective, and thus could be considered to be "phenocopies." The power of our genetic investigations will be reduced if we classify the symptom-free and spectrum-disorder individuals in the figure as being unaffected, and including phenocopies as "affected" can seriously undermine the prospects for the success of our genetic analyses.

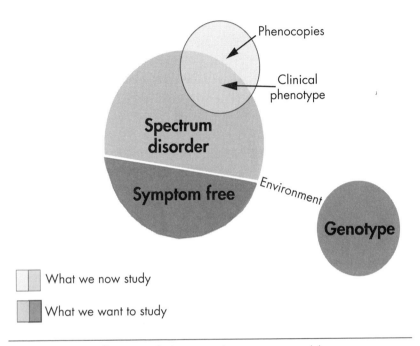

FIGURE 9–1. Genetic and phenotypic heterogeneity model.

Consistent with the heterogeneous list of genes that may contribute to the susceptibility for or expression of schizophrenia, many phenotypes have been proposed to reflect or contribute to liability for the disorder. The most common basis for identifying such phenotypes involves the presence of statistically significant differences between nonpsychotic adult relatives of individuals with schizophrenia and relevant control subjects (Faraone et al. 1995a, 2001). Considerable effort remains, however, to determine which phenotypes will be useful in distinguishing individuals who are more likely to express psychosis from those who are not, and which ones should be included formally in a syndrome of liability. There are several considerations to assess in addition to the probability of significant group differences between relative and control groups. These include, among others, the extent to which a measure's statistical sensitivity and specificity is adequate (Faraone et al. 1995a, 2001) and the degree to which a predictor (e.g., inattention, social withdrawal, substance abuse) is specific for schizophrenia (Dazzan et al. 2004). A related consideration is that no single factor predicts schizophrenia (so far), even in high-risk groups (Dazzan et al. 2004). This latter finding likely is at least in part a consequence of a multifactorial, polygenic model in which multiple vulnerability factors of small or moderate effect contribute to the overall risk of developing psychosis. For this reason, multiple measures or combinations of measures often show more predictive power than individual ones (Erlenmeyer-Kimling 2000).

Measures of neuropsychological function are among those that have been particularly informative. Cognitive deficits are widely considered to be core components of schizophrenia that contribute to functional outcome of the illness (e.g., Green 1996; Green et al. 2000; Heinrichs 2005). Cognitive deficits are found in subjects with schizophrenia and related "spectrum" conditions (e.g., schizoaffective disorder and schizotypal personality disorder), and in clinical (e.g., prodromal) and genetic (e.g., the children of parents with schizophrenia) high-risk subjects (Heinrichs and Zakzanis 1998; Snitz et al. 2006; Stone et al. 2005).

In a series of studies over the past 20 years, we documented widespread cognitive deficits in schizophrenia (Faraone et al. 2001; Kremen and Hoff 2004). Moreover, Faraone et al. (1995b) assessed neuropsychological functioning in 35 nonpsychotic adult relatives of schizophrenia patients and 72 healthy control subjects. We used linear combinations of neuropsychological tests to create scales assessing 10 neuropsychological functions: abstraction/executive function, verbal ability, spatial ability, verbal memory, visual memory, learning, perceptual–motor speed, mental control/encoding, motor ability, and auditory attention/vigilance. On the basis of previous neuropsychological studies of schizophrenia patients and our review of family studies, we predicted that relatives of persons with schizophrenia would exhibit deficits in abstraction/executive function, learning, and memory, as well as several components of attention (perceptual–motor speed, mental control/encoding, and auditory attention/vigilance). A multivariate analysis of variance found the neuropsychological profile of the relatives to be significantly more impaired than the control profile (Figure 9–2).

The relatives performed significantly more poorly than controls and had greater variability on 3 neuropsychological functions: abstraction/executive function, verbal memory, and auditory attention/vigilance. They had lower mean scores but similar variability on verbal ability and mental control/encoding. They showed more variability, but not lower mean scores, on learning and motor ability. The two groups did not differ on spatial ability, visual memory, or perceptual–motor function. The deficits observed could not be accounted for by psychopathology in the relatives, educational attainment, or parental social class. These results remained significant when the original sample was increased to 54 nonpsychotic relatives, with the additional finding of significantly impaired visual memory (Toomey et al. 1998).

In a 4-year follow-up study, we showed that executive function, declarative memory, and working memory deficits in adult relatives of patients with schizo-

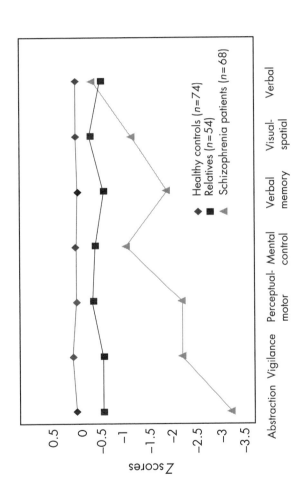

FIGURE 9–2. Neuropsychological profiles in schizophrenia patients, relatives, and healthy control subjects.

phrenia were stable traits (Faraone et al. 1999). In addition to stable working memory deficits, the most robust indicators of impairment were verbal declarative memory functions (e.g., story recall). Support for the importance of verbal learning and memory deficits—in particular, impaired semantic clustering—was confirmed in an independent sample of relatives of patients with schizophrenia (Lyons et al. 1995).

The identification of cognitive deficits in relatives of schizophrenia patients raises the question of individual differences. In particular, what factors influence cognitive performance among relatives? We addressed this issue by comparing a sample of relatives in which one family member was affected with schizophrenia ("simplex" families) with a sample in which two members were affected ("multiplex" families), with the assumption that the multiplex group had the higher genetic risk for schizophrenia (Faraone et al. 2000). Relatives from multiplex families performed significantly worse than simplex relatives and control subjects on verbal declarative memory, while relatives from simplex families performed significantly worse than control subjects on verbal and visual memory. Together, these results suggest strongly that particular neuropsychological impairments (including verbal declarative memory impairments) are stable and core features in schizophrenia that occur relatively independently of psychosis, as emphasized in studies of nonpsychotic relatives.

Moreover, neuropsychological impairments are related to other dimensions of dysfunction. One such dimension involves abnormalities in brain structure, which we and other investigators have documented both in patients with schizophrenia and in their close biological relatives (Faraone et al. 2003; Seidman and Wencel 2003; Seidman et al. 2003, 2004). We assessed relationships between brain structure and neuropsychological performance in the simplex and multiplex samples described above, as well as in patients with schizophrenia (Seidman et al. 2002). The subjects in this study included 45 nonpsychotic adult first-degree relatives from multiplex ($n = 17$) or simplex ($n = 28$) families with schizophrenia, 18 patients with schizophrenia, and 48 healthy control subjects. Volumes of the total cerebrum and the hippocampus were measured. Relatives from multiplex families and patients with schizophrenia demonstrated significantly smaller left hippocampi compared with controls. Interestingly, verbal memory and left hippocampal volumes were significantly and positively correlated. Within families, hippocampal volumes did not differ between patients with schizophrenia and their nonpsychotic relatives. These results support the hypothesis that the vulnerability to schizophrenia includes smaller left hippocampi and verbal memory deficits, and that the degree of genetic liability to schizophrenia influences both the nature and the magnitude of the deficits.

COHERENCE OF COGNITIVE AND CLINICAL DEFICITS IN RELATIVES INTO A SYNDROME OF LIABILITY

Individuals who have an elevated risk for schizophrenia, such as adolescent or young adult (nonpsychotic) first-degree biological relatives of people with schizophrenia, can manifest this liability overtly. One way to do so is to meet DSM-IV (American Psychiatric Association 1994) diagnostic criteria for a related but milder condition, such as schizotypal personality disorder (SPD). Although most individuals with SPD do not develop schizophrenia (Faraone et al. 2001; Tsuang et al. 1999a), characterizations of these individuals' liability are important, partly as a way to develop interventions that target clinical manifestations. Moreover, the study of nonpsychotic, nonschizotypal adult relatives of schizophrenic patients who carry the risk, but do not develop schizophrenia, can also clarify the liability to develop the disorder. As the accuracy of prediction increases, the potential for early intervention becomes increasingly realistic.

Multiple sources, over a period of 100 years, contribute to our current notions about the nature of liability to, and protection from, psychosis. Among the sources that have guided our conceptualization and assessment is the well-established view that schizophrenia has a significant genetic component (Gottesman 2001; Gottesman and Gould 2003; Kendler 2001). Based in part on the frequent observation that some nonpsychotic relatives of people with schizophrenia show eccentric or odd behaviors, and on Rado's (1953, 1960) suggestion that "schizotypes" result from a genetic liability to schizophrenia, Paul Meehl (1962, 1989) proposed a model in which a "schizogene" produces a "neural integrative defect" that he referred to as "schizotaxia." He concluded that this deficit could not be observed directly through behavior, although its underlying neurobiology would be defined eventually. Instead, the neural defect produced a phenotype called "schizotypy," which is a type of personality organization that interacts with environmental variables (e.g., social learning) and other, polygenic factors (e.g., a predisposition to high or low anxiety, or to various features related to temperament). These latter genes differed from the major schizogene that causes schizotaxia in that they were more likely to include common genes of small or moderate effect. In relatively favorable environmental and genetic circumstances, the resulting phenotype would involve only minor clinical symptoms (e.g., "compensated schizotypy"), but less favorable genetic and/or environmental circumstances would result in more severe, decompensated phenotypes, such as schizophrenia.

For about 40 years, schizotaxia was used by researchers to conceptualize the premorbid, neurological liability for, and basis of, schizophrenia. Unlike schizotypy, however, which entered the psychiatric nomenclature in the form of schizotypal personality disorder, schizotaxia remained defined operationally during that period. The possibility that schizotaxia is both a definable and meaningful clinical syndrome emerged from growing empirical literature showing that some first-degree nonpsychotic relatives of people with schizophrenia demonstrate abnormalities in cognition, brain structure and function, affect, and social functioning compared with healthy control subjects.

Recently, we reformulated the term *schizotaxia* to integrate newer data. Although our conception is consistent with Meehl's view of schizotaxia as the underlying liability among people predisposed to schizophrenia, some aspects of his theory were modified. For example, we proposed that the syndrome resulted from a combination of genes and adverse biological consequences of environmental events (e.g., pregnancy or delivery problems such as maternal diabetes or preeclampsia) in most cases, rather than from a major gene. On the basis of evidence of abnormal function in several dimensions, as described above, Tsuang et al. (1999b) proposed a set of research criteria for schizotaxia. The initial research criteria involved a subset of theoretically important symptoms/deficits that had been relatively well studied at the time. They included a clinical variable (negative symptoms) and specific deficits in neuropsychological functioning. At least moderate levels of negative symptoms (defined as at least 6 items on the Schedule for the Assessment of Negative Symptoms [SANS; Andreasen 1983] rated 3 or higher) and neuropsychological deficits (defined as performance deficits in specific measures of attention, verbal declarative memory, and/or executive function that are at least 2 standard deviations lower than expected in one of the three domains, and at least 1 standard deviation below expectation in a second domain) were required for a diagnosis of schizotaxia in never-psychotic first-degree adult relatives of patients with schizophrenia. Additional inclusion and exclusion criteria (e.g., a history of a head injury or other neurological disorder known to impair cognitive function or to increase negative symptoms; a current substance abuse diagnosis; very low levels of overall cognitive ability) were intended to minimize false-positive diagnoses (Tsuang et al. 1999b).

One corollary of defining schizotaxia on the basis of these neuropsychological deficits is that a large proportion of "unaffected" relatives of patients will demonstrate core features of the proposed syndrome. We estimated that 20%–50% of first-degree relatives might demonstrate such features, largely on the basis of our studies of neuropsychological deficits in this group (Faraone et al. 1995a, 1995b). Because neither schizophrenia nor schizotypal personality disorder occurs at such high rates (Faraone et al. 2001; Tsuang et al. 1999a, 2002), a significant clinical implication of the revised formulation is that schizotaxia does not lead to either schizotypal personality disorder or to schizophrenia in most people. Instead, it may be a stable syndrome in most cases. This view is consistent with our finding that neuropsychological deficits in these areas were stable over a period of 4 years, as described above (Faraone et al. 1999).

Although the proposed syndrome of schizotaxia coheres conceptually, its utility can be established only through empirical validation. Nevertheless, there are several reasons for cautious optimism. First, our initial pilot studies demonstrated that 8 of 27 first-degree relatives met our criteria for schizotaxia (Stone et al. 2001), in agreement with earlier estimates of its likely rate of 20%–50% (Faraone et al. 1995a, 1995b).

Second, 6 of the 8 schizotaxic individuals agreed to participate in an open-label drug trial with a low dose of risperidone (0.25–2.0 mg). We reasoned that if relatives shared genes and psychopathological features with their ill relatives, they might also respond to the same type of treatment (i.e., one of the newer antipsychotic medications) that benefits many individuals with schizophrenia. The findings were consistent with this prediction, as 5 out of 6 subjects improved on a demanding test of working memory (Figure 9–3) and showed 25%–50% reductions in negative symptoms (Figure 9–4). Notably, the one subject who did not improve demonstrated an IQ score that was well below average and also below that of the other subjects, a finding that may have implications for the limits of pharmacological treatment.

Third, a validation study performed with the same subjects showed that relatives who met criteria for schizotaxia performed worse on several independent measures of clinical function than did relatives who did not meet the diagnostic criteria (Stone et al. 2001). Several measures were employed, including some that involved self-ratings (including the Social Adjustment Scale—Self-Report [SAS-SR; Weissman and Bothwell 1976], the Symptom Checklist–90–Revised [SCL-90-R; Derogatis 1983], and the Physical Anhedonia Scale [Chapman et al. 1976]) and one that was rated blindly by the investigators (DSM-IV Global Assessment of Functioning [GAF] scale). The groups did not differ in age, education, paternal education, IQ, or number of ill relatives. At the time these clinical data were collected, neither the raters nor the subjects knew their clinical status (i.e., schizotaxic vs. nonschizotaxic). This study was the first to show evidence of concurrent validation for the proposed syndrome.

Fourth, Chen et al. (1998) showed that deficits in cognition (i.e., sustained attention) were more associated with negative and disorganized symptoms of schizotypy than they were with positive symptoms in nonpsychotic relatives of

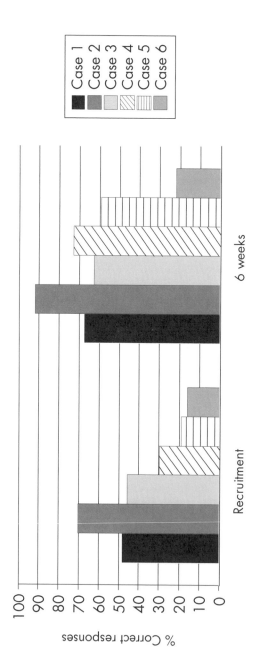

FIGURE 9–3.   Changes in performance on a working memory test (an auditory continuous performance test) in six relatives before and after 6 weeks of treatment with risperidone.

Higher scores are associated with improvement.

Source.   Reprinted from Tsuang MT, Stone WS, Seidman LJ, et al.: "Treatment of Nonpsychotic Relatives of Patients With Schizophrenia: Four Case Studies." *Biological Psychiatry* 41:1412–1418, 1999b. Used with permission.

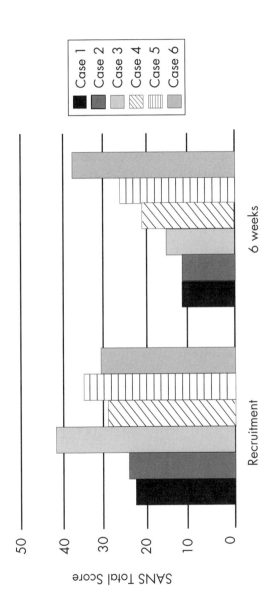

FIGURE 9–4. Changes in Assessment of Negative Symptoms (SANS) total scores in six relatives before and after treatment with risperidone for 6 weeks.

Lower scores are associated with improvement.

Source. Reprinted from Tsuang MT, Stone WS, Seidman LJ, et al.: "Treatment of Nonpsychotic Relatives of Patients With Schizophrenia: Four Case Studies." *Biological Psychiatry* 41:1412–1418, 1999b. Used with permission.

individuals with schizophrenia. This study, although not conducted in subjects with schizotaxia per se, provides evidence that the major clinical components of schizotaxia co-aggregate with one another in relatives. It is also consistent with our own findings that deficits in neuropsychological domains that are often impaired in schizotaxia co-aggregate with each other in relatives more than they do in control subjects (Toomey et al. 1998).

The validation of schizotaxia in its current form, while promising, is an interim measure. Our conception of schizotaxia will expand to include other measures of cognitive and clinical function, and also other dimensions. Abnormalities in brain structure and function, for example, are a likely direction, as is dysfunction in other physiological systems, such as glucose and other types of metabolic regulation (Ryan and Thakore 2002; Stone et al. 2004). One of the most important avenues for future research will involve the attempt to define the genetic liability for schizotaxia/schizophrenia. The following discussion focuses on our current efforts in this domain.

GENE-BASED VERSUS GENOME-BASED RESEARCH

There are two general approaches to discovering genes responsible for a disease: 1) *gene-based* research, which examines specific genes, focusing on a specific section of the total genome; and 2) *genome-based* research, which examines the expression levels of all of the genes in the organism (this concept is also known as "system biology"). Gene-based research allows us to view the genome through "windows" the width of several genes. Genome-based research opens a complete window on all genes in the organism.

Microarray Analysis

Because schizophrenia is a highly heritable disorder, many candidate-gene association studies have been conducted to identify its underlying etiological factors. However, candidate genes found to be associated with the disorder in one study have not been replicated in others. Unlike candidate-gene approaches that test the influence on disease risk of one gene at a time, microarray analysis is a tool that can be used to measure the expression of hundreds or thousands of genes simultaneously (Eisen and Brown 1999). Thus, relative to traditional candidate-gene studies predicated on existing disease models, microarray analysis is a less constrained strategy that could foster the discovery of novel risk genes that otherwise would not come under study. Using mRNA and cDNA microarrays, researchers have established differential gene expression profiles between individuals with and without various disorders (Satagopan and Panageas 2003). Because gene expression can reflect both genetic and environmental influences, it may be particularly useful for identifying risk factors for a complex disorder such as schizophrenia, which is thought to have a multifactorial, polygenic etiology, in which many genes and environmental factors interact. Although microarray technology has several applications, the one most relevant to our interests is gene identification, which relates to the detection of overexpressed and underexpressed gene subsets from a given biological sample. A probe can be applied, and its fluorescent intensity gives an indication of the amount of mRNA produced by specific genes and thus provides a measure of that gene's expression (Eisen and Brown 1999).

Altered patterns of gene expression have been implicated in the development of various psychiatric disorders. The study of neuropsychiatric disease presents significant challenges to microarray techniques due to the desirability of examining central nervous system (CNS) DNA, although microarray analysis has been applied to several neurological diseases, including HIV-associated dementia, Alzheimer's disease, multiple sclerosis, and schizophrenia (Marcotte et al. 2003; Minagar et al. 2004). Because of the recurrent interaction of gene expression products (mRNA and proteins) with the environment, which shapes the ongoing activity of the nervous system, the measurement of gene expression in the postmortem brain has severe limitations (Gladkevich et al. 2004). Gene and protein expression levels are not static, and the very nature of learning and adaptation requires a rapid turnover in gene and protein expression in the brain as compared with other tissues (Marcotte et al. 2003). Nonetheless, a number of such studies have been performed (DeLisi 2000; Mirnics et al. 2001). One intriguing set of findings identified differential expression of key myelin-related genes in postmortem schizophrenia brains compared with control brains (Hakak et al. 2001; Tkachev et al. 2003).

Using Blood for Microarray Analyses

Circulating blood is a notably dynamic environment involving the turnover of approximately one trillion blood cells daily, including 200 billion red blood cells (RBCs) and 70 billion neutrophilic leukocytes. Circulating blood may act as a "sentinel tissue" that can reflect the state of health or disease within the body. Using blood as a source material allows the collection of larger sample sizes, better standardization of technical procedures, and the ability to relatively noninvasively profile human subjects. Blood-based diagnostics could be applied to the study of psychiatric disorders for which human brain tissue biopsy samples are unavailable.

Gladkevich et al. (2004) argued that cDNA from lymphocytes extracted from blood may be an acceptable proxy for CNS DNA, given that 1) lymphocytic function has been demonstrated to be altered in neuropsychiatric disorders (Ganguli et al. 1995; Inglot et al. 1994); 2) neuroactive proteins and processes are expressed in lymphocytes (Felten et al. 1987; Gladkevich et al. 2004); and 3) similarities of hormonal effects on nervous system processes and lymphocyte physiology have been reported (Muller and Ackenheil 1998). Furthermore, genes whose expression levels are influenced by genetic polymorphisms in their promoter regions or transcriptional regulatory sites might be expected to have similar levels of expression in all tissues, depending more on the presence or absence of such polymorphisms than on the tissue in which they are being measured. Although application of microarray technology using lymphocytes in live patients with psychiatric disorders is relatively new, it has been successfully used in investigations of the effects of various antidepressants in Alzheimer's disease patients (Palotas et al. 2004a, 2004b). The expression profiles of Alzheimer's lymphocytes differed in magnitude from those of control lymphocytes, and sequences that were differentially expressed after antidepressant treatment could be identified. Recently, peripheral blood cell–derived gene expression patterns were also used to differentiate trauma-exposed individuals who would go on to develop posttraumatic stress disorder from those who showed no lasting ill effects of their traumatic exposure (Segman et al. 2005).

Gladkevich et al. (2004) and Muller and Ackenheil (1998) concluded that disturbances in the major CNS neurotransmitter systems (dopaminergic, noradrenergic, and serotonergic) and in the HPA axis such as those observed in psychiatric disorders are concomitant with altered functioning and metabolism of lymphocytes. The similarities in the receptor properties and transduction processes of lymphocytes and the CNS suggest that lymphocytes may serve as a tool in the investigation of CNS pathology in psychiatric disorders. An early confirmatory result by our group (Tsuang et al. 2005) demonstrated the ability to discriminate between patients with schizophrenia, patients with bipolar disorder, and healthy controls with 95%–97% accuracy on the basis of the expression levels of as few as six genes. It should be noted that this work is preliminary and that additional replications need to be done. Vawter et al. (2004), using lymphocytic data from a high-density multiplex schizophrenia pedigree, applied microarray analysis to 1,128 brain-focused genes. They found two genes that were significantly downregulated and one that was significantly upregulated in comparison with family controls. These authors suggest screening a larger set of genes in additional schizophrenic families.

One potential concern in gene expression studies with relatives is whether or not the variation represents disease manifestations or family resemblance. Maas et al. (2005) examined gene transcript levels in unaffected first-degree relatives of patients with autoimmune disease and concluded that variations in transcript levels were associated with family resemblance rather than manifestations of disease. Aune et al. (2004), also studying autoimmune disease, found that lymphocytes from probands and unaffected first-degree relatives shared a common gene expression profile. These results suggest that the expression levels of certain genes may be under genetic control (i.e., they are heritable); however, the degree to which familial resemblance in expression levels translates into heritability is unknown. Furthermore, it remains to be determined if any disease-related genes also show heritable variation in affected and unaffected members of the same family.

Pilot Study of Gene Expression Profiles of Schizophrenia From Peripheral Blood

In the first study of its kind, we assessed the sensitivity and specificity of mRNA expression patterns in circulating peripheral blood samples from patients with DSM-IV–defined schizophrenia ($n = 30$) or bipolar disorder ($n = 16$) and control subjects ($n = 28$) (Tsuang et al. 2005) Approximately 10 mL of whole blood was collected from each subject, after which each blood sample was separated into plasma, buffy coat, and red blood cell (RBC) layers by centrifugation. Plasma was discarded, RBCs were ruptured, and each mixture was centrifuged to yield a pellet of white blood cells. Approximately 5 mg of mRNA was extracted from each reduced and purified blood sample and then profiled on either the Affymetrix U133A or the U133 Plus 2.0 GeneChip. Signal intensities of the gene expression images were trimmed, scaled, and normalized, and data were filtered so that only genes called present or marginal in at least 80% of the samples per group were used for further analysis. Sets of differentially expressed genes were identified by a combination of parametric and nonparametric tests with a threshold P value of 0.05 or less. Because of the relatively large number of significant genes, more stringent thresholds were also used to identify genes with even greater reliability. Unsupervised hierarchical cluster analysis was then performed to determine correlations between samples based on the identified sets of differentially expressed genes. Samples were grouped together according to the similarity of the expression levels of these genes.

This procedure identified 567 genes ($P<0.005$) that were differentially expressed between schizophrenia or bipolar disorder patients and controls. From this set of genes, eight of the best candidate biomarker genes (based on the magnitude of their fold-change difference between schizophrenia patients and controls) were then selected for verification by real-time quantitative reverse transcriptase polymerase chain reaction (QRT-PCR). Differential expression of each of these genes in the discrete subject groups was successfully demonstrated with this more sensitive and accurate mRNA quantification technique. Next, we evaluated the diagnostic accuracy (i.e., the probability of true vs. false-positive and true vs. false-negative calls) of our QRT-PCR data for these eight genes by receiver operating characteristic (ROC) curve analysis. Expression levels of these eight genes performed exceedingly well in classifying a separate sample of schizophrenia or bipolar disorder patients and controls. Figure 9–5 illustrates the ROC curves obtained for the optimal combination of these eight genes in differentiating schizophrenia patients from control subjects (panel A) and bipolar disorder patients (panel B). These ROC curves yielded areas under the curve ranging from 0.95 to 0.97, which corresponds to near-perfect diagnostic accuracy. We acknowledge that this exceptional performance was derived from the optimal combination of these markers and that such results may not be expected to generalize as well to samples from other populations; however, they certainly demonstrate the great potential utility of our methods, especially in comparison with other potential endophenotypic biomarkers for schizophrenia that are currently being pursued.

Subsequently, we reexamined these data with a more sophisticated approach, employing CORGON and MADCAP algorithms to limit the number of putative biomarker designations and to identify biological processes and molecular functions that are carried out by these differentially expressed genes (Glatt et al. 2005). Microarray analyses such as these are susceptible to false-positives, but CORGON yields a type I error rate of 4.4%; this is a substantial advance over the rates of 29% and 15% attained by other widely accepted methods (Affymetrix MicroArray Suite 5.0 and the method of Li et al. [2001], respectively). Application of the CORGON algorithm reduced the number of differentially expressed genes between schizophrenia patients and control subjects from 567 to 123. In addition, numerous ontological functions were significantly overrepresented among the differentially expressed genes in the peripheral blood of schizophrenia patients and controls, which is useful for suggesting possible etiological mechanisms beyond the single-gene level.

To validate these results, we sought comparable gene expression changes in the dorsolateral prefrontal cortex. By using the same conservative analytic strategy employing the CORGON and MADCAP algorithms, we identified 177

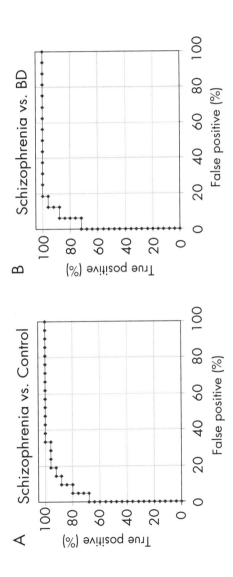

FIGURE 9–5. ROC curve analysis for pairwise comparisons of subject groups, showing that optimal combinations of eight genes differentiates subjects with schizophrenia from controls and from subjects with bipolar disorder (BD).

BD = bipolar disorder; ROC = receiver operating characteristic.

Source. Reprinted from Tsuang MT, Nossova N, Yager T, et al.: "Assessing the Validity of Blood-Based Gene Expression Profiles for the Classification of Schizophrenia and Bipolar Disorder: A Preliminary Report." *American Journal of Medical Genetics B: Neuropsychiatric Genetics* 133:1–5, 2005. Used with permission.

genes that were differentially expressed in postmortem dorsolateral prefrontal cortex (DLPFC) tissue between 19 schizophrenia cases and 27 nonpsychiatric control subjects in the National Brain Databank maintained by the Harvard Brain Tissue Resource Center. Of note, six genes (BTG1, GSK3A, HLA-DRB1, HNRPA3, SELENBP1, and SFRS1) were differentially expressed in both peripheral blood and postmortem DLPFC tissue from two entirely different samples of subjects. The strongest finding was for SELENBP1, which was significantly upregulated in both blood and brain in the schizophrenia patients. This constitutes a double replication, because we obtained the same finding in *two independent samples* in which we assessed *two different tissue compartments*. We also examined the protein expression pattern of SELENBP1 (which codes for selenium binding protein 1) and determined that the intensity and ratio of glial to neuronal SELENBP1-antibody staining was noticeably increased in DLPFC tissue from at least three of four schizophrenia patients. This gene also maps to chromosome 1q21–1q22, which has been implicated by linkage analysis as a strong candidate locus for harboring a risk gene for schizophrenia (Badner and Gershon 2002; Brzustowicz et al. 2000). The exact function of this gene is unknown, but our data, if replicated, suggest that it may be considered a high-likelihood putative biomarker for the illness that is worthy of functional characterization. This result in particular highlights a major benefit of our objective approach, which facilitates the identification of unconventional candidate risk genes for a complex polygenic disorder such as schizophrenia.

Thus, our results indicate that blood cell–derived mRNA profiles can differentiate schizophrenia and bipolar disorder patients and healthy control subjects with excellent sensitivity and specificity. These data support our hypothesis that blood cell–derived mRNA may allow identification of differentially expressed genes that are involved in the pathophysiology of the disorder. Although potential limitations of blood-based mRNA profiling of schizophrenia have been noted, our use of state-of-the-art data analytic and bioinformatics approaches offers several innovations to overcome these restrictions. In summary, this work demonstrates the vast potential utility of blood-based mRNA profiling as an objective approach to candidate risk-gene identification, which may be particularly advantageous for the study of schizophrenia because brain tissue biopsies are not obtainable from human subjects. Our evidence that peripheral blood cell gene expression patterns can accurately reflect aspects of gene expression in the brain strongly supports the further exploitation of this method for identifying components of the underlying pathology and pathophysiology of schizophrenia. It is also important to note the possibility that medication effects account for the schizophrenia–control differences in gene expression.

FUTURE DIRECTIONS

For more than 35 years, our research program has focused on understanding the nature, extent, and etiology of schizophrenia. As summarized in Table 9–1, the first phase of this research involved exploration of the nosology of schizophrenia, its familiality, its outcomes, and its forms of expression (e.g., its subtypes). The second phase focused on the heterogeneity of the disorder, including the nature of gender differences, neuropsychological weaknesses, range of treatment responses, and effects of adverse environmental events. The third phase expanded our horizon by focusing on brain-based abnormalities in schizophrenia and on the nature of the liability to develop the disorder. We are now well into the fourth phase of our work, which focuses further on the nature of the liability to schizophrenia, and in so doing, on the clinical implications of our research. As we learn to identify the nature of the liability to schizophrenia, we can focus our efforts in clinical intervention at earlier and earlier time points. In so doing, we contribute to the possibility that at some point, the course of schizophrenia may be attenuated, or even prevented.

Our continued ability to progress in this direction will involve multidisciplinary explorations and collaborations. One of the key components of these efforts will include a greater understanding of how genes interact with the environment to produce liability to, and protection from, major mental illness. In the near future, progress toward the ultimate goal of prevention is likely to reflect progress in interim goals, which include the following:

1. **Investigate gene expression patterns of first-degree relatives**—analyze the gene expression patterns of "normal" relatives of schizophrenia patients to circumvent the problems associated with the effects of the medications.
2. **Apply bioinformatics methodologies**—incorporate the vast amounts of information being generated in the fields of bioinformatics, especially proteomics and the fledgling field of metabolomics, to complement our genetic epidemiology studies.
3. **Focus on prevention**—obtain increased genetic and epidemiological information to allow us to move ever closer to our ultimate goal of prevention.

CLINICAL IMPLICATIONS

There is considerable evidence that the biological relatives of schizophrenic patients are at increased risk for schizophrenia and related disorders, but molecu-

Table 9–1. Stages in the study of schizophrenia directed by Ming T. Tsuang, M.D., Ph.D., over the last 35 years

Phase I	Phase II	Phase III	Phase IV
Nosology 1972–	Heterogeneity 1982–	Genes and brain 1992	Prevention 1998
Family studies	Neurophysiology	Structural MRI	High-risk children
Outcome	Gender differences	Functional MRI	Schizotaxia
Subtyping	Treatment response	Working memory	Early detection and intervention
Risk factors	Obstetric complications	Vulnerability markers	Development of innovative preventive treatments
	Negative/positive symptoms	Linkage and candidate genes	Genomics, proteomics, and metabolomics

lar genetic studies have been slow to identify susceptibility genes that contribute large proportions of vulnerability. If we are to make progress in identifying clinically relevant genetic influences, we will need to use informative measures of the relevant clinical phenomena.

We propose that the vulnerability to schizophrenia results from a combination of genes and adverse biological consequences of environmental events (e.g., pregnancy or delivery problems such as maternal diabetes or preeclampsia) in most cases, rather than from a major gene. Because schizophrenia is at least in part an outcome of a multifactorial, polygenic process in which multiple vulnerability factors of small or moderate effect contribute to the overall risk of developing psychosis, multiple phenotypic measures or combinations of measures should provide more predictive power than individual ones. Among the most promising approaches for identifying clinically useful measures is neuropsychological functioning. One of the most important avenues for future research will involve the attempt to define the potentially multifactorial manifestations of this genetic liability and to relate these manifestations directly to the responsible genes.

REFERENCES

American Psychiatric Association: Diagnostic and Statistical Manual of Mental Disorders, 4th Edition. Washington, DC, American Psychiatric Association, 1994

Andreasen NC: The Scale for the Assessment of Negative Symptoms (SANS). Iowa City, University of Iowa, 1983

Aune TM, Parker JS, Maas K, et al: Co-localization of differentially expressed genes and shared susceptibility loci in human autoimmunity. Genet Epidemiol 27:162–172, 2004

Badner JA, Gershon ES: Meta-analysis of whole-genome linkage scans of bipolar disorder and schizophrenia. Mol Psychiatry 7:405–411, 2002

Brzustowicz LM, Hodgkinson KA, Chow EW, et al: Location of a major susceptibility locus for familial schizophrenia on chromosome 1q21–q22. Science 288:678–682, 2000

Chapman LJ, Chapman JP, Raulin ML: Scales for physical and social anhedonia. J Abnorm Psychol 87:374–407, 1976

Chen WJ, Liu SK, Chang CJ, et al: Sustained attention deficit and schizotypal personality features in nonpsychotic relatives of schizophrenic patients. Am J Psychiatry 155:1214–1220, 1998

Dazzan P, Kravariti E, Fearon P, et al: Is the development of schizophrenia predictable? In Early Clinical Intervention and Prevention in Schizophrenia. Edited by Stone WS, Faraone SV, Tsuang MT. Totowa, NJ, Humana Press, 2004, pp 225–252

DeLisi LE: Critical overview of current approaches to genetic mechanisms in schizophrenia research. Brain Res Rev 31:187–192, 2000

Derogatis L: SCL-90-R Manual II. Towson, MD, Clinical Psychometric Research, 1983

Eisen MB, Brown PO: DNA arrays for analysis of gene expression. Methods Enzymol 303:179–205, 1999

Eisen MB, Spellman PT, Brown PO, et al: Cluster analysis and display of genome wide expression patterns. Proc Natl Acad Sci U S A 95:14863–14868, 1998

Erlenmeyer-Kimling L: Neurobehavioral deficits in offspring of schizophrenic parents: liability indicators and predictors of illness. Am J Med Genet (Neuropsychiatr Genet) 97:65–71, 2000

Faraone SV, Kremen WS, Lyons MJ, et al: Diagnostic accuracy and linkage analysis: how useful are schizophrenia spectrum phenotypes? Am J Psychiatry 152:1286–1290, 1995a

Faraone SV, Seidman LJ, Kremen WS, et al: Neuropsychological functioning among the nonpsychotic relatives of schizophrenic patients: a diagnostic efficiency analysis. J Abnorm Psychol 104:286–304, 1995b

Faraone SV, Seidman LJ, Kremen WS, et al: Neuropsychological functioning among the nonpsychotic relatives of schizophrenic patients: a four-year follow-up study. J Abnorm Psychol 108:176–181, 1999

Faraone SV, Seidman LJ, Kremen WS, et al: Neuropsychological functioning among the nonpsychotic relatives of schizophrenic patients: the effect of genetic loading. Biol Psychiatry 48:120–126, 2000

Faraone SV, Green AI, Seidman LJ, et al: "Schizotaxia": clinical implications and new directions for research. Schizophr Bull 27:1–18, 2001

Faraone SV, Seidman LJ, Kremen WS, et al: Structural brain abnormalities among relatives of patients with schizophrenia: implications for linkage studies. Schizophr Res 60:125–140, 2003

Felten D, Felten S, Bellinger D, et al: Noradrenergic sympathetic neural interactions with immune system: structure and function. Immunol Rev 100:225–226, 1987

Ganguli R, Brar JS, Chengappa KR, et al: Mitogen-stimulated interleukin-2 production in never-medicated first episode schizophrenic patients. The influence of age at onset and negative symptoms. Arch Gen Psychiatry 52:668–672, 1995

Gladkevich A, Kauffman HF, Korf J: Lymphocytes as a neural probe: potential for studying psychiatric disorders. Prog Neuropsychopharmacol Biol Psychiatry 28:559–576, 2004

Glatt SJ, Everall IP, Kreman WS, et al: Comparative gene expression analysis of blood and brain provides concurrent validation of SELENBP1 up-regulation in schizophrenia. Proc Natl Acad Sci U S A 102:15533–15538, 2005

Gottesman II: Psychopathology through a life-span genetic prism. Am Psychol 56:864–878, 2001

Gottesman II, Gould TD: The endophenotype concept in psychiatry: etymology and strategic intentions. Am J Psychiatry 160:636–645, 2003

Green MF: What are the functional consequences of neurocognitive deficits in schizophrenia. Am J Psychiatry 153:321–330, 1996

Green MF, Kern RS, Braff DL, et al: Neurocognitive deficits and functional outcome in schizophrenia: are we measuring the "right stuff"? Schizophr Bull 26:119–136, 2000

Hakak Y, Walker JR, Li C, et al: Genome-wide expression analysis reveals dysregulation of myelination-related genes in chronic schizophrenia. Proc Natl Acad Sci U S A 98:4746–4751, 2001

Harrison PJ, Weinberger DR: Schizophrenia genes, gene expression, and neuropathology: on the matter of their convergence. Mol Psychiatry 10:40–68, 2005

Heinrichs RW: The primacy of cognition in schizophrenia. Am Psychol 60:229–242, 2005

Heinrichs RW, Zakzanis KK: Neurocognitive deficit in schizophrenia: a quantitative review of the evidence. Neuropsychology 12:426–445, 1998

Inglot AD, Leszek J, Piasecki E, et al: Interferon responses in schizophrenia and major depressive disorders. Biol Psychiatry 35:464–473, 1994

Kendler KS: Twin studies of psychiatric illness: an update. Arch Gen Psychiatry 58:1005–1014, 2001

Kremen WS, Hoff AL: Neurocognitive deficits in the biological relatives of individuals with schizophrenia, in Early Clinical Intervention and Prevention with Schizophrenia. Edited by Stone WS, Faraone SV, Tsuang MT. Totowa, NJ, Humana Press, 2004, pp 133–158

Li T, Underhill J, Liu XH, et al: Transmission disequilibrium analysis of HLA class II DRB1, DQA1, DQB1 and DPB1 polymorphisms in schizophrenia using family trios from a Han Chinese population. Schizophr Res 49:73–78, 2001

Lyons MJ, Toomey R, Seidman LJ, et al: Verbal learning and memory in relatives of schizophrenics: preliminary findings. Biol Psychiatry 37:750–753, 1995

Maas K, Chen H, Shyr Y, et al: Shared gene expression profiles in individuals with autoimmune disease and unaffected first-degree relatives of individuals with autoimmune disease. Hum Mol Genet 14:1305–1314, 2005

Marcotte ER, Srivastava LK, Quirion R: cDNA microarray and proteomic approaches in the study of brain diseases: focus on schizophrenia and Alzheimer's disease. Pharmacol Ther 100:63–74, 2003

Meehl PE: Schizotaxia, schizotypy, schizophrenia. Am Psychol 17:827–838, 1962

Meehl PE: Schizotaxia revisited. Arch Gen Psychiatry 46:935–944, 1989

Minagar A, Shapshak P, Duran EM, et al: HIV-associated dementia, Alzheimer's disease, multiple sclerosis, and schizophrenia: gene expression review. J Neurol Sci 224:3–17, 2004

Mirnics K, Middleton FA, Lewis DA, et al: Analysis of complex brain disorders with gene expression microarrays: schizophrenia as a disease of the synapse. Trends Neurosci 24:479–486, 2001

Muller N, Ackenheil M: Psychoneuroimmunology and the cytokine action in the CNS: implications for psychiatric disorders. Prog Neuropsychopharmacol Biol Psychiatry 22:1–33, 1998

Palotas A, Puskas LG, Kitajka K, et al: Altered response to mirtazapine on gene expression profile of lymphocytes from Alzheimer's patients. Eur J Pharmacol 497:247–254, 2004a

Palotas A, Puskas LG, Kitajka K, et al: The effect of citalopram on gene expression profile of Alzheimer lymphocytes. Neurochem Res 29:1563–1570, 2004b

Rado S: Dynamics and classification of disordered behavior. Am J Psychiatry 110:406–416, 1953

Rado S: Theory and therapy: the theory of schizotypal organization and its application to the treatment of decompensated schizotypal behavior, in The Outpatient Treatment of Schizophrenia. Edited by Scher SC, Davis HR. New York, Grune & Stratton, 1960, pp 87–101

Ryan MCM, Thakore JH: Physical consequences of schizophrenia and its treatment: the metabolic syndrome. Life Sci 71:239–257, 2002

Satagopan JM, Panageas KS: Tutorial in biostatistics: a statistical perspective on gene expression data analysis. Stat Med 22:481–499, 2003

Segman RH, Shefi N, Goltser-Dubner T, et al: Peripheral blood mononuclear cell gene expression profiles identify emergent post-traumatic stress disorder among trauma survivors. Mol Psychiatry 10:500–513, 2005

Seidman LJ, Wencel HE: Genetically mediated brain abnormalities in schizophrenia. Curr Psychiatry Rep 5:135–144, 2003

Seidman LJ, Faraone SV, Goldstein JM, et al: Left hippocampal volume as a vulnerability indicator for schizophrenia: a magnetic resonance imaging morphometric study of nonpsychotic first-degree relatives. Arch Gen Psychiatry 59:839–849, 2002

Seidman LJ, Pantelis C, Keshavan MS, et al: A review and a new report of medial temporal lobe dysfunction as a vulnerability indicator for schizophrenia: a MRI morphometric family study of the parahippocampal gyrus. Schizophr Bull 29:803–808, 2003

Seidman LJ, Wencel HE, McDonald C, et al: Neuroimaging studies of nonpsychotic first-degree relatives of people with schizophrenia, in Early Clinical Intervention and Prevention in Schizophrenia. Edited by Stone WS, Faraone SV, Tsuang MT. Totowa, NJ, Humana Press, 2004, pp 179–210

Snitz BE, Macdonald AW 3rd, Carter CS: Cognitive deficits in unaffected first-degree relatives of schizophrenia patients: a meta-analytic review of putative endophenotypes. Schizophr Bull 32:179–194, 2006

Stone WS, Faraone SV, Seidman LJ, et al: Concurrent validation of schizotaxia: a pilot study. Biol Psychiatry 50:434–440, 2001

Stone WS, Glatt SJ, Faraone SV: The biology of schizotaxia, in Early Clinical Intervention and Prevention of Schizophrenia. Edited by Stone WS, Faraone SV, Tsuang MT. Totowa, NJ, Humana Press, 2004, pp 339–353

Stone WS, Faraone SV, Seidman LJ, et al: Searching for the liability to schizophrenia: concepts and methods underlying genetic high-risk studies of adolescents. J Child Adolesc Psychopharmacol 15:403–417, 2005

Tkachev D, Mimmack ML, Ryan MM, et al: Oligodendrocyte dysfunction in schizophrenia and bipolar disorder. Lancet 362:798–805, 2003

Toomey R, Faraone SV, Seidman LJ, et al: Association of vulnerability markers in relatives of schizophrenic patients. Schizophr Res 31:89–98, 1998

Tsuang MT, Stone WS, Faraone SV: Schizophrenia: a review of genetic studies. Harv Rev Psychiatry 7:185–207, 1999a

Tsuang MT, Stone WS, Seidman LJ, et al: Treatment of nonpsychotic relatives of patients with schizophrenia: four case studies. Biol Psychiatry 41:1412–1418, 1999b

Tsuang MT, Stone WS, Tarbox SI, et al: An integration of schizophrenia with schizotypy: identification of schizotaxia and implications for research on treatment and prevention. Schizophr Res 54:169–175, 2002

Tsuang MT, Nossova N, Yager T, et al: Assessing the validity of blood-based gene expression profiles for the classification of schizophrenia and bipolar disorder: a preliminary report. Am J Med Genet B Neuropsychiatr Genet 133:1–5, 2005

Vawter MP, Ferran E, Galke B, et al: Microarray screening of lymphocyte gene expression differences in a multiplex schizophrenia pedigree. Schizophr Res 67:41–52, 2004

Weissman M, Bothwell S: Assessment of social adjustment by patient self-report. Arch Gen Psychiatry 33:1111–1115, 1976

Part IV

NIH Perspectives on Prevention

10

Prospects for the Prevention of Mental Illness

Integrating Neuroscience and Behavior

Cheryl A. Boyce, Ph.D.
Robert Heinssen, Ph.D.
Courtney B. Ferrell, Ph.D.
Richard K. Nakamura, Ph.D.

The President's New Freedom Commission on Mental Health (2003) (hereafter called the President's Commission) encouraged the field to "accelerate research to promote recovery and resilience, and ultimately to cure and prevent mental illness" (p. 21). The urgency for increased prevention efforts seems evident with reports from the World Health Organization (2002) that mental illness is the primary cause of disease burden in the United States and Canada among those in our population that should be the healthiest and most productive, 15- to 44-year-olds. In fact, one mental illness, unipolar depression, is ranked as the number-one cause of disability among all ages, with bipolar disorder and schizophrenia also among the top 10 causes (World Health Organization 2002). Other estimates for both younger and older populations in the United States provoke similar concerns about the extent of mental illness and the burden it places on individuals and society (National Institute of Mental Health 1999, 2003).

From both an economic and a social-capital perspective, prevention of illness is clearly more desirable than treatment of diseases that have a course that is often chronic or with repeated episodes. Health economists have modeled and projected the effects of prevention across the life span and have estimated the economic burden of mental illness (Ringel and Sturm 2001). Estimates of the direct costs of mental illness are about 79 billion dollars in the United States. The public sector (i.e., Medicaid, Medicare, state and local government) bears responsibility for more than 50% of all mental health expenditures (President's Commission 2003). In addition to increased health care costs, the indirect costs of mental illness are large. For example, due to the negative impact of serious mental illness on employment capacity, individuals with serious mental illnesses represent the single largest diagnostic group (35%) of social security disability benefit recipients (President's Commission 2003). Benefits of prevention relate not only to the personal and economic costs of mental illness but also to the effects of mental illness on mortality. The vast majority of suicide deaths (90%) involve a mental disorder (Institute of Medicine 2002); in 2002 there were 31,655 suicide deaths, compared with 17,638 homicide deaths (Centers for Disease Control and Prevention 2006b). In 2001, suicide was the third leading cause of death among adolescent and young adult populations 15–24 years of age (Centers for Disease Control and Prevention 2006a). It is too rarely recognized that mental illnesses are nearly unique among diseases in creating a level of pain and suffering that can cause individuals to end their lives.

Identifying individuals at risk for mental disorders and their recurrence as early as possible is the key to successful prevention efforts. To reduce the personal, economic, and social burdens of mental illness, the President's Commission (2003) recommended "early detection, assessment and links with treatment and supports" (p. 9) to help prevent mental health problems from worsening. Similarly, in 2005 the U.S. Preventive Services Task Force recommended preventive services, including screening in the primary care setting by clinicians, for mental health conditions and substance abuse. In addition to these general recommendations for increased mental health prevention efforts, the Office of the Surgeon General formally issued a "call to action" for increased suicide prevention efforts (U.S. Public Health Service 1999). The Surgeon General has also identified prevention of child maltreatment, a risk factor for mental illness, as a priority area (U.S. Department of Health and Human Services 2005).

In this chapter we describe a framework for prevention of mental illness that has evolved from recent scientific discoveries on multiple levels, from the cellular, systems, and individual levels to the community environment. Innovative prospects for the prevention of mental illness have emerged from the environmental context and from neuroscience research that will have an important public health impact. Multidisciplinary, translational research perspectives offer exciting new directions for the prevention of mental illness across the developmental life span. National Institute of Mental Health (NIMH) prevention efforts have focused on pre-onset phenomena, but there are opportunities to establish translational links between emerging findings from the basic sciences, and describing potential applications in contemporary prevention science.

EVOLUTION OF A FRAMEWORK FOR PREVENTION OF MENTAL ILLNESS

Prevention traditionally refers to interventions that are applied before the onset of a clinically diagnosable disorder with the aim of reducing the number of new cases of that disorder (Muñoz et al. 1996). Preventive methods can be viewed as any attempt to prevent entry to, or progression along, the pathway toward a severe, debilitating psychological disorder (Mrazek and Haggerty 1994). An earlier report from the Institute of Medicine (1994) on the prospects for preventing mental illness proposed a tight definition of prevention that distinguished prevention efforts from treatment interventions. However, as knowledge about the causes, prevention, and treatment of mental illness has expanded, the definition of prevention has also expanded. The NIMH definition of prevention research is somewhat broader than those presented above. In addition to interest in preventing onset, NIMH emphasizes the importance of preventing relapse, disability, and comorbidity among persons already diagnosed with a mental disorder. The landmark Workgroup Report on Prevention from the National Advisory Mental Health Council in 1998 (National Advisory Mental Health Council Workgroup on Mental Disorders Prevention Research 2001) expanded the continuum of mental health interventions to include preventive measures for at-risk populations, acute treatment for persons with newly diagnosed disorders, and maintenance care for those with established mental illness. The goal of the report was to minimize gaps between prevention and basic risk-factor research at one end of the spectrum, and between prevention and treatment at the other end.

Universal preventive interventions for mental disorders are targeted to the general public or to a whole-population group that has not been identified on the basis of risk. There are few examples of universal interventions to prevent occurrence of mental disorders or behavioral problems with strong scientific evidence. *Selective* preventive interventions are targeted to individuals belonging to subgroups of the population whose risk of developing mental disorders is significantly higher than average. The risk may be an imminent risk or a lifetime risk. Generally, selective interventions do not exceed a moderate level of cost. Examples of selective interventions include classroom-based social skills programs for all children attending elementary schools within a high-crime area (Schmidt and Vasey 2002), nurse home-visitation programs for pregnant adolescents (Olds 2002), and classroom management training for teachers working in schools that have a high proportion of disruptive students (Horne et al. 1999). Such interventions reduce the occurrence of externalizing disorders, high-risk behaviors, and substance abuse.

Indicated preventive interventions are targeted to high-risk individuals who are identified as having minimal but detectable signs or symptoms that foreshadow mental disorder. For example, low-dose antipsychotic pharmacotherapy or cognitive-behavioral therapy (CBT) for persons in the prodromal phase of schizophrenia have been demonstrated to be effective indicated preventive intervention strategies (McGorry et al. 2002). Most prevention research in mental health has involved selective and indicated interventions. The cost for universal interventions that target a large group may initially be very expensive when compared with selected or indicated preventive interventions, although the long-term benefits may be substantial.

NIMH goals for prevention research are to support evidence-based approaches that improve our ability to 1) detect mental illness risk across all stages of human development, 2) chart the nonlinear progression of risk to active illness, 3) neutralize causal risk factors with effective interventions, 4) adapt highly controlled prevention methods for real-world settings, and 5) disseminate and implement effective programs in the community. We can expand the effectiveness of known efficacious interventions for use with additional populations, new settings, and people with comorbid disorders by integrating the strong evidence on environmental context and new discoveries in neuroscience.

INTEGRATING NEUROSCIENCE PERSPECTIVES

New prospects for the prevention of mental illness have emerged not only from research evidence from traditional psychosocial models of risk factors and preventive interventions but also from advances in neuroscience. The complex integration of environmental context and neuroscience has yet to be explored to its full potential for prevention research. This broadening of prevention to include neuroscience and behavior must be developed. The key insight is that the brain is not the static structure that it was thought to be until the discovery of adult neurogenesis in humans in 1998 (Eriksson et al. 1998). The brain is now known to respond to changes in behavior and the environment with changes in its physical structure and molecular dynamics. The development of the brain in infancy and childhood is also known to be heavily dependent on the interaction of the inherited genes with behavior and the environment, with lifelong consequences. The challenge remains for neuroscientists not only to theorize about models of mental illness from new discoveries, but also to use prevention designs to truly test their hypotheses (Reiss 2001). There are promising interactive methods from neuroscience that can lead to prevention, including the plasticity of the genotype, dynamic phenotype, functional imaging, and animal models of brain and behavior. The discovery of permanent genetic modification through environmental manipulations can provide new information not only to understand mental disorders but also to reduce risk for mental illness.

Our genes specify a general plan with many options. The brain changes its physical structure through behavior and interactions with the environment. Various mechanisms of neural plasticity may affect behavior and cognition: neurogenesis, apoptosis, epigenetics, gene promoters and repressors, synapse modification (i.e., vesicle control and receptor changes), and microRNAs.

Although born with genetic vulnerabilities and/or resilience, children and adolescents have developmental plasticity and can adapt to changes in the environment with positive or negative mental health outcomes. Mental disorders such as autism, schizophrenia, and bipolar disorder have high heritability. Prevention for these mental disorders is challenging and requires the integration of genetic knowledge with disease etiology to develop efficacious preventive interventions. Early results from interventions in the prodrome of schizophrenia—which suggest the potential efficacy of CBT to significantly prevent or delay onset of frank psychosis—are very promising (Morrison et al. 2004).

Mapping of the human genome was completed in 2003 and this is just the first step toward understanding how genes relate to the complex disease process of mental disorders. Although the most common mental illnesses are not Mendelian, already there are promising results in identifying potential vulnerability genes for depression (*5-HTT, MAOA*) (Online Mendelian Inheritance in Man: Depression 2006), anxiety (*MAOA*) (Online Mendelian Inheritance in Man: Anxiety 2006), and schizophrenia (*neuregulin-1, COMT*) (Online Mendelian Inheritance in Man: Schizophrenia 2006). We expect that further identification of vulnerability genes will permit a better understanding of individual variation that could be important for targeted prevention efforts. Confirmed vulnerability genes will lead to an iterative process that will stratify patient populations and permit further identification of disease processes through the understanding of gene function and participation within neural circuits.

In the next phase of genomic research, the International HapMap Project, additional common patterns of human genetic variation or the human haplotype map will be explored (International HapMap Consortium 2005). However, mental disorders such as Alzheimer's disease and schizophrenia are caused by many genetic variants and common variations that individually have a relatively weak contribution to the disorder and a small effect on susceptibility, but together can increase the risk of illness (Insel 2005a). It is not expected that the HapMap will reveal genes for mental disorders, single genes of large effect, or a revolution in the diagnosis of mental disorder (Insel 2005b). However, genes channel behavior, and understanding their influence is crucial for unlocking the mechanisms and targets for preventive interventions. Once we have identified genes that confer vulnerability, research to identify the detailed functions of those genes is expected to yield major clues to the elusive etiology of mental disorder.

In some instances, the environment can change gene activity. Paradigms in which animals are cross-fostered to experience different maternal behaviors than would be expected as original offspring demonstrate that an epigenomic state of a gene can be affected by behavioral programming (Meaney and Szyf 2005). Active licking and grooming of rat pups by their dams can permanently modify the activity of the glucocorticoid receptor gene in the pups, making them more resilient to subsequent stressors.

Treatments for mood and anxiety disorders are thought to work, in part, by helping patients control the stresses in their lives. A study in rats provides insight into the brain mechanisms likely involved. When a stressor is perceived to be controllable, an executive hub in the frontal lobes of the brain suppresses an alarm center deep in the brain stem, preventing the adverse behavioral and physiological effects of uncontrollable stress (Amat et al. 2005). Other recent evidence suggesting that antidepressants may act by triggering the birth of new neurons in the adult hippocampus, the brain's memory hub, has heightened interest in adult neurogenesis (Henn and Vollmayr 2004). New neurons may also sprout in the parts of the adult brain involved in the thinking and mood disturbances of depression and anxiety. Scientists have found newly born neurons that communicate via the chemical messenger gamma-aminobutyric acid (GABA) in the adult rat cortex. This is the site of higher-order executive functions and, in the striatum, the site of habits, reward, and motor skill learning. In the cortex, the new neurons appear to arise from previously unknown precursor cells native to the area, rather than from cells migrating from another area (Dayer et al. 2005).

Our ability to visualize brain changes reflecting the neurocircuitry underlying behavior, as well as reflecting changes in the environment or disease states, is also increasing dramatically. The ability of a key anterior cingulate structure in the frontal lobe to suppress fear and anxiety in both rape victims and veterans of war trauma has been a critical insight and enables both pharmaceutical firms and psychotherapists to target this circuit for both therapy and prevention of disorders such as posttraumatic stress disorder (PTSD) (Lanius et al. 2004).

Environmental and other nongenetic factors also contribute to the risk and expression of mental disorders and make it more difficult to identify genetic factors. Promising epidemiological research studies from New Zealand by Caspi et al. (2002) have examined the interaction of genotype with environment for the development of depression and antisocial personality disorder. Here, a large sample of male children was followed from birth to adulthood, which has allowed insight into why some children who are maltreated grow up to develop antisocial behavior, whereas others do not. A functional polymorphism in the gene encoding the neurotransmitter-metabolizing enzyme monoamine oxidase A (*MAOA*) was found to moderate the effect of maltreatment. Maltreated children with a genotype conferring high levels of *MAOA* expression were less likely to develop antisocial behavior. These findings may partly explain why not all victims of maltreatment grow up to victimize others, and they provide epidemiological evidence that genotypes can moderate children's sensitivity to environmental insults, and strongly suggest that interventions that reduce early maltreatment can reduce vulnerability to disorder.

Another study by the same research team (Caspi et al. 2003) examined the interaction of genes and environment in depression. A functional polymorphism in the promoter region of the serotonin transporter gene (*5-HTT*) was found to modulate the influence of stressful life events. Those individuals with one or two copies of the short allele of the *5-HTT* promoter polymorphism exhibited more depressive symptoms, diagnosable depression, and suicidality in relation to stressful life events than did individuals who were homozygous for the long allele. Individuals with this specific genotype who experienced more than four episodes of life stress were more likely than those with other genotypes to develop major depressive disorder. Genotype interacted with stress in the environmental context to increase the risk for depression. Together, these studies suggest the importance of identifying risk and preventive interventions for the reduction of serious mental illness and behavioral disorders. These findings provide evidence of a gene–environment interaction in which an individual's response to environmental insults is moderated by his or her genetic makeup.

Neuroscience innovations can provide evidence of treatment-specific effects for pharmacological as well as behavioral prevention therapies. For example, CBT has been shown to modulate the functioning of sites in the limbic and cortical regions of the brain, similar to other antidepressant treatments (Goldapple et al. 2004). There may be varying mechanisms and effects on regions of the brain according to the treatment modality. In this example, neuroscience technologies provided evidence for the support of behavioral research.

INCORPORATING ENVIRONMENTAL CONTEXT

Given the continued focus on the prevention of mental illness, it is important to recognize the progress that has been made thus far in regard to prevention research. Rigorous scientific trials have been conducted showing the efficacy of psychosocial prevention programs for both externalizing disorders such as conduct problems (e.g., Berrento-Clement et al. 1984; Brown et al., Chapter 15, this volume) and internalizing disorders such as depression (e.g., Muñoz et al. 1987). Examining the environmental context and identifying potential risk factors in the development of disorders has been the stronghold of prevention research. Current shifts in the prevention literature have highlighted the notion that there does not appear to be one single pathway in the development of mental disorders, nor does there appear to be one single risk factor associated with outcome. Instead, there is greater acknowledgement regarding the contribution of both genetic predisposition and environmental context in the development of mental disorders.

Disruptive Behavioral Disorders

NIMH has been supporting research on disruptive behavior problems for several decades. To a great extent, this work has focused on the identification of powerful and malleable risk factors and on interventions to reduce disruptive behavior problems. There have been a number of activities that involve a careful examination of research progress and gaps in knowledge in areas relevant to childhood behavior problems. For example, the report "Taking Stock of Risk Factors for Child/Youth Externalizing Behavior Problems" (Hann 2001) summarized what is known about risk factors and interventions for disruptive behavior disorders of youth, and "Youth Violence: A Report of the Surgeon General" (U.S. Public Health Service 2001) reviewed violence risk and intervention research findings. Research has led to the development of several psychosocial and behavioral intervention strategies effective for reducing child and adolescent behavioral problems and improving social, emotional, and academic skills. These interventions tend to be multifaceted, targeting multiple risk and protective factors (e.g., academic and social skills, cognitive biases, discipline, association with delinquent peers), and have relevance at different points in development and in different settings—and, thus, involve different targets (e.g., parents, teachers, youth), service sectors, and providers.

In October 2004, the National Institutes of Health (NIH) convened a state-of-the-science conference, "Preventing Violence and Related Health-Risking Social Behaviors in Adolescents," to examine and summarize the progress within prevention science for externalizing disorders in youth. Leading investigators in the field examined current risk factors, developmental psychopathology, and intervention literatures and concluded that the following elements were essential in creating successful prevention programs: 1) awareness of multiple, overlapping risk factors as predictors of violence and conduct problems; 2) integrative conceptual models that emphasize transactional relationships among risk factors; and 3) developmentally based, multicomponent prevention programs and sustained prevention efforts across developmental periods.

Relative to other prevention targets, the literature that addresses prevention of externalizing disorders is fairly mature. Successful prevention research for externalizing disorders has moved beyond the efficacy and effectiveness stages. Existing multicomponent programs are now poised for dissemination and implementation research (for details, see Chambers et al. 2005).

Depressive and Anxiety Disorders

The internalizing prevention research literature is similar to the externalizing research literature in that more than one pathway or set of risk factors is associated with the development of disorders. However, the examination of these pathways is primarily new in comparison with the studies conducted within the externalizing literature. Evidence for the biomedical and behavioral influences for depressive and anxiety disorders suggest new targets for early prevention.

Depressive Disorders

Numerous etiological models have described a diathesis-stress model for the development of depression (Garber 2006). This integrative model proposed that there are overlapping risk factors that interact over time. Specifically, an individual's genetic vulnerability predicts his or her response to stressors. Environmental factors can also influence the individual's response to stressors, which in turn can lead to symptoms associated with internalizing disorders. Given this framework, prevention programs for depressive disorders tend to be more focused on a narrower set of targets (e.g., family treatment at the environmental level; CBT at the individual diathesis level). In addition, programs designed to prevent depression are often time-limited and therefore not sustainable across developmental periods. NIMH has recognized that additional work is needed to examine 1) depressive risk factors over developmental periods and 2) the efficacy of multicomponent prevention programs for depression.

The picture appears more complex for the prevention of bipolar disorder. Although individuals with bipolar disorder are at high risk for poor functioning and other negative outcomes, prevention is primarily at the tertiary level. Although there is some disagreement by scientists on the exact phenomenology of bipolar disorder among children, the first longitudinal cohorts of children of parents with bipolar disorder suggest that they are at increased risk for depressive and anxiety disorders and may benefit from preventive interventions. Other research suggests that bipolar disorder that begins in childhood or early adolescence may be more severe and more likely to be comorbid with attentional and behavioral disorders compared with bipolar disorder with an onset in late adolescence or adulthood (Carlson et al. 1998; Geller and Luby 1997). As we learn more about early risk for specific types of depressive disorders, preventive efforts can incorporate proven psychopharmacology and behavioral and functioning outcomes.

Anxiety Disorders

Preventive interventions for anxiety have encompassed the full range of prevention programs, from universal to indicated (Feldner et al. 2004). For example, universal programs have been designed to reduce nonspecific anxiety symptoms (e.g., Barrett and Turner 2001), selected interventions have targeted anxiety sensitivity (e.g., Schmidt and Vasey 2002), and indicated programs have focused on anxiety symptoms while aiming to prevent the development of nonspecific psychopathology (e.g., Dadds et al. 1999). Results from these programs indicate that preventive interventions are effective in reducing anxiety symptoms, especially the development of nonspecific anxiety symptoms. Anxiety prevention studies are at the stage of testing and replicating prevention programs. However, more work needs to be done in the area of pointed prevention programs that focus on specific anxiety disorders. Specifically, current prevention programs are generally modifications of existing intervention strategies and, therefore, often lack the ability to target specific or theorized risk factors (Feldner et al. 2004).

More recently, a focus within the anxiety literature has been on examining the role of the brain in the fear response and anxiety disorders. For example, studies of both animals and humans suggests that the amygdala is implicated in the fear response. Specifically, greater activation of the amygdala in the presence of novel versus familiar faces has been reported with adults (Schwartz et al. 2003). Findings such as these have great implications for further prevention development, as the amygdala's role is to prepare the body for quick action before the cognitive aspects of the brain are capable of processing feared stimuli. Targeted prevention programs could focus on increasing cognitive control over the amygdala so as to interrupt the "act now, think later" process, rather than to continue to focus on nonspecific anxiety symptoms as means of preventive intervention. Alternatively, since the amygdala response can be controlled by the medial prefrontal cortex (MPC), perhaps the MPC responses could be strengthened via behavioral or medication intervention (Milad and Quirk 2002; Shin et al. 2001).

Aside from anxiety symptoms in general, some work has been done in examining specific anxiety disorders with respect to avenues for prevention work. For example, within the literature on PTSD, building on prior studies that examined the role of stress and catecholamines, new research is examining whether chemicals such as propranolol, which block abnormal stress responses after a trauma, can prevent the development or reduce the severity of PTSD (e.g., Vaiva et al. 2003; see also Pitman and Delahanty, Chapter 16, this volume). Other studies are focusing on the anticonvulsant gabapentin, which has primarily been used to prevent seizures in epilepsy, in improving PTSD symptomatology, particularly sleep difficulties (e.g., Hamner et al. 2001). Brain regions such as the amygdala are areas of interest for PTSD studies and suggest the possibility of predicting which individuals may be at risk for PTSD in real-world settings.

Converging multidisciplinary studies have already led to the development and testing of new preventive and treatment interventions for PTSD. There is much that remains to be clarified, such as the exact causes of lowered cortisol levels in people and recently reported neuroanatomical differences in people with PTSD. Nonetheless, research directions for the future point to exciting pathways of discovery and improved treatment and prevention of PTSD, especially with adult populations.

Neurodevelopmental Disorders

As mentioned previously, a large part of prevention research involves the identification of risk factors associated with the development of disorders. With respect to the etiology of neurodevelopmental disorders, most of the focus has been on identifying biological risk factors. Most notably, research on schizophrenia and autism has focused on examining biological markers because of the high degree of heritability associated with each disorder. However, it is becoming increasingly evident that these disorders do not develop from genetic abnormalities alone. Accordingly, current attention has shifted to examine not only the biological risk factors but also the environmental risk factors and the interplay between them. For example, it is now becoming recognized that environment, both prenatal and postnatal, plays a role in shaping brain development and subsequent behavior (National Advisory Mental Health Council Blueprint for Change 2001). In addition, further investigation into how environmental exposures during prenatal development can cause changes in the neurobiology of this process may lead to areas of future prevention development.

Autism

Prevention research for autism is in its infancy as a result of the complexities associated with establishing the disorder's etiology. Given the high degree of heritability of autism, much of the early preventive efforts have focused on attempting to identify particular genes that may be implicated in the development of this disorder. To date, several studies, including studies funded by NIH, have shown that there is in fact a genetic component associated with autism (Veenstra-Vanderweele and Cook 2003). Specifically, the genetic basis of autism has been supported by family and twin studies at Studies to Advance Autism Research and Treatment (STAART) centers funded by NIH. However, no specific gene or brain region has been implicated in the development of autism, and the growth of prevalence rates suggest that environmental influences may play a role in the development of autism (Lawler et al. 2004).

Although autism prevalence rates have soared almost 10 times in recent decades (Rutter 2005), debate continues as to whether this is a true increase in prevalence or an artifact. New theories have been proposed regarding the etiology of autism as a result. It is now suspected that autism may be a disease of very early fetal development, and that environmental complications during pregnancy could cause or contribute to autism (London 2000). Several large, population-based studies have shown that pregnancy complications and adverse birth outcomes are associated with an increased risk of autism (Hultman et al. 2002).

Further investigation into perinatal factors has shown that increased autism risk may involve the interaction of a genetic vulnerability and adverse environmental events during early development (Glasson et al. 2004; Larsson et al. 2005).

The literature examining pre- and perinatal environmental influences in relation to risk for the development of autism is growing and could therefore serve as an opportunity for future prevention research. If evidence continues to support adverse pre- or perinatal events as risk factors in the development of autism, then such events could serve as potential targets in prevention and intervention efforts (Newschaffer and Cole 2005). Under the leadership and direction of NIMH, the Interagency Autism Coordinating Committee has developed a research matrix for prioritizing research in autism, and among the major elements of the research matrix is a call for research on genetic and nongenetic causes of autism and their interactions.

Schizophrenia

Prevention efforts are still in the earliest stages for the most serious mental disorders such as schizophrenia, but some exciting developments in psychopathology research raise hope for the future. Although the empirical literature on prevention of schizophrenia is very limited, emerging research on the earliest prepsychotic phases of this disorder is occurring worldwide. Since 2000, NIMH has funded seven investigations as part of the North American Prodromal Longitudinal Study (NAPLS; see http://www.nimh.nih.gov/publicat/schizresfact.cfm#initiatives_cognition) to identify high-risk individuals before psychotic symptoms emerge. This research collaboration includes research sites in both the United States and Canada. The aims are to discover new information on the clinical and neurobiological features of the prodromal phase of schizophrenia, including environmental events that may trigger progression to psychosis. Together, these studies are designed not only to identify risk factors proximal to the onset of psychosis, but also to discover new targets relevant to the delay or prevention of psychotic episodes.

In 2004, NIMH provided leadership to methodologically integrate these studies of high-risk individuals before psychotic symptoms emerge, with the goal of creating the world's largest data set for exploring the behavioral, social, and environmental factors associated with the onset of schizophrenia. The collaborative effort that ensued will compare the longitudinal course of approximately 400 high-risk adolescents and young adults with that of 400 control subjects. Results from this project promise to identify reliable predictors of illness onset, to detect risk factors related to functional impairment, and to specify targets for indicated prevention. Furthermore, recent data suggest that the prodromal phase of schizophrenia can be reliably identified. Some evidence exists as to the predictive validity for the risk of developing schizophrenia following a year of the emergence of prodromal symptoms (Lee et al. 2005). As emphasis continues to be placed on examining the prodromal phase of schizophrenia, measures have been developed with the ability to combine knowledge of environmental risk factors with data on endophenotypes associated with schizophrenia. The ultimate aim of these types of measures is to have the ability to assess individuals in the prodromal stage of schizophrenia in order to find ways to intervene prior to the development of the disorder (Seeber and Cadenhead 2005).

The behavioral, environmental, and molecular components of schizophrenia have long been studied without major treatment advances in recent years. Individuals and families continue to suffer the effects of this serious mental illness. Psychopharmacology has advanced its methodologies. For persons with schizophrenia, the medication clozapine received the first-ever U.S. Food and Drug Administration indication for effectiveness in preventing suicide attempts among persons with schizophrenia (Meltzer et al. 2003).

Although the diagnosis of schizophrenia is usually made much later than autism, knowledge gained from emerging multisite research collaborations for both of these neurodevelopmental disorders can inform prevention for mental disorders at various levels of prevention and developmental stages. Unlike previous research attempts through smaller studies, both the STAART centers for autism and the NAPLS for schizophrenia have the research design and technology from advances in neuroscience to unlock the mysteries of brain and behavior.

TRANSLATIONAL RESEARCH PRIORITIES

Although emerging findings from basic science hold great promise for informing the next era of prevention research, innovations in prevention science will come from basic, clinical, and behavioral interdisciplinary translational collaborations. Prevention science remains a high priority at NIMH, and, along with development of novel pharmacological and psychosocial treatment approaches, it is an important element in the research program of translational clinical research. Research on pathophysiology, genomics, and new clinical and behavioral interventions across the translational spectrum will identify innovative prospects for the prevention of mental illness from "bench to bedside."

It is important to note that the reorganization of NIMH extramural programs has been designed to optimize the translation of new discoveries from genomics, neuroscience, and behavioral science into more effective services for individuals diagnosed with mental and behavioral disorders, as well as those at greatest risk for developing these conditions. The reorganization of NIMH presents opportunities, as well as several challenges, for prevention research. Prevention research has been integrated within refocused and expanded extramural research programs within NIMH. Moreover, current research priorities at NIMH have direct relevance to prevention science across multiple scientific disciplines, including areas of neuroscience such as neurogenesis and epigenetics that were not traditionally viewed as areas of opportunity for the prevention of mental illness (National Institute of Mental Health 2004).

Exciting prospects for the prevention of mental illness include the identification of genetic, biological, behavioral, and/or environmental mechanisms and their interactions that confer vulnerability to childhood and adult psychiatric illnesses. The development of biological markers for detecting vulnerability and risk states, diagnosing illness onset, and charting the progression of mental disorders is another area of promise for prevention. Early interventions can be pharmacological and/or psychosocial to prevent the incidence and severity of psychopathology. We can expand the effectiveness of known efficacious interventions for use in additional populations, new settings, and comorbid mental disorders.

Larger efforts at NIH through the Roadmap initiative also have the potential to develop innovations in prevention (see http://nihroadmap.nih.gov/initiatives.asp). As researchers are encouraged to seek new pathways to discovery, they may uncover genetic and/or biological risks and targets for preventive efforts. The Roadmap initiative to build multidisciplinary research teams of the future can reflect the translational focus required to build innovative teams for the prevention of mental illness. The reengineering of the clinical research enterprise call for in the Roadmap may suggest cost-effective, efficacious preventive interventions for mental illness alone, as well as for co-occurring physical health problems and substance abuse. Using public health interventions, real-world relevance, services research, and dissemination, we can indeed move from bedside to practice.

PROSPECTS FOR FUTURE RESEARCH TO PREDICT AND PREVENT MENTAL ILLNESS

The need for increased mental health prevention efforts for diverse populations and across the life span is clear. However, this involves serious challenges. First among these is the "family myth," which proposes that interventions targeting the environment cannot influence disease. However, scientific evidence strongly suggests that there is an interaction of genetic risk with environment that can affect mental health outcomes (e.g., Caspi et al. 2002, 2003). Another challenge for preventive interventions is funding. Universal interventions, which could affect large groups of individuals, are often the most expensive. The integration of biological and behavioral approaches to prevention proposed in this chapter can be expensive as well, especially at this exploratory stage of science. Even when a preventive intervention does demonstrate a strong effect, its sustainability may require new funding or a shifting of fiscal priorities within service systems.

Nonetheless, there may be key developmental transitions where the interaction of brain, behavior, and environmental context is ripe for the prevention of mental illness and an increased investment. Early interventions with parents for social-emotional and cognitive development among young children, targeting brain development plasticity during early childhood developmental transitions and adolescence, and suicide prevention in primary care settings for the elderly are examples of promising avenues for prevention.

Over the next 20 years, the vision for mental health care and the prevention of mental illness is ambitious. For the next decade, we can build upon technologies such as clinical genomics, neuroimaging, proteomics, molecular diagnostics, and preventive interventions to move from diagnosis by symptoms and treatment of episodes of mental illness through pathophysiology to biodiagnostics and treatment of core pathology (Insel 2005b). The promise of prevention through mind, body, and behavior will need the integration of neuroscience and environmental context. The hope is that this complex integration of biomedical and behavioral influences will lead to the earliest preventive efforts for personalized care based on determined risk without stigma. If this promise is fulfilled, it can reduce the overwhelming economic and personal costs of mental illness for individuals, their families, and society.

CLINICAL IMPLICATIONS

The dividing line between prevention and clinical intervention is not always perfectly distinct. *Prevention* traditionally refers to interventions that are applied before the onset of a clinically diagnosable disorder, with the aim of reducing the number of new cases of that disorder, but it may also be considered to include attempts to prevent entry to, or progression along, the pathway toward a severe mental disorder. The Workgroup Report on Prevention from the National Advisory Mental Health Council in 1998 described a continuum of mental health interventions, which included preventive measures for at-risk populations, acute treatment for persons with newly diagnosed disorders, and maintenance care for those with established mental illness. Early interventions in the prodrome of schizophrenia have also suggested the potential efficacy of CBT to significantly prevent or delay onset of frank psychosis (McGorry et al. 2002). Treatments for mood and anxiety disorders may work, in part, by helping patients control their stress. A study in rats has suggested brain mechanisms likely to be involved: When a stressor is perceived to be controllable, an executive hub in the frontal lobes suppresses an alarm center in the brain stem, preventing adverse behavioral and physiological effects (Amat et al. 2005). It is not always clear where "prevention" ends and "clinical treatment" begins.

REFERENCES

Amat J, Baratta MV, Bland ST, et al: Medial prefrontal cortex determines how stressor controllability affects behavior and dorsal raphe nucleus. Nat Neurosci 8:365–371, 2005

Barrett P, Turner C: Prevention of anxiety symptoms in primary school children: preliminary results from a universal school-based trial. Br J Clin Psychol 40:399–410, 2001

Berrento-Clement JR, Schweinhart LJ, Barnett WS, et al: Changed Lives: The Effects of the Perry Preschool Program on Youths Through Age 19. Ypsilanti, MI, High/Scope Press, 1984

Carlson GA, Loney J, Salisbury H, et al: Young referred boys with DICA-P manic symptoms vs. two comparison groups. J Affect Disord 121:113–121, 1998

Caspi A, McClay J, Moffitt TE, et al: Role of genotype in the cycle of violence in maltreated children. Science 297:851–854, 2002

Caspi A, Sugden K, Moffitt T, et al: Influence of life stress on depression: moderation by a polymorphism in the 5-HTT gene. Science 301:386–389, 2003

Centers for Disease Control and Prevention: National Center for Injury Prevention and Control: Suicide Fact Sheet. Available at: http://www.cdc.gov/ncipc/factsheets/suifacts.htm. Accessed September 22, 2006a.

Centers for Disease Control and Prevention: National Center for Health Statistics: All injuries. Available at: http://www.cdc.gov/nchs/fastats/injury.htm. Accessed September 22, 2006b.

Chambers DA, Ringeisen H, Hickman EE: Federal, state, and foundation initiatives around evidence-based practices for child and adolescent mental health. Child Adolesc Psychiatr Clin N Am 14:307–327, ix, 2005

Dadds MR, Holland DE, Laurens KR, et al: Early intervention and prevention of anxiety disorders in children: results at 2-year follow-up. J Consult Clin Psychol 67:145–150, 1999

Dayer A, Cleaver K, Abouantoun T, et al: New GABAergic interneurons in the adult neocortex and striatum are generated from different precursors. J Cell Biol 168: 415–427, 2005

Eriksson PS, Perfilieva E, Bjork-Eriksson T, et al: Neurogenesis in in the adult human hippocampus. Nat Med 4: 1313–1317. 1998

Feldner MT, Zvolensky MJ, Schmidt NB: Prevention of anxiety psychopathology: a critical review of the empirical literature. Clinical Psychology: Science and Practice 11:405–424, 2004

Garber J: Depression in children and adolescents: linking risk research and prevention. Am J Prev Med 31 (6 suppl 1):104–125, 2006

Geller B, Luby J: Child and adolescent bipolar disorder: a review of the past 10 years. J Am Acad Child Adolesc Psychiatry 36:1168–1176, 1997

Glasson EJ, Bower C, Petterson B, et al: Perinatal factors and the development of autism: a population study. Arch Gen Psychiatry 61:618–627, 2004

Goldapple K, Segal Z, Garson C, et al: Modulation of cortical-limbic pathways in major depression: treatment specific effects of cognitive behavior therapy compared to paroxetine. Arch Gen Psychiatry 61:34–41, 2004

Hamner MB, Brodrick PS, Labbate LA: Gabapentin in PTSD: a retrospective, clinical series of adjunctive therapy. Ann Clin Psychiatry 13:141–146, 2001

Hann DM (ed): Taking Stock of Risk Factors for Child/Youth Externalizing Behavior Problems. 2001. Available at: http://www.tourettesyndrome.net/Files/takingstock.pdf. Accessed September 22, 2006.

Henn FA, Vollmayr B: Neurogenesis and depression: etiology or epiphenomenon? Biol Psychiatry 56:146–150, 2004

Horne AM, Baker JA, Kamphaus RW: Project ACT Early—school-based linked early intervention for children at risk. Paper presented at the American Psychological Association National Convention, San Francisco, CA, August 1999

Hultman CM, Spare´n P, Cnattingius S: Perinatal risk factors for infantile autism. Epidemiology 13:417–423, 2002

Insel TR: Predict and prevent: a vision of mental disorders in 2025. Paper presented at the annual meeting of the Society for Prevention Research, Washington, DC, May 2005a

Insel TR: Implications of genetics for prevention. Paper presented at the annual meeting of the Society for Prevention Research, Washington, DC, May 2005b

Institute of Medicine: Reducing Risks for Mental Disorders: Frontiers for Preventive Intervention Research. Washington, DC, National Academy Press, 1994

Institute of Medicine: Reducing Suicide: A National Imperative. Washington, DC, National Academy Press, 2002

International HapMap Consortium: A haplotype map of the human genome. Nature 436:1299–1320, 2005

Lanius R, Williamson P, Densmore M, et al: Comparison of rape victims with and without subsequent PTSD. Am J Psychiatry 161:36–44, 2004

Larsson H, Eaton W, Madsen K, et al: Risk factors for autism: perinatal factors, parental psychiatric history, and socioeconomic status. Am J Epidemiol 161:916–925, 2005

Lawler C, Croen L, Grether J, et al: Identifying environmental contributions to autism: provocative clues and false leads. Ment Retard Dev Disabil Res Rev 10:292–302, 2004

Lee C, McGlashan TH, Woods SW: Prevention of schizophrenia: can it be achieved? CNS Drugs 19:193–206, 2005

London E: The environment as an etiologic factor in autism: a new direction for research. Environ Health Perspect 108 (suppl 3):401–404, 2000

McGorry PD, Yung AR, Phillips LJ, et al: Randomized controlled trial of interventions designed to reduce the risk of progression to first-episode psychosis in a clinical sample with subthreshold symptoms. Arch Gen Psychiatry 59:921–928, 2002

Meaney M, Szyf M: Maternal care as a model for experience-dependent chromatin plasticity? Trends Neurosci 28:456–463, 2005

Meltzer HY, Alphs L, Green AI, et al: International Suicide Prevention Trial Study Group. Clozapine for suicidality in schizophrenia: International Suicide Prevention Trial (InterSePT). Arch Gen Psychiatry 60:82–89, 2003

Milad MR, Quirk GJ: Neurons in medial prefrontal cortex signal memory for fear extinction. Nature 420: 70–74, 2002

Morrison AP, French P, Walford, L et al : Cognitive therapy for the prevention of psychosis in people at ultra high risk. Br J Psychiatry 185: 291–297, 2004

Mrazek PJ, Haggerty RJ (eds): Reducing Risks for Mental Disorders: Frontiers for Preventive Intervention Research. Washington, DC, National Academy Press, 1994

Muñoz RF, Ying YW, Armas R, et al: The San Francisco depression prevention research project: a randomized trial with medical outpatients, in Depression Prevention: Research Directions. Edited by Muñoz RF. Washington, DC, Hemisphere Press, 1987, pp 119–215

Muñoz R, Mrazek P, Haggerty R: Institute of Medicine report on prevention of mental disorders: summary and commentary. Am Psychol 51:1116–1122, 1996

National Advisory Mental Health Council Workgroup on Child and Adolescent Mental Health Intervention Development and Deployment: Blueprint for change: research on child and adolescent health. 2001. Available at: http://www.nimh.nih.gov/publicat/nimhblueprint.pdf. Accessed September 22, 2006.

National Advisory Mental Health Council Workgroup on Mental Disorders Prevention Research: Priorities for prevention research at NIMH. Prevention and Treatment. 2001. Available at: http://journals.apa.org/prevention/volume4/pre0040017a.html. Accessed September 22, 2006.

National Institute of Mental Health: Depression Research at the National Institute of Mental Health (NIH Publication No. 00-4501). Bethesda, MD, National Institute on Mental Health, 1999

National Institute of Mental Health: Older Adults: Depression and Suicide Facts (NIH Publication No. 03-4593). Bethesda, MD, National Institute of Mental Health, 2003

National Institute of Mental Health: Research Funding: NIMH Reorganized Programs Effective October 2004. October 2004. Available at: http://www.nimh.nih.gov/researchfunding/reorganization.cfm. Accessed September 22, 2006.

National Institute of Mental Health: Division of Pediatric Translational Research and Treatment Development (DPTR). Available at: http://www.nimh.nih.gov/dptr/dptr.cfm. Accessed September 22, 2006.

Newschaffer C, Cole S: Invited commentary: Risk factors for autism—perinatal factors, parental psychiatric history, and socio-economic status. Am J Epidemiol 161:926–928, 2005

Olds DL: Prenatal and infancy home visiting by nurses: from randomized trials to community replication. Prev Sci 3:153–172, 2002

Online Mendelian Inheritance in Man. Anxiety. Available at: http://www.ncbi.nlm.nih.gov/entrez/query.fcgi?CMD=searchandDB=omim. Accessed September 22, 2006.

Online Mendelian Inheritance in Man. Depression. Available at: http://www.ncbi.nlm.nih.gov/entrez/query.fcgi?CMD=searchandDB=OMIM. Accessed September 22, 2006.

Online Mendelian Inheritance in Man. Schizophrenia. Available at: http://www.ncbi.nlm.nih.gov/entrez/query.fcgi?CMD=searchandDB=omim. Accessed September 22, 2006.

Reiss D: Priorities for prevention research at NIMH: will expanding the definition of prevention research reduce its impact? Prevention and Treatment 4: Article 19, 2001. Available at: http://journals.apa.org/prevention/volume4/pre0040019c.html. Accessed September 22, 2006.

Ringel J, Sturm R: Expenditures for children in 1998. J Behav Health Serv Res 28:319–333, 2001

Rutter M: Autism research: lessons from the past and prospects for the future. J Autism Dev Disord 35:241–257, 2005

Schmidt NB, Vasey M: Primary prevention of psychopathology in a high risk youth population, in New Research in Mental Health, 15. Edited by Roth D. Columbus, OH, Ohio Department of Mental Health, 2002, pp 203–209

Schwartz C, Wright C, Shin L, et al: Differential amygdalar response to novel versus newly familiar neutral faces: a functional MRI probe developed for studying inhibited temperament. Biol Psychiatry 53:854–862, 2003

Seeber K, Cadenhead KS: How does studying schizotypal personality disorder inform us about the prodrome of schizophrenia? Curr Psychiatry Rep 7:41–50, 2005

Shin LM, Whalen PJ, Pitman RK, et al: An fMRI study of anterior cingulated function in posttraumatic stress disorder. Biol Psychiatry 50: 932–942, 2001

U.S. Department of Health and Human Services: Surgeon General's Workshop Making Prevention of Child Maltreatment a National Priority: Implementing Innovations of a Public Health Approach. Washington, DC, U.S. Department of Health and Human Services, 2005

U.S. Public Health Service: The Surgeon General's Call to Action to Prevent Suicide. Washington, DC, U.S. Department of Health and Human Services, 1999

U.S. Public Health Service: Youth Violence: A Report of the Surgeon General. 2001. Available at: http://www.surgeongeneral.gov/library/youthviolence. Accessed September 22, 2006.

Vaiva G, Ducrocq F, Jezequel K, et al: Immediate treatment with propranolol decreases posttraumatic stress disorder two months after trauma. Biol Psychiatry 54:947–949, 2003

Veenstra-Vanderweele J, Cook E: Genetics of childhood disorders: autism. J Am Acad Child Adolesc Psychiatry 42:116–118, 2003

World Health Organization: Report. 2002. Available at http://www.who.int/healthinfo/bodestimates/en. Accessed September 22, 2006.

11

Drugs and Alcohol

Treating and Preventing Abuse, Addiction, and Their Medical Consequences

Nora D. Volkow, M.D., Ph.D.
Ting-Kai Li, M.D.

O̲ur views on the biological bases of drug and alcohol addiction have changed profoundly in recent years. To translate the new understanding into more effective prevention and treatment programs, the scientific and nonscientific communities will need to 1) coordinate efforts to curb the prevalence and high cost associated with alcohol and drug addiction, 2) study and reduce the phenomenon of early onset, 3) foster wider acceptance of the concept of substance addiction as a chronic relapsing brain disease, 4) engage pharmaceutical industry participa-

This chapter was previously published in the journal *Pharmacology and Therapeutics* (Volume 108, Issue 1, pages 3–17, October 2005).

The authors thank Dr. Ruben Baler for his valuable help with this manuscript.

263

tion in the research and development of new and effective treatments for substance addiction, and 5) facilitate reimbursement of treatment costs by private medical insurance companies.

PREVALENCE, TRENDS, AND COSTS OF SUBSTANCE ABUSE IN THE UNITED STATES

According to 2003 data from the National Survey on Drug Use and Health (Substance Abuse and Mental Health Services Administration 2004b), 9.1% of the total population, or an estimated 21.6 million people age 12 years or older, can be classified with dependence or abuse of psychoactive substances (alcohol or illicit addictive drugs). Recent data also show that abuse of illegal drugs and of nicotine in young individuals has apparently begun to decline. According to Monitoring the Future (MTF), a survey that monitors drug use among high school students, current (past month) use of illicit drugs has declined 17% from 2001 to 2004 in this group (Johnston et al. 2005). At the same time, MTF and other surveys also reveal disturbingly high levels of nonmedical use of prescription drugs (stimulant medications, opiate analgesics, and benzodiazepines), the rise of which has been most dramatic in the painkillers category. This is likely to reflect multiple factors, including the increase in the number of prescriptions for some of these medications, their frequent presence in the media, and their relatively easy and private access via Web sites that do not require prescriptions (Lineberry and Bostwick 2004). Another factor that is likely to contribute is a new pattern of drug abuse that is initiated not by the desire to get "high" but by the desire to improve performance. For example, stimulant medications are increasingly being abused by high school students to improve their scores on college entrance exams, by girls to achieve a body image that conforms to unrealistic standards, and by adults trying to cope in highly competitive environments.

Despite generally positive trends, the prevalence of substance abuse remains unacceptably high. Moreover, the economic impact of substance abuse is enormous. The estimated costs associated with illicit drugs are approximately $280 billion (including costs from crime, loss in productivity, health care, incarceration, and drug enforcement operation costs; Harwood 2004); for alcohol, around $185 billion (Harwood 2000); and for nicotine, approximately $158 billion (Centers for Disease Control and Prevention 2005a, 2005b, 2005c). This brings the grand total estimated economic impact of substance abuse in the United States to more than half a trillion dollars.

OBSTACLES IN THE TREATMENT OF ADDICTION

Despite the fact that there are effective treatments for drug addiction, less than 15% of those addicted receive treatment (Gerada 2005). This is likely a reflection not only of the addicted person's denial of there being a problem but also of the fear of stigmatization for being labeled an addict, as well as the lack of access to an acceptable treatment program. In this respect, the lack of reimbursement by private insurance companies hinders a wider involvement of the medical community in the early evaluation and treatment of drug addiction.

Another obstacle pertains to the limited range of medications currently available for the treatment of addiction. This reflects, in part, the limited participation of the pharmaceutical industry in the development of addiction medications. Understandably, the stigma associated with drug addiction, the lack of insurance reimbursement for drug abuse treatment, and the perceived relatively small size of the users' market create an environment that is not conducive to active collaborations with industry.

Recognizing the impact of this gap, the Institute of Medicine has recommended the implementation of a program of targeted incentives for the pharmaceutical industry (Fulco et al. 1995). In the meantime, we continue to pursue collaborations with pharmaceutical companies in an effort to move their novel and promising compounds forward and into the process of clinical evaluations for the treatment of addictive disorders.

Whenever we are able to access and reevaluate medications developed to target other diseases (i.e., antiepileptics and antidepressants) for their potential application to addiction, much valuable research and preliminary safety testing has already taken place, resulting in substantial savings of time and resources.

DRUG ABUSE AND HIV

Drug abuse and HIV/AIDS are intertwined epidemics (McCoy et al. 2004; Schuster 1992). Injection drug use (IDU) accounts for approximately one-third of all the AIDS cases in the United States (Figure 11–1), and more than 90% of HIV-infected injection drug users are also infected with hepatitis C (Amin et al. 2004). However, that is only one part of the problem of HIV transmission, because non-IDU drug abusers also show much higher rates of HIV infection than the general population (McCoy et al. 2004). There are many factors that contribute to such high rates, but chief among them is the risky sexual behaviors that many drug and alcohol abusers engage in due to changes in their mental state from drug intoxication. Basic research shows that certain drugs of abuse can also compromise the immune system (Safdar and Schiff 2004; Yu et al. 2003; Zhu et al. 2000), putting users at greater risk of contracting the illness or suffering a more severe course. It is also reasonable to expect a synergistic, deleterious interaction between centrally acting psychoactive drugs and neurotoxic substances released during the course of an HIV infection (Nath et al. 2002).

Addiction treatment has been shown to be an effective way to prevent the spread of diseases, such as HIV/AIDS and hepatitis. Drug injectors who do not enter treatment, for example, are up to 6 times more likely to become infected with HIV than are injectors who enter and remain in treatment (National Institute on Drug Abuse 2000). Participation in treatment also offers good opportunities for screening, counseling, and referral for additional services, all of which can help reduce the spread of diseases to the general population.

National Institute on Drug Abuse (NIDA) research has shown that screening can be a cost-effective way to prevent and treat diseases, such as HIV/AIDS. When broad screening for HIV in health care settings is provided, early detection and active antiretroviral therapy result in increased life expectancy and reduced transmission rates (Paltiel et al. 2005; Sanders et al. 2005). For example, screening a person at 30 years of age could increase his/her life expectancy by almost 2 years. Furthermore, by screening larger segments of the population, HIV transmission rates can be decreased by about 20%.

The HIV/AIDS epidemic has taken a disproportionate toll on racial and ethnic minority populations. The Centers for Disease Control and Prevention (CDC) reports that during 2000–2003, HIV/AIDS rates for African American males were 7 times those for white males, and African American females had 19 times the rates for white females, exceeding the rates for males of all races/ethnicities other than African Americans (Centers for Disease Control and Prevention 2004a). NIDA has launched an initiative that is focused specifically on reducing HIV rates among African Americans, including conducting more studies in geographic areas where rates are highest and developing interventions that are ethnically appropriate. Furthermore, because African American males are nearly 8 times more likely to be incarcerated than white males, supporting research on the intersection of drug use and criminal justice consequences in the African American population is a high priority.

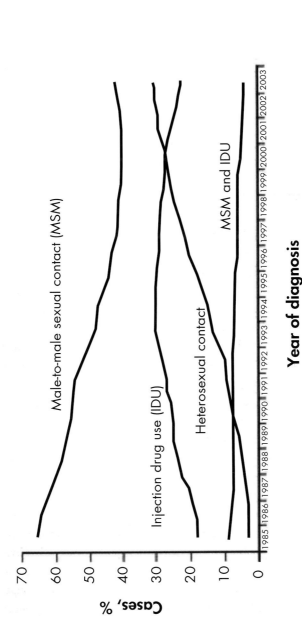

Year of diagnosis

FIGURE 11–1. Proportion of AIDS cases among adults and adolescents, by exposure category and year of diagnosis: United States, 1985–2003.

Source. Centers for Disease Control and Prevention 2005a.

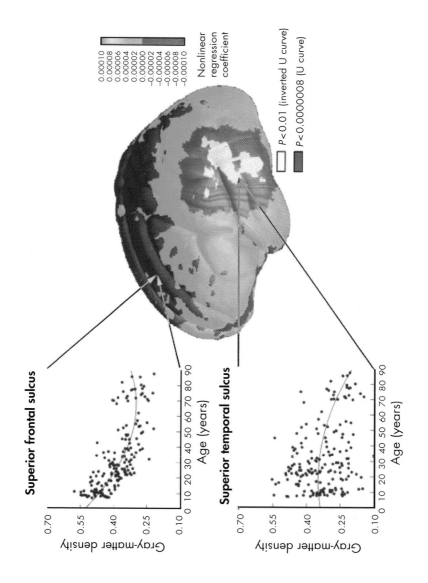

FIGURE 11–2. *(opposite)* Nonlinear effects of age on gray-matter density (GMD) on the lateral brain surface.

This statistical map *(left frontal view)* shows the effects of age on GMD on the lateral surface of the brain between childhood and old age. Regions shown in either *red* or *white* correspond to regression coefficients that have significant positive or negative nonlinear age effects, respectively. Representative scatterplots of age effects with the best-fitting quadratic regression line are shown for sample surface points in the superior frontal sulcus and the superior temporal sulcus. See original article for more details.

Source. Reprinted from Sowell ER, Thompson PM, Toga AW: "Mapping Changes in the Human Cortex Throughout the Span of Life." *Neuroscientist* 10:372–392, 2004. Used with permission.

NEUROBIOLOGY OF SUBSTANCE ABUSE AND ADDICTION

Developmental Aspects

In addressing the neurobiology of drug abuse and addiction, it is critical to consider the influence of specific developmental stages. Experimentation with illicit use of addictive substances during childhood and adolescence is not only dangerous but also disturbingly common (Johnston et al. 2005). To a large degree, initiation for most youth results from the convergence of social influences and the typically rebellious behaviors that appear around the preteen and teenage years. Research shows that periods of enhanced risk for seeking drugs coincide with major transitions in children's lives (National Institute on Drug Abuse 2003). As children navigate through these developmental stages, they face not only increased social, emotional, and educational challenges but also greater access to addicting substances.

Overlaying these behavioral and social risk factors is the recent finding showing that brain development continues well beyond childhood and adolescence (Figure 11–2; Sowell et al. 2004). The adolescent brain is characterized by vigorous changes in growth and connectivity. The continuous pruning and fine-tuning that eventually create the adult brain coincide with the commonly observed shifts in adolescent behavior and thought processes that compromise the early adolescent's ability to consistently carry through with intended and planned choices (Luna and Sweeney 2004). Recent imaging data revealed that one of the last areas of the brain to mature is the prefrontal cortex (Gogtay et al. 2004), which is an area involved in judgment, decision making, and control of emotional responses. It is reasonable to hypothesize a link between the immaturity of the adolescent brain, the ensuing high level of risk taking and novelty seeking, and the increased morbidity and mortality observed in adolescence when compared with adults (Kelley et al. 2004; Resnick et al. 1997).

Exposure to drugs of abuse at such active developmental stages may increase a child's vulnerability to the effects of drugs and may adversely impact brain development. Exposure of young animals to nicotine, for example, has been found to induce changes in their brains that lead to an increased effect of nicotine later in life (Belluzzi et al. 2004). Epidemiological evidence also shows that youth who begin abusing substances early in their lives constitute the group at highest risk for later development of chronic addiction to drugs (Spear 2000) and alcohol (Grant et al. 2001).

Both NIDA and the National Institute on Alcohol Abuse and Alcoholism (NIAAA) are studying the effects of drugs and alcohol on brain development in a variety of ways. We support basic research with animals to directly examine the effects that early exposure to drugs and alcohol can have on brain development and behavior. Both NIDA and NIAAA support research in adolescents, focusing on cognition (e.g., learning, judgment, and decision making) and emotion (e.g., social reinforcers, motivation, and stress responses), which should enhance our ability to create effective messages and interventions to discourage teens from abusing alcohol and drugs.

NIDA participates, along with the National Institute of Child Health and Human Development (NICHD), National Institute of Mental Health (NIMH), and National Institute of Neurological Disorders and Stroke (NINDS), in the National Institutes of Health Magnetic Resonance Imaging Study of Normal Brain Development, the goal of which is to determine the path of normal brain development and its relationship to cognitive and behavioral maturation. The hope is to capitalize on the findings of research to facilitate the investigation of how drugs and alcohol affect developmental trajectories.

Substance Abuse in Pregnancy

By extension, it is equally important to evaluate the specific vulnerabilities and risks associated with earlier stages in life. Indeed, alcohol and drug use by pregnant women are known to pose significant risks to brain development; 4.3% of pregnant women between the ages of 15 and 44 years report past-month use of illicit drugs (Substance Abuse and Mental Health Services Administration 2004b), while the prevalence of any alcohol use among pregnant women was about 10% (Centers for Disease Control and Prevention 2004b). While these rates are significantly lower than those among the nonpregnant, child-bearing age female population (10% and 53%, respectively), extrapolation from CDC pregnancy rate data (Ventura et al. 2004) reveals the disturbing fact that close to 800,000 fetuses in the United States could be exposed to the harmful effects of alcohol and drugs every year. Similarly, the rate of pregnant women who smoke during pregnancy, estimated to be about 18% (Substance Abuse and Mental Health Services Administration 2004b), is still unacceptably high. Therefore, the identification and measurement of each substance's contribution to potentially adverse cognitive, emotional, and behavioral outcomes are top priorities.

Suspected early consequences of drug and alcohol use during pregnancy include brain growth alterations and withdrawal symptoms. Subsequent behavior, development, and neurological function may also suffer from prenatal and/or childhood exposure. Also, medical complications during delivery are much more frequent in mothers who use drugs during pregnancy (Huestis and Choo 2002).

As new experimental tools become available, we are gaining more confidence in our ability to assess scientifically the effects of substance abuse on the developing brain. Thanks to these tools, we now know, for example, that the neuronal loss underlying fetal alcohol syndrome (FAS) is more severe and much more widespread (affecting many brain regions, spinal cord, and retina) than previously thought. Animal studies clearly show that such deficits hinge on ethanol's ability to enter the fetal brain and disrupt synaptogenesis, a process whose blockage activates a cellular cascade that drives a large number of neurons to undergo unscheduled programmed cell death (Olney 2004). This finding could explain the smaller brains and the neurobehavioral and cognitive disturbances associated with the well-studied human FAS (Ikonomidou et al. 2000). A related mechanism is also likely to underlie the observed disruption of brain surface and gray matter density asymmetry patterns in adolescents that have been prenatally exposed to large quantities of alcohol (Sowell et al. 2002).

Many other psychoactive drugs traverse the placental and fetal brain barriers unimpeded and potentially affect the developing brain directly (Figure 11–3; Benveniste et al. 2005). This possibility, which has been the focus of prospective epidemiological studies, remains hard to assess in humans. Results must be interpreted in light of multiple confounding factors, such as a drug users' tendency to use combinations of various substances (e.g., alcohol, tobacco, marijuana). Additional risks can result from exposure to deleterious environmental factors, such as toxins and poor nutrition, often linked to low socioeconomic status and known to influence various parameters of cognitive development.

In contrast, complementary and properly controlled studies using nonhuman primates have produced some evidence of the potential harmful effects of alcohol and drugs on the developing fetus. For example, a recent review of several such studies, in 4 different rhesus monkey models, indicates possible detriments in overall growth in newborns exposed to relatively high levels of cocaine in utero. The primate models of oral cocaine administration demonstrate that prenatal exposure can result in detectable neurobehavioral deficits, but only when

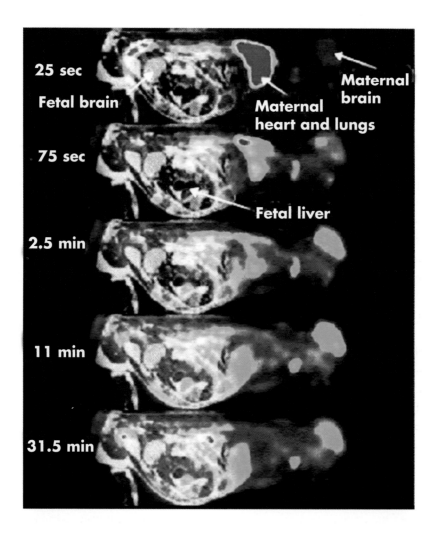

FIGURE 11–3. Time series of ^{11}C-cocaine positron emission tomography (PET) scans from third-trimester pregnant *Macaca radiata*.

Each PET frame is coregistered to a corresponding magnetic resonance image. Early PET frames (25 seconds, 75 seconds, and 2.5 minutes) clearly show early ^{11}C uptake in placental vessels and maternal heart, lungs, and kidneys. Later time frames demonstrate uptake in fetal liver.

Source. Reprinted from Benveniste H, Fowler JS, Rooney W, et al.: "Maternal and Fetal 11C-Cocaine Uptake and Kinetics Measured In Vivo by Combined PET and MRI in Pregnant Nonhuman Primates." *Journal of Nuclear Medicine* 46:312–320, 2005. Used with permission.

assessed beyond the first week after birth (postnatal weeks 2 and 4; Lidow 2003). Intriguingly, one study showed a delayed and long-lasting impaired ability to adapt to new environmental contingencies in monkeys that had been prenatally exposed to cocaine 6 years earlier, yet no other discernible cognitive effects were observed (Chelonis et al. 2003). This result is reminiscent of a human study that found no significant effects of prenatal cocaine exposure on the growth, intellectual ability, academic achievement, or teacher-rated classroom behavior of 6-year-olds, although deficits in their ability to sustain attention on a computerized vigilance task were detected (Richardson et al. 1996). Similarly, one prospective report showed no association between prenatal cocaine exposure and lower IQ scores but hinted at persistent attentional and other cognitive deficits as the exposed children grew older (Singer et al. 2004). Interestingly, the same study showed that the quality of the caregiving environment could have a significant compensatory effect. It seems reasonable to hypothesize that the ultimate impact of prenatal cocaine will reflect the combined influence of many factors, including the dose and pattern of exposure as well as the postpartum environment in which the child will be raised.

Use of methamphetamine during pregnancy is of particular concern, because of the drug's prevalent use among women of child-bearing age (Substance Abuse and Mental Health Services Administration 2004a). Moreover, methamphetamine's ability to cause long-lasting changes in brain function in chronic users (Hanson et al. 2004) and its neurotoxic effects on selected dopaminergic and serotonergic terminals in the rat brain (Cadet et al. 2003) suggest that its use during pregnancy could have serious implications for fetal brain development.

In a recent study, structural abnormalities were observed in regions of the brain associated with cognition and emotion in methamphetamine abusers (Thompson et al. 2004). Moreover, prenatal methamphetamine exposure has been associated with abnormal brain metabolism (Smith et al. 2001), and a group of methamphetamine- and cocaine-exposed newborns displayed significantly reduced visual recognition memory, compared with unexposed controls (Hansen et al. 1993). Another magnetic resonance imaging (MRI) study provided evidence of an association between prenatal methamphetamine exposure and smaller volumes in discrete subcortical structures, which correlated with poorer performance on sustained attention and delayed verbal memory (Chang et al. 2004).

Clearly, more research is needed to establish the individual contributions of all the factors influencing the long-term impact of substance abuse, by pregnant women, on the developing brain. NIDA is currently funding longitudinal studies with children who have been prenatally exposed to marijuana, cocaine, and nicotine to gain information about their cognitive and emotional development, as well as their vulnerability to drug abuse and addiction later in life. Additionally, NIDA has recently launched the first large-scale study of the developmental consequences of methamphetamine exposure, which includes seven hospitals in Iowa, Oklahoma, California, and Hawaii.

The long-term effects of prenatal alcohol exposure throughout pregnancy have been well documented and reviewed (Day and Richardson 2004; Nordstrom-Klee et al. 2002). A current emphasis of NIAAA is the exploration of behavioral methodologies that could improve the neurocognitive performance of children diagnosed as having fetal alcohol spectrum disorder (FASD).

Neural Substrates of Substance Abuse and Addiction

All compounds with abuse potential have the ability to disrupt the processing of information in the brain by subverting one or more of the common neurotransmitter systems (i.e., gamma-aminobutyric acid [GABA], glutamate, acetylcholine, dopamine, serotonin, and opioid peptides). However, an (early) increase in dopamine signaling has been one of the most consistent observations across studies of the reinforcing effects of drugs of abuse.

Not surprisingly, acute drug intoxication is accompanied by highly localized and dynamic patterns of brain activation and deactivation (Breiter et al. 1997; Stein et al. 1998), as well as complex cascades of transcriptional reprogramming (Yuferov et al. 2003; Zhang et al. 2002). These changes are rapid and robust and can dramatically alter the function of regions neuroanatomically connected with dopamine systems known to be involved in reward, memory, motivation, drive, and self-control. Dopaminergic involvement is likely an equally important factor in the progression to alcohol addiction, since the reinforcing properties of ethanol appear to rely on increased opioid neurotransmission, which can indirectly enhance dopamine release (Oswald and Wand 2004).

Imaging technologies, such as MRI and positron emission tomography (PET), now allow us to investigate the anatomical and functional changes that characterize the process of drug addiction in the human brain (Figure 11–4). The result has been a growing series of studies that largely corroborates the widely held notion that disruption of dopaminergic neurotransmission is a key event in the initiation and maintenance of the adverse effects stemming from substance abuse, both acute and chronic.

Paradoxically, it has also been shown that, in contrast to the increases in dopamine neurotransmission observed in the brain reward centers during initial acute administration, chronic drug use leads to measurable decreases in dopaminergic activity (Volkow et al. 1997), which can persist for months after detoxification and are associated with dysregulation of frontal brain regions (Volkow et al. 2004). Furthermore, preclinical studies show that chronic drug exposure can dramatically change the expression (Zhang et al. 2005) and activity (Hu et al. 2005) of various proteins involved in dopamine signaling.

Thus, the current understanding of the addiction cycle as a behavioral process gone awry can explain much of the reinforcing properties of addictive substances during initiation and early use. It also provides testable hypotheses regarding the specific structural changes in the brain associated with the impaired decision-making that facilitates substance abuse even in the face of serious adverse consequences (Volkow et al. 2002).

Imaging and behavioral studies suggest the involvement of at least four interacting brain circuits in mediating the three states of the drug addiction process: intoxication, craving, and withdrawal. The first circuit is located in the nucleus accumbens (Di Chiara 2002) and the ventral pallidum and mediates the reward process (Volkow et al. 2003). A second circuit that maps onto the orbitofrontal cortex and the subcallosal cortex is responsible for the generation of motivation and emotional responses. The third circuit, in the amygdala and hippocampus, spawns memories and supports conditioned learning. The last circuit is in charge of high-level cognitive control and executive function and is located in the prefrontal cortex and the anterior cingulate gyrus (Volkow et al. 1993). In addition, imaging studies are providing increasing evidence of the involvement of the temporal insula in addiction (Franklin et al. 2002; Wang et al. 1999). Given that the insula is a cortical region involved in the processing of autonomic responses, it may serve to underlie the strong peripheral responses that occur during drug craving (Wang et al. 1999).

The four underlying circuits receive direct innervation from dopamine neurons but are also connected with one another through direct or indirect projections that are mostly glutamatergic (Kalivas 2004a). Predictably, there are experimental data that support a significant glutamatergic contribution to the orchestration of maladaptive responses to drugs and alcohol. Animal studies show that glutamatergic pathways play an important role in mediating drug craving and relapse (Kalivas 2004b). This finding is consistent with the drug-dependent modulation of glutamatergic transmission in the prefrontal cortex, nucleus accumbens (McFarland et al. 2003), and amygdala (Lu et al. 2005), as well as with the drug-induced deregulation of proteins involved in pre- and postsynaptic glutamate transmission (Kalivas et al. 2005).

Thus, excitatory networks, as embodied in cortical and corticofugal glutamatergic projections, may play a more important role in substance abuse–dependent neuroadaptation processes than previously thought (Kalivas 2004b).

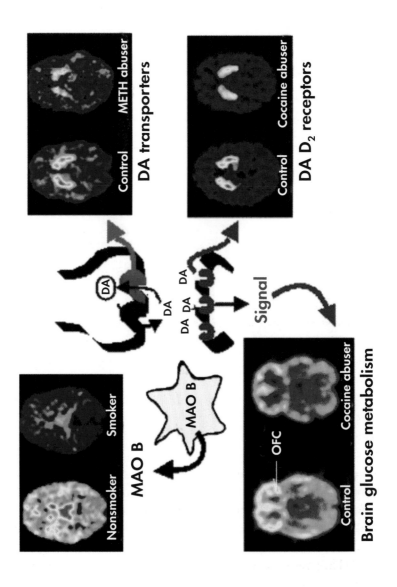

FIGURE 11–4. *(opposite)* Effects of chronic drug exposure on dopamine neurotransmission and brain function.

Brain-imaging tools such as positron emission tomography (PET) allow for an unprecedented view of the pathological process to which an addicted brain is subjected. The images provide solid evidence for the deleterious functional (i.e., enzymes, transporters, and receptors) and metabolic effects of various drugs of abuse. DA = dopamine; MAO = monoamine oxidase; METH = methamphetamine; OFC = orbitofrontal cortex.

Source. Reprinted from Volkow ND, Fowler JS, Wang GJ: "The Addicted Human Brain: Insights From Imaging Studies." *Journal of Clinical Investigation* 111:1444–1451, 2003. Used with permission.

Unfortunately, the lack of radiotracers for imaging glutamate function in the human brain has prevented the assessment of glutamatergic pathways in drug-addicted subjects.

Genes, Environment, and Their Interactions

There is little doubt that genetic factors play an important part in determining vulnerabilities to drug seeking and addictive behavior. The fact is that not everyone who takes drugs becomes addicted, and both NIDA and NIAAA are funding research to understand why some individuals become addicted while others do not.

Evidence for the involvement of genes in the process of drug addiction comes from classical epidemiological and genetic approaches. Twin studies, for example, have shown robust genetic components in alcohol, opiate, cocaine, and tobacco addictions (Kreek et al. 2004; True et al. 1999). On the other hand, studies with various knockout mouse strains have illuminated the role of specific gene products, such as *Homer2* (Szumlinski et al. 2004), opioid receptors (Chefer et al. 2004), and alpha$_4$ nicotinic receptors (Tapper et al. 2004), in conferring either protection from or increased risks of falling prey to drug addiction.

However, the contribution of single genes is only a small part of the picture. Genes exert their effects in the context of genetic networks, which are typically under the influence of environmental factors. As a result, the assignment of strong linkages between genetic polymorphisms and enhanced vulnerabilities to the addictive properties of drugs has proven to be a difficult goal to achieve.

Fortunately, the genetic research landscape is undergoing a radical transformation, and our efforts to better define the genetic underpinnings of substance abuse will likely benefit as a result. The newer screening techniques provide us with powerful tools to explore global transcriptional changes in response to drug administration (Nestler 2004) and allow for the rapid identification of candidate genes whose modulation may signal the induction of long-lasting changes in the brain (McClung et al. 2004). By the same token, completion of the human genome project will permit an unbiased search for candidate genes from among all possible human coding sequences. When this data set is combined with the massive throughput screening techniques now available, it will be possible to scan through millions of single nucleotide polymorphisms, in hundreds of samples. The first genetic screens taking advantage of such an approach demonstrate unprecedented power and sensitivity (Hinds et al. 2005).

Better designs in primary data collection, combined with increased computing power, will make it possible to develop genetic risk analysis tools that take into account specific environmental risks and protective factors, long established to affect the trajectory of drug addiction. With this approach in mind, we plan to embark on cooperative efforts to identify genes associated with abuse to specific substances, evaluate their contributions to a persistent addictive behavior, and assess how they might interact with other genes and the environment.

Comorbidity With Mental Illness

The challenge of drug abuse research, particularly in the context of genetic screening, becomes even more daunting when the high incidence of comorbid mental illnesses is taken into account. For persons who abuse drugs, other than nicotine and alcohol, mood disorders were found to be 4.7 times more prevalent than in the entire population (Regier et al. 1990). On the other hand, abuse of other drugs, including cocaine, sedative-hypnotics, and opioids, is also greater in individuals with depression compared with those without it, and those with the highest risk seem to be the ones with comorbid anxiety disorders (Goodwin et al. 2002). Similarly, the comorbidity between mental illness and nicotine addiction is alarmingly high (Lasser et al. 2000). NIAAA and NIDA have also joined forces to establish and deploy the National Epidemiologic Survey on Alcohol and Related Conditions (NESARC), designed to determine the extent of alcohol use disorders and their associated disabilities in the general population (Grant et al. 2004).

Both epidemiological and preclinical studies suggest that developmental factors are likely to play an important role in establishing these comorbidity linkages. The preliminary evidence suggests that early exposure to substances of abuse, during periods in which the brain is still undergoing significant changes, could lead to neurobiological changes associated with depression, enhanced sensitivity to stress, and decreased sensitivity to natural reinforcers (Volkow 2004).

Genes and environment are key contributors to the connections between substance abuse and other mental disorders. Genetic components linking substance abuse and vulnerability to depression and to anxiety disorders were suggested by human (e.g., adoption, twin) and animal (e.g., using genetically altered strains of mice) studies. On the other hand, several environmental factors, such as family disruption, poor parental monitoring, acute and chronic stress, and low social class of rearing, have all been found, predictably, to contribute to the manifestation of substance abuse and certain comorbid mental illnesses (Tarter et al. 1995).

The neurobiological substrate for comorbid phenomena is likely to reside in or involve various limbic and paralimbic structures. Drug-induced changes in these regions have been implicated in the induction of the negative emotional symptoms that often occur during early phases of withdrawal from many psychoactive substances. Similarly, it is likely that a significant anatomical overlap exists with brain regions mediating the diverse symptoms of depression. Brain imaging studies of human depression as well as of substance abusers have demonstrated changes in the activity of numerous areas, including regions involved in mood regulation (e.g., ventral cingulate gyrus), cognitive operations (e.g., prefrontal cortex), memory (e.g., hippocampus), reward (e.g., ventral striatum), and arousal (e.g., thalamus; Drevets 2001; Liotti and Mayberg 2001).

We recognize the real obstacles that we confront in this area: the difficulty in describing complex phenotypes and the typically unknown sequence of events that lead to their manifestation. Yet, we will continue to support the research needed to tease apart the contribution of specific vulnerabilities to the occurrence of comorbid conditions.

STRATEGIES TO OPTIMIZE THE USE OF SCIENTIFIC RESEARCH

The knowledge derived from research in substance abuse has the potential to impact the lives of millions of individuals. However, in order to focus these efforts, it is important to ensure that the products of research are not just useful (effective) but also accepted and used by the community. Blending research with practice is one of the main goals of both our Institutes, which are working in concert with other organizations and federal agencies.

Prevention

Epidemiological data show consistently that the longitudinal trends of drug abuse and perceived risk of harm maintain a close inverse correlation, namely, the use of addicting substances tends to rise whenever the perception of their harmfulness drops. In addition, 25 years of epidemiological research has clearly identified distinct socioeconomic and cultural factors that can either compromise or enhance a person's ability to reject the use of addictive drugs. It follows that prevention should be at the forefront of our strategies to mitigate the personal and societal burden of drug addiction.

To be efficacious, prevention must be rooted in scientific evidence: The multifaceted nature of the vulnerabilities for addiction, the high frequency of comorbid conditions, and the long-lasting neurobehavioral impact of drugs of abuse on the brain all play a critical role in shaping our prevention efforts.

The ability to investigate the motivational processes at work in the adolescent brain can provide valuable information regarding the drive and decision to drink and to use drugs, as well as unique opportunities to evaluate and select intervention strategies that are more likely to succeed. Accordingly, both NIDA and NIAAA allocate significant resources on prevention programs that target children and adolescents.

The Adolescents Training and Learning to Avoid Steroids (ATLAS) and Athletes Targeting Healthy Exercise and Nutrition Alternatives (ATHENA) programs, two examples of evidence-based prevention strategies, have demonstrated that sport teams are effective vehicles for delivering gender-specific, peer-led curricula that promote a healthy lifestyle. These interventions have been very successful at reducing steroid and other drug use among high school athletes (Elliot et al. 2004; Goldberg et al. 1996).

As children become adolescents, the role of their peer groups in influencing their behavior becomes more prominent. Those who begin using substances early become part of a culture that engages in illegal activities, pitting themselves squarely against the criminal justice system. The ethos associated with drug abuse often encourages other forms of risky behaviors, including sexual activities that can expose youth to HIV, hepatitis, and sexually transmitted diseases. Indeed, it is estimated that about half of new cases of HIV crop up in people younger than age 25 years (Centers for Disease Control and Prevention 2005b).

NIDA-supported researchers also found that many of the risk-taking behaviors of adult women who contract HIV were associated with childhood sexual abuse (Klein and Chao 1995), suggesting that early learned behaviors, negative or positive, can impact later disease outcomes. Early exposure to stress or trauma is also known to be a risk factor for both substance abuse and mental health disorders (Kendler et al. 2000). For these reasons, it is critical that we devote more resources to developing preventive interventions geared toward protecting children and adolescents who may be at high risk for comorbid disorders.

The HIV epidemic and drug addictive disorders disproportionately affect incarcerated individuals. This is an unfortunate but well-established fact, which NIDA recognizes as a unique opportunity for the optimization of effective interventions. Several NIDA-supported projects have been initiated to develop and test models for an integrated approach for the treatment of criminal offenders suffering from HIV infection and/or drug addiction.

Pharmacotherapies

Clinical trials to assess the effectiveness of medications or of behavioral interventions should be based on the conceptualization of addiction as a chronic disease (McLellan et al. 2000). As for patients with other chronic diseases, most addicted subjects will require some type of continued therapeutic support (McLellan et al. 2005).

The evolving view of the neurobiological basis of the effects of substance abuse on the brain is continuously expanding the list of potential targets for intervention. The following medications are good examples of effective or promising treatments that emerged from a better understanding of the molecular and physiological bases of the reward, craving, withdrawal, and relapse phases of addiction.

Buprenorphine (Fudala et al. 2003) is a relatively recent addition to the list of effective medications for the treatment of heroin addiction. Because it is a partial opioid agonist, buprenorphine has the additional advantage that it is more difficult to overdose with it unintentionally. And, because it is the first office-based treatment option for opiate dependence, buprenorphine shows great promise as a detoxifying and treatment agent. The NIDA Clinical Trials Network sponsored two clinical trials assessing buprenorphine–naloxone for short-term opioid detoxification. These trials provided an unprecedented field test of its use in 12 diverse community-based treatment programs.

Modafinil, a novel medication for the treatment of narcolepsy, is also being tested as a potential treatment for cocaine and methamphetamine dependence. Though the mechanism of action of modafinil is not properly understood, it is believed that it has both dopaminergic as well as glutamatergic effects. Hence, it has been proposed that modafinil could help counteract the cocaine-induced neuroadaptations on dopamine and glutamate reward circuits that, in turn, could help alleviate cocaine withdrawal symptoms (Dackis et al. 2003).

While cocaine administration primarily stimulates the central "reward system," many of its behavioral effects rely upon cortical circuits, making them attractive targets for pharmacological intervention. Topiramate, an anticonvulsant that facilitates GABAergic neurotransmission and inhibits glutamatergic activity, can affect these circuits and has recently shown potential usefulness for the treatment of alcohol and opiate addiction. In a small pilot trial (Kampman et al. 2004), topiramate offered an efficacious and safe way to treat cocaine addiction as well.

Gamma vinyl-GABA (GVG, vigabatrin) is another antiepileptic medication used in Europe and other nations (but not in the United States) that increases the amount of GABA in the brain. Preclinical studies with GVG revealed that it interferes with drug-induced increases in dopamine in the nucleus accumbens in the brain (Schiffer et al. 2003). A preliminary open clinical trial in cocaine-addicted subjects reported that their cravings for cocaine disappeared within 2–3 weeks after starting GVG treatment (Brodie et al. 2003).

Baclofen, a GABA$_B$ agonist, was shown to reduce acquisition of cocaine self-administration (Campbell et al. 2002) and to attenuate the reinforcing effects of the psychostimulant D-amphetamine in rats (Brebner et al. 2005). Recent clinical reports show that baclofen treatment could block craving in alcoholic individuals (Addolorato et al. 2000) and improve abstinence in drug-abusing patients (Shoptaw et al. 2003). These preclinical and limited clinical findings have prompted further studies of baclofen in human addiction. Although in their early stages, some studies in cocaine populations suggest a promising future for this and other GABA$_B$ agonists (Brebner et al. 2002).

Disulfiram (Antabuse), originally marketed for the treatment of alcoholism, was tested as a strategy to reduce alcohol use among cocaine users (Higgins et al. 1993). It later became evident that the drug appeared to facilitate maintenance of cocaine abstinence in humans, showing promise for reducing cocaine use and addiction, particularly when combined with cognitive-behavioral treatment (Carroll et al. 1998).

Naltrexone is an opioid antagonist that blocks the subjective effects of opioids. Its potential as an effective treatment for alcoholism and opiate addiction derives from the fact that, compared with other maintenance therapies, naltrexone is nonaddicting, has only subtle adverse effects, and is seldom traded in the illicit drug market (Greenstein et al. 1997). In spite of its demonstrated effectiveness (Kirchmayer et al. 2003), naltrexone success has been rather limited to patients who are highly motivated to rein in their addiction. For other patients who lack a strong external incentive to stop using drugs, noncompliance has been a significant obstacle to naltrexone achieving its full potential. However, evidence consistently suggests that behavioral therapies can significantly improve the retention of patients treated for either opiate (Carroll et al. 2001) or alcohol (Balldin et al. 2003) dependence.

During the past decade, the understanding of the cellular, molecular, and genetic mechanisms underlying alcohol addictive behavior has increased rapidly. It is now known that alcohol-seeking behavior and drinking is influenced by an array of neurotransmitter systems as well as neuromodulators, hormones, and several intracellular signal transduction pathways. As a result, multiple molecular targets have been identified for novel drug development (Litten et al. 2005). A diversity of new medications is now being tested clinically for alcoholism treatment. These include the anticonvulsants topiramate, valproate, and gabapentin, agents that facilitate GABA and inhibit glutamine activities; the 5-HT$_3$ antagonist ondasterone; the GABA$_B$ agonist baclofen; aripiprazole, a partial dopamine D$_2$ agonist; and kudzu, a medicinal plant used in traditional Chinese medicine (Litten et al. 2005). In addition, there are many promising targets that are being investigated preclinically in the hope of developing new lead compounds. These targets include corticotropin-releasing factor receptors CRF$_1$ and CRF$_2$; neuropeptide Y receptors NPY$_1$, NPY$_2$, and NPY$_5$; adenosine A$_1$ and A$_2$ receptors; cholinergic nicotinic and muscarinic receptors; and nociceptin and neurokinin receptors (Litten et al. 2005). Finally, research efforts are also focused on identifying neurocircuits responsible for different aspects of alcoholism, such as craving, positive reward, protracted withdrawal symptoms, impaired control, tolerance, and psychological and cognitive components. Targeting specific sites within these circuits may lead to novel compounds that could alleviate certain aspects of alcoholism.

The fast pace of discoveries has also led to the identification of novel pharmacotherapeutic targets. For example, research on the cannabinoid receptor system has demonstrated its involvement in reward, learning, and memory. Research on the cannabinoid system has not only provided new insights into how marijuana disrupts memory traces, but has also led to the recognition of connections between the cannabinoid system and the neuronal processes underlying reward. The new science of cannabinoid (CB) receptor biology has triggered the development of rimonabant, the first CB$_1$ receptor–specific antagonist, and a potential medication for the treatment of a variety of ailments, including obesity and the metabolic syndrome (Van Gaal et al. 2005), pain, and addictive disorders. Rimonabant blocks the subjective high elicited by marijuana and may also be useful in preventing relapse to other drug use (Le Foll and Goldberg 2005).

The related CB$_2$ receptor was identified in a recent study as an exciting pharmacotherapeutic target (Ibrahim et al. 2005). Activation of the CB$_2$ receptor was found to inhibit acute, inflammatory, and neuropathic pain responses, but the absence of CB$_2$ receptors in the brain prevents any unwanted effects in the central nervous system (CNS). This discovery heralds the possibility of a potent pain medication without addiction liability.

The last example comes from recent examination of the connections between stress and substance addiction. It has been hypothesized that compounds that can dampen the stress response could be useful because of the important role that stress plays during a relapse to abusing drugs, alcohol, and nicotine. Such medications are currently being developed for the treatment of anxiety disorders and depression, but they may also have a role in the treatment of drug addiction. Indeed, several compounds, known as CRF receptor antagonists, have recently been shown to block the initiation of the stress response in the brain. These compounds have also shown a remarkable ability to block the initiation of drug taking in animals and the stress-induced reinstatement of drug-seeking behavior for a number of drugs of abuse (Koob 1999). These positive observations have prompted NIDA to move Antalarmin, the most promising among these, through preclinical development.

Behavioral Therapies

Many years of field experience show that substance abuse treatment programs can significantly increase treatment adherence and help the patients remain abstinent. By offering group and individual counseling opportunities and encouraging them to participate in complementary 12-Step programs, such as Alcoholic or Narcotics Anonymous, these intervention opportunities can produce impressive gains in treatment outcomes (Fiorentine and Hillhouse 2003). Historically, the concept and principles of 12-Step programs have strongly influenced the development of modern substance abuse treatments. However, as of today, there have not been any large clinical trials done to assess the active components relevant to the therapeutic effectiveness of these programs.

Studies clearly indicate that social context can affect brain dopaminergic function and the probability of succumbing to the addictive allure of psychoactive substances (Morgan et al. 2002; Shively et al. 1997). It is not surprising then that behavioral therapies have evolved to the point of offering effective treatment for the uncontrollable craving and frequent relapse characteristic of many alcohol and drug addicts.

In behavioral approaches, patients are typically ushered into a process that motivates them to initiate a personal recovery. The details and stringency of the strategies vary among the different modalities, which include cognitive, motivational, family, and couple therapies. Controlled studies have clearly shown the extent to which these therapies can help addicted individuals. In the late 1990s, for example, four different intensive psychosocial interventions for cocaine-dependent patients were compared by NIDA in the Collaborative Cocaine Treatment Study, and all treatments were found to be efficacious and to significantly reduce cocaine use by about 70% at 12-month follow-up (Crits-Christoph et al. 1999).

A similar outcome was obtained from Project MATCH (Matching Alcoholism Treatments to Client Heterogeneity), an NIAAA-sponsored large clinical trial designed to assess if different kinds of alcohol-dependent individuals fared better when assigned to different kinds of treatments (Babor and Del Boca 2002).

The Matrix model (Rawson et al. 1995) is another success story: an outpatient integrated therapeutic approach developed in the 1980s in response to an overwhelming demand for stimulant abuse treatment services. More than 5,000 cocaine addicts and more than 1,000 methamphetamine users were treated by therapists who fostered a positive, encouraging relationship with the patient and used that relationship to reinforce positive behavioral changes. The model has been extended more recently to include alcohol- and opiate-addicted individuals. NIDA-funded projects (Rawson et al. 1995, 2002) have demonstrated that participants treated with the Matrix model show statistically significant reductions in drug and alcohol use, improvements in psychological indicators, and reduced risky sexual behaviors associated with HIV transmission. Currently, projects are being conducted in 12 states and 4 countries employing this approach in treatment settings for stimulant, opiate, and alcohol users.

A commonly encountered obstacle to the successful treatment of people addicted to but trying to remain abstinent from heroin, alcohol, or other drugs of abuse is that they often fail to stay in treatment. Contingency management is a new empirically based treatment, based on positive reinforcement approaches, that has been specifically developed to address this issue. Contingency management can interface with an array of substance addiction treatment programs already in place in the community. The implementation of contingency management programs involves the collaboration of scientifically oriented researchers and clinicians from NIDA's Clinical Trials Network. Contingency management has been attracting a lot of attention lately as studies have begun to produce scientific evidence for its efficacy in the treatment of diverse drug abusing populations (Higgins et al. 2002; Petry 2000).

Because of the multiplicity of brain circuits underlying the various substance addiction syndromes, a multimodal approach, when validated, has emerged as the modality of choice, offering the best chance to successfully treat drug addiction. Consequently, and in the context of increasingly more effective interventions, psychosocial therapies ought to be regarded as critical components of a comprehensive substance abuse treatment (Substance Abuse and Mental Health Services Administration 1999).

Both NIDA and NIAAA will continue to support research on the synergistic interactions between medications and behavioral interventions that target different underlying causes so that subjects could benefit from mutually enhancing effects.

Treating Comorbidity

As mentioned earlier, a great number of individuals simultaneously suffer from substance abuse and mental illness, as well as other medical or physical disorders, such as chronic pain, hepatitis C, and AIDS. Unfortunately, our current health care system is not designed to identify and optimally address co-occurring drug and health problems.

The high prevalence of comorbidity between drug abuse and mental illness suggests common contributing factors. Thus, both NIDA and NIAAA are committed to support more research on the neurobiological underpinnings of co-occurring disorders and the risk and protective factors that influence these phenomena.

We are interested, for example, in assessing whether some mentally ill patients might enter the cycle of drug and alcohol addiction as a result of self-medication practices. On the other hand, it is critical to carefully evaluate whether any currently used medication has the potential to put a patient at increased risk of developing an addiction problem. The first line of treatment for noncomorbid attention-deficit/hyperactive disorder (ADHD), for example, consists of psychomotor stimulants, such as methylphenidate (Ritalin) and dextroamphetamine (Adderall), which are drugs that have reinforcing potential and can lead to addiction and abuse. These psychostimulants are prescribed with increasing frequency and for longer periods of time, so that understanding their long-term effects, both adverse and beneficial, has become an urgent priority. Specifically, do ADHD medications pose increased risks of substance abuse later in life? Interestingly, a recent meta-analysis concluded that adolescents treated for ADHD with methylphenidate appear to be 50% less likely to later develop drug abuse problems, compared with untreated individuals (Wilens et al. 2003). This is likely to reflect, in part, the protection afforded by associated changes in school performance, criminality levels, and self-worth (Fone and Nutt 2005). More research is needed to assess the true direct impact of psychostimulant drugs on the vulnerability toward drug addiction later in life, particularly in those individuals that may have been misdiagnosed as ADHD and treated with stimulant medications.

It is hard to overestimate the importance of accurately assessing the demographics and prevalence of co-occurring diseases, such as HIV/AIDS, mental illness, chronic pain, or hepatitis C in guiding research, prevention, and intervention programs. The co-occurrence of drug addiction together with many other disorders greatly enhances the vulnerability of at-risk populations, particularly the very young. Accordingly, there is a pressing need to support research on the development of more evidence-based strategies to address the problem of comorbidity.

MEETING THE CHALLENGES

Ultimately, our efforts should reduce the number of people entering the cycle of drug and alcohol addiction and increase the number of treatment options to help afflicted individuals recover from their disease and reclaim a life free of hurtful stigmas. While it is essential that we keep supporting the production of new knowledge to achieve these goals, it is clearly not sufficient. Our Institutes' outreach efforts are designed to maximize the transfer of knowledge back into society and educate the public about the emerging model of drug addiction as a chronic disease and the best strategies to prevent and treat addiction.

This goal appears more urgent than ever, as we enter an era when gaining a competitive edge is an end that justifies any means. Increasingly, medications such as steroids or stimulants are being used not just to cure ailments, but to improve perceived deficiencies, delay the effects of aging, and enhance cognitive and physical performance. NIDA will rise to the challenge of constantly updating its dissemination efforts, which must remain relevant in the face of changing patterns of drug abuse across the nation.

In this context, we hope that the implementation of cooperative initiatives with state authorities, community treatment centers, and the Substance Abuse and Mental Health Services Administration (SAMHSA) will also help us deliver a much more focused and accurate message.

Our efforts to meet the challenges identified in this article are being multiplied by our participation in cross-institutional programs for the development of tools and strategies designed to benefit all neuroscience-related diseases. NIDA and NIAAA are engaged in active collaborations toward the implementation of the National Institutes of Health Neuroscience Blueprint and Roadmap initiatives, and in the continuous monitoring of population survey figures and community derived epidemiological information, for the identification of emerging alcohol and drug-related threats to public health.

CONCLUSION

Recent research has increased our knowledge of how drugs can affect gene expression and neural circuitry in the brain, and how these changes ultimately alter human behavior. It has shed new light on the relationship between drug abuse and mental illness and the roles played by heredity, age, and other factors in increasing vulnerability to addiction. One of the main corollaries of such research efforts has been the clear understanding that substance addiction is a chronic and relapsing brain disease. At the individual level, this paradigm shift suggests that therapy approaches should be multipronged and attempt to 1) reduce the drug's rewarding effects, 2) enhance the rewarding effects of alternative reinforcers, 3) block drug-associated conditioned learning, and 4) engage cognitive and motivational control in treatment. At a higher level, the new concept should elicit society's commitment to destigmatize drug and alcohol addictions.

In spite of the tremendous progress made so far, much remains to be done. We are still delineating the brain's circuits involved in making addicted individuals more vulnerable to the effects of addictive substances. Thanks to the increased availability of high-resolution brain-imaging technologies and growing genetic databases, addiction researchers will be able to define, in ever increasing detail, the critical issues surrounding the maladaptive processes leading to addiction, craving, and relapse. We are beginning to explore the complex interactions among genes, and between genes and the environment, that influence the trajectory of the addiction process and the underlying factors that predispose to comorbid conditions. The information gained from these efforts should revolutionize the way clinicians approach the prevention and treatment of addiction and accelerate the development of individually tailored interventions that take into account socioeconomic, cultural, age, gender, and genetic factors.

CLINICAL IMPLICATIONS

Recent advances in the fields of genetics, molecular biology, behavioral neuropharmacology, and brain imaging have dramatically changed our understanding of the addictive process and why relapse occurs even in the face of catastrophic consequences. Addiction is now recognized as a chronic brain disease that involves complex interactions between repeated exposure to drugs, biological (i.e., genetic and developmental), and environmental (i.e., drug availability, social, and economic variables) factors. Its treatment, therefore, requires, in general, not only a long-term intervention but also a multipronged approach that addresses the psychiatric, medical, legal, and social consequences of addiction. Also, because addiction usually starts in adolescence or early adulthood and is frequently comorbid with mental illness, we need to expand our treatment interventions in this age group both for substance abuse and psychiatric disorders.

REFERENCES

Addolorato G, Caputo F, Capristo E, et al: Ability of baclofen in reducing alcohol craving and intake, II: preliminary clinical evidence. Alcohol Clin Exp Res 24:67–71, 2000

Amin J, Kaye M, Skidmore S, et al: HIV and hepatitis C coinfection within the CAESAR study. HIV Med 5:174–179, 2004

Babor TF, Del Boca FK: Treatment Matching in Alcoholism. International Research Monographs in the Addictions Series. Cambridge, UK, Cambridge University Press, 2002

Balldin J, Berglund M, Borg S, et al: A 6-month controlled naltrexone study: combined effect with cognitive behavioral therapy in outpatient treatment of alcohol dependence. Alcohol Clin Exp Res 27:1142–1149, 2003

Belluzzi JD, Lee AG, Oliff HS, et al: Age-dependent effects of nicotine on locomotor activity and conditioned place preference in rats. Psychopharmacology (Berl) 174:389–395, 2004

Benveniste H, Fowler JS, Rooney W, et al: Maternal and fetal 11C-cocaine uptake and kinetics measured in vivo by combined PET and MRI in pregnant nonhuman primates. J Nucl Med 46:312–320, 2005

Brebner K, Childress AR, Roberts DC: A potential role for GABA(B) agonists in the treatment of psychostimulant addiction. Alcohol Alcohol 37:478–484, 2002

Brebner K, Ahn S, Phillips AG: Attenuation of d-amphetamine self-administration by baclofen in the rat: behavioral and neurochemical correlates. Psychopharmacology (Berl) 177:409–417, 2005

Breiter HC, Gollub RL, Weisskoff RM, et al: Acute effects of cocaine on human brain activity and emotion. Neuron 19:591–611, 1997

Brodie JD, Figueroa E, Dewey SL: Treating cocaine addiction: from preclinical to clinical trial experience with gamma-vinyl GABA. Synapse 50:261–265, 2003

Cadet JL, Jayanthi S, Deng X: Speed kills: cellular and molecular bases of methamphetamine-induced nerve terminal degeneration and neuronal apoptosis. FASEB J 17:1775–1788, 2003

Campbell UC, Morgan AD, Carroll ME: Sex differences in the effects of baclofen on the acquisition of intravenous cocaine self-administration in rats. Drug Alcohol Depend 66:61–69, 2002

Carroll KM, Nich C, Ball SA, et al: Treatment of cocaine and alcohol dependence with psychotherapy and disulfiram. Addiction 93:713–727, 1998

Carroll KM, Ball SA, Nich C, et al: Targeting behavioral therapies to enhance naltrexone treatment of opioid dependence: efficacy of contingency management and significant other involvement, Arch Gen Psychiatry 58:755–761, 2001

Centers for Disease Control and Prevention: Diagnoses of HIV/AIDS—32 states, 2000–2003. MMWR Weekly 53:1106–1110, 2004a

Centers for Disease Control and Prevention: Alcohol consumption among women who are pregnant or who might become pregnant. MMWR Weekly 53:1178–1181, 2004b

Centers for Disease Control and Prevention: AIDS Surveillance—General Epidemiology L178 Slide Series (slide 9). Atlanta, GA, Division of HIV/AIDS Prevention, National Center for HIV, STD, and TB Prevention, Centers for Disease Control and Prevention, 2005a

Centers for Disease Control and Prevention: HIV Prevention Strategic Plan Through 2005. Atlanta, GA, Division of HIV/AIDS Prevention, National Center for HIV, STD, and TB Prevention, Centers for Disease Control and Prevention, 2005b

Centers for Disease Control and Prevention: Targeting Tobacco Use: The Nation's Leading Cause of Death. Atlanta, GA, National Center for Chronic Disease Prevention and Health Promotion, Centers for Disease Control and Prevention, 2005c

Chang L, Smith LM, LoPresti C, et al: Smaller subcortical volumes and cognitive deficits in children with prenatal methamphetamine exposure. Psychiatry Res 132:95–106, 2004

Chefer VI, Kieffer BL, Shippenberg TS: Contrasting effects of mu opioid receptor and delta opioid receptor deletion upon the behavioral and neurochemical effects of cocaine. Neuroscience 127:497–503, 2004

Chelonis JJ, Gillam MP, Paule MG: The effects of prenatal cocaine exposure on reversal learning using a simple visual discrimination task in rhesus monkeys. Neurotoxicol Teratol 25:437–446, 2003

Crits-Christoph P, Siqueland L, Blaine J, et al: Psychosocial treatments for cocaine dependence: National Institute on Drug Abuse Collaborative Cocaine Treatment Study. Arch Gen Psychiatry 56:493–502, 1999

Dackis CA, Lynch KG, Yu E, et al: Modafinil and cocaine: a double-blind, placebo-controlled drug interaction study. Drug Alcohol Depend 70:29–37, 2003

Day NL, Richardson GA: An analysis of the effects of prenatal alcohol exposure on growth: a teratologic model. Am J Med Genet Part C Semin Med Genet 127:28–34, 2004

Di Chiara G: Nucleus accumbens shell and core dopamine: differential role in behavior and addiction. Behav Brain Res 137:75–114, 2002

Drevets WC: Neuroimaging and neuropathological studies of depression: implications for the cognitive–emotional features of mood disorders. Curr Opin Neurobiol 11:240–249, 2001

Elliot DL, Goldberg L, Moe EL, et al: Preventing substance use and disordered eating: initial outcomes of the ATHENA (Athletes Targeting Healthy Exercise and Nutrition Alternatives) program. Arch Pediatr Adolesc Med 158:1043–1049, 2004

Fiorentine R, Hillhouse MP: Why extensive participation in treatment and twelve-step programs is associated with the cessation of addictive behaviors: an application of the addicted-self model of recovery. J Addict Dis 22:35–55, 2003

Fone KC, Nutt DJ: Stimulants: use and abuse in the treatment of attention deficit hyperactivity disorder. Curr Opin Pharmacol 5:87–93, 2005

Franklin TR, Acton PD, Maldjian JA, et al: Decreased gray matter concentration in the insular, orbitofrontal, cingulate, and temporal cortices of cocaine patients. Biol Psychiatry 51:134–142, 2002

Fudala PJ, Bridge TP, Herbert S, et al: Office-based treatment of opiate addiction with a sublingual-tablet formulation of buprenorphine and naloxone. N Engl J Med 349:949–958, 2003

Fulco CE, Liverman CT, Earley LE: Development of Medications for the Treatment of Opiate and Cocaine Addictions: Issues for the Government and Private Sector. Washington, DC, National Academy Press, 1995

Gerada C: Drug misuse: a review of treatments. Clin Med 5:69–73, 2005

Gogtay N, Giedd JN, Lusk L, et al: Dynamic mapping of human cortical development during childhood through early adulthood. Proc Natl Acad Sci U S A 101:8174–8179, 2004

Goldberg L, Elliot D, Clarke GN, et al: Effects of a multidimensional anabolic steroid prevention intervention. The Adolescents Training and Learning to Avoid Steroids (ATLAS) Program. JAMA 276:1555–1562, 1996

Goodwin RD, Stayner DA, Chinman MJ, et al: The relationship between anxiety and substance use disorders among individuals with severe affective disorders. Compr Psychiatry 43:245–252, 2002

Grant BF, Stinson FS, Harford TS: Age at onset of alcohol use and DSM-IV alcohol abuse and dependence: a 12-year follow-up. J Subst Abuse 13:493–504, 2001

Grant BF, Dawson DA, Stinson FS, et al: The 12-month prevalence and trends in DSM-IV alcohol abuse and dependence: United States, 1991–1992 and 2001–2002. Drug Alcohol Depend 74:223–234, 2004

Greenstein RA, Fudala PJ, O'Brien CP: Alternative Pharmacotherapies for Opiate Addiction. New York, Williams & Wilkins, 1997

Hansen RL, Struthers JM, Gospe SM Jr: Visual evoked potentials and visual processing in stimulant drug-exposed infants. Dev Med Child Neurol 35:798–805, 1993

Hanson GR, Rau KS, Fleckenstein AE: The methamphetamine experience: a NIDA partnership. Neuropharmacology 47:92–100, 2004

Harwood H: Updating Estimates of the Economic Costs of Alcohol Abuse in the United States: Estimates, Update Methods, and Data. Bethesda, MD, Report prepared by The Lewin Group for the National Institute on Alcohol Abuse and Alcoholism, National Institutes of Health, 2000

Harwood H: The Economic Costs of Drug Abuse in the United States: 1992–2002. Report prepared by The Lewin Group for the Office of National Drug Control Policy (ONDCP), 2004

Higgins ST, Budney AJ, Bickel WK, et al: Disulfiram therapy in patients abusing cocaine and alcohol. Am J Psychiatry 150:675–676, 1993

Higgins ST, Alessi SM, Dantona RL: Voucher-based incentives: a substance abuse treatment innovation. Addict Behav 27:887–910, 2002

Hinds DA, Stuve LL, Nilsen GB, et al: Whole genome patterns of common DNA variation in three human populations. Science 307:1072–1079, 2005

Hu XT, Ford K, White FJ: Repeated cocaine administration decreases calcineurin (PP2B) but enhances DARPP-32 modulation of sodium currents in rat nucleus accumbens neurons. Neuropsychopharmacology 30:916–926, 2005

Huestis MA, Choo RE: Drug abuse's smallest victims: in utero drug exposure. Forensic Sci Int 128:20–30, 2002

Ibrahim MM, Porreca F, Lai J, et al: CB2 cannabinoid receptor activation produces antinociception by stimulating peripheral release of endogenous opioids. Proc Natl Acad Sci U S A 102:3093–3098, 2005

Ikonomidou C, Bittigau P, Ishimaru MJ, et al: Ethanol induced apoptotic neurodegeneration and fetal alcohol syndrome. Science 287:1056–1060, 2000

Johnston LD, O'Malley PM, Bachman JG, et al: Monitoring the Future. National Results on Adolescent Drug Use: Overview of Key Findings, 2004, National Institute on Drug Abuse, 2005

Kalivas PW: Glutamate systems in cocaine addiction. Curr Opin Pharmacol 4:23–29, 2004a

Kalivas PW: Recent understanding in the mechanisms of addiction. Curr Psychiatry Rep 6:347–351, 2004b

Kalivas PW, Volkow N, Seamans J: Unmanageable motivation in addiction: a pathology in prefrontal-accumbens glutamate transmission. Neuron 45:647–650, 2005

Kampman KM, Pettinati H, Lynch KG, et al: A pilot trial of topiramate for the treatment of cocaine dependence. Drug Alcohol Depend 75:233–240, 2004

Kelley AE, Schochet T, Landry CF: Risk taking and novelty seeking in adolescence: introduction to part I. Ann N Y Acad Sci 1021:27–32, 2004

Kendler KS, Bulik CM, Silberg J, et al: Childhood sexual abuse and adult psychiatric and substance use disorders in women: an epidemiological and co-twin control analysis. Arch Gen Psychiatry 57:953–959, 2000

Kirchmayer U, Davoli M, Verster A: Naltrexone maintenance treatment for opioid dependence, in The Cochrane Database of Systematic Reviews, Issue 2. Chichester, UK, John Wiley & Sons, 2003

Klein H, Chao BS: Sexual abuse during childhood and adolescence as predictors of HIV related sexual risk during adulthood among female sexual partners of injection drug users. Violence Against Women 1:55–76, 1995

Koob GF: Stress, corticotropin-releasing factor, and drug addiction. Ann N Y Acad Sci 897:27–45, 1999

Kreek MJ, Nielsen DA, LaForge KS: Genes associated with addiction: alcoholism, opiate, and cocaine addiction. Neuromol Med 5:85–108, 2004

Lasser K, Boyd JW, Woolhandler S, et al: Smoking and mental illness: a population-based prevalence study. JAMA 284:2606–2610, 2000

Le Foll B, Goldberg SR: Cannabinoid CB1 receptor antagonists as promising new medications for drug dependence. J Pharmacol Exp Ther 312:875–883, 2005

Lidow MS: Consequences of prenatal cocaine exposure in nonhuman primates. Brain Res Dev Brain Res 147:23–36, 2003

Lineberry TW, Bostwick JM: Taking the physician out of "physician shopping": a case series of clinical problems associated with Internet purchases of medication. Mayo Clin Proc 79:1031–1034, 2004

Liotti M, Mayberg HS: The role of functional neuroimaging in the neuropsychology of depression. J Clin Exp Neuropsychol 23:121–136, 2001

Litten RZ, Fertig J, Mattson M, et al: Development of medications for alcohol use disorders: Recent advances and ongoing challenges. Expert Opin Emerg Drugs 10:323–343, 2005

Lu L, Hope BT, Dempsey J, et al: Central amygdala ERK signaling pathway is critical to incubation of cocaine craving. Nat Neurosci 8:212–219, 2005

Luna B, Sweeney JA: The emergence of collaborative brain function: fMRI studies of the development of response inhibition. Ann N Y Acad Sci 1021:296–309, 2004

McClung CA, Ulery PG, Perrotti LI, et al: DeltaFosB: a molecular switch for long-term adaptation in the brain. Brain Res Mol Brain Res 132:146–154, 2004

McCoy CB, Lai S, Metsch LR, et al: Injection drug use and crack cocaine smoking: independent and dual risk behaviors for HIV infection. Ann Epidemiol 14:535–542, 2004

McFarland K, Lapish CC, Kalivas PW: Prefrontal glutamate release into the core of the nucleus accumbens mediates cocaine-induced reinstatement of drug-seeking behavior. J Neurosci 23:3531–3537, 2003

McLellan AT, Lewis DC, O'Brien CP, et al: Drug dependence, a chronic medical illness: implications for treatment, insurance, and outcomes evaluation. JAMA 284:1689–1695, 2000

McLellan AT, McKay JR, Forman R, et al: Reconsidering the evaluation of addiction treatment: from retrospective follow-up to concurrent recovery monitoring. Addiction 100:447–458, 2005

Morgan D, Grant KA, Gage HD, et al: Social dominance in monkeys: dopamine D2 receptors and cocaine self-administration. Nat Neurosci 5:169–174, 2002

Nath A, Hauser KF, Wojna V, et al: Molecular basis for interactions of HIV and drugs of abuse. J Acquir Immune Defic Syndr 31:S62–S69, 2002

National Institute on Drug Abuse: Principles of Drug Addiction Treatment: A Research-Based Guide (NIH Publication No. 00-4180). Bethesda, MD, National Institute on Drug Abuse, National Institutes of Health, 2000

National Institute on Drug Abuse: Preventing Drug Abuse Among Children and Adolescents (NIH Publication No. 03-4212[B]). Bethesda, MD, National Institute on Drug Abuse, National Institutes of Health, 2003

Nestler EJ: Molecular mechanisms of drug addiction. Neuropharmacology 47:24–32, 2004

Nordstrom-Klee B, Delaney-Black V, Covington C, et al: Growth from birth onwards of children prenatally exposed to drugs: a literature review. Neurotoxicol Teratol 24:481–488, 2002

Olney J: Fetal alcohol syndrome at the cellular level. Addict Biol 9:137–149, 2004

Oswald LM, Wand GS: Opioids and alcoholism. Physiol Behav 81:339–358, 2004

Paltiel AD, Weinstein MC, Kimmel AD, et al: Expanded screening for HIV in the United States—an analysis of cost-effectiveness. N Engl J Med 352:586–595, 2005

Petry NM: A comprehensive guide to the application of contingency management procedures in clinical settings. Drug Alcohol Depend 58:9–25, 2000

Rawson RA, Shoptaw SJ, Obert JL, et al: An intensive outpatient approach for cocaine abuse treatment. The Matrix model. J Subst Abuse Treat 12:117–127, 1995

Rawson RA, Huber A, Brethen P, et al: Status of methamphetamine users 2–5 years after outpatient treatment. J Addict Dis 21:107–119, 2002

Regier DA, Farmer ME, Rae DS, et al: Comorbidity of mental disorders with alcohol and other drug abuse. Results from the Epidemiologic Catchment Area (ECA) Study. JAMA 264:2511–2518, 1990

Resnick MD, Bearman PS, Blum RW, et al: Protecting adolescents from harm. Findings from the National Longitudinal Study on Adolescent Health. JAMA 278:823–832, 1997

Richardson GA, Conroy ML, Day NL: Prenatal cocaine exposure: effects on the development of school-age children. Neurotoxicol Teratol 18:627–634, 1996

Safdar K, Schiff ER: Alcohol and hepatitis C. Semin Liver Dis 24:305–315, 2004

Sanders GD, Bayoumi AM, Sundaram V, et al: Cost-effectiveness of screening for HIV in the era of highly active antiretroviral therapy. N Engl J Med 352:570–585, 2005

Schiffer WK, Marsteller D, Dewey SL: Sub-chronic low-dose gamma-vinyl GABA (vigabatrin) inhibits cocaine-induced increases in nucleus accumbens dopamine. Psychopharmacology (Berl) 168:339–343, 2003

Schuster CR: Drug abuse research and HIV/AIDS: a national perspective from the US. Br J Addict 87:355–361, 1992

Shively CA, Grant KA, Ehrenkaufer RL, et al: Social stress, depression, and brain dopamine in female cynomolgus monkeys. Ann N Y Acad Sci 807:574–577, 1997

Shoptaw S, Yang X, Rotheram-Fuller EJ, et al: Randomized placebo-controlled trial of baclofen for cocaine dependence: preliminary effects for individuals with chronic patterns of cocaine use. J Clin Psychiatry 64:1440–1448, 2003

Singer LT, Minnes S, Short E, et al: Cognitive outcomes of preschool children with prenatal cocaine exposure. JAMA 291:2448–2456, 2004

Smith LM, Chang L, Yonekura ML, et al: Brain proton magnetic resonance spectroscopy in children exposed to methamphetamine in utero. Neurology 57:255–260, 2001

Sowell ER, Thompson PM, Peterson BS, et al: Mapping cortical gray matter asymmetry patterns in adolescents with heavy prenatal alcohol exposure. Neuroimage 17:1807–1819, 2002

Sowell ER, Thompson PM, Toga AW: Mapping changes in the human cortex throughout the span of life. Neuroscientist 10:372–392, 2004

Spear LP: The adolescent brain and age-related behavioral manifestations. Neurosci Biobehav Rev 24:417–463, 2000

Stein EA, Pankiewicz J, Harsch HH, et al: Nicotine induced limbic cortical activation in the human brain: a functional MRI study. Am J Psychiatry 155:1009–1015, 1998

Substance Abuse and Mental Health Services Administration: SAMHSA/CSAT Treatment Improvement Protocol (TIP) 35: Enhancing Motivation for Change in Substance Abuse Treatment (SMA 99 3354). Rockville, MD, Center for Substance Abuse Treatment, Substance Abuse and Mental Health Services Administration, 1999

Substance Abuse and Mental Health Services Administration: Drug and Alcohol Services Information System (DASIS) Report: Pregnant Women in Substance Abuse Treatment: 2002. Rockville, MD, Office of Applied Studies, Substance Abuse and Mental Health Services Administration, 2004a

Substance Abuse and Mental Health Services Administration: Results From the 2003 National Survey on Drug Use and Health (NSDUH Series H-25). Rockville, MD, Office of Applied Studies, Substance Abuse and Mental Health Services Administration, 2004b

Szumlinski KK, Dehoff MH, Kang SH, et al: Homer proteins regulate sensitivity to cocaine. Neuron 43:401–413, 2004

Tapper AR, McKinney SL, Nashmi R, et al: Nicotine activation of alpha4 receptors: sufficient for reward, tolerance, and sensitization. Science 306:1029–1032, 2004

Tarter RE, Blackson T, Brigham J, et al: The association between childhood irritability and liability to substance use in early adolescence: a 2-year follow-up study of boys at risk for substance abuse. Drug Alcohol Depend 39:253–261, 1995

Thompson PM, Hayashi KM, Simon SL, et al: Structural abnormalities in the brains of human subjects who use methamphetamine. J Neurosci 24:6028–6036, 2004

True WR, Xian H, Scherrer JF, et al: Common genetic vulnerability for nicotine and alcohol dependence in men. Arch Gen Psychiatry 56:655–661, 1999

Van Gaal LF, Rissanen AM, Scheen AJ, et al: Effects of the cannabinoid-1 receptor blocker rimonabant on weight reduction and cardiovascular risk factors in overweight patients: 1-year experience from the RIO-Europe study. Lancet 365:1389–1397, 2005

Ventura SJ, Abma JC, Mosher WD, et al: Estimated pregnancy rates for the United States, 1990–2000: an update. National Vital Statistics Report 52:1–9, 2004

Volkow ND: The reality of comorbidity: depression and drug abuse. Biol Psychiatry 56:714–717, 2004

Volkow ND, Fowler JS, Wang GJ, et al: Decreased dopamine D2 receptor availability is associated with reduced frontal metabolism in cocaine abusers. Synapse 14:169–177, 1993

Volkow ND, Wang GJ, Fowler JS, et al: Decreased striatal dopaminergic responsiveness in detoxified cocaine-dependent subjects. Nature 386:830–833, 1997

Volkow ND, Fowler JS, Wang GJ, et al: Role of dopamine, the frontal cortex and memory circuits in drug addiction: insight from imaging studies. Neurobiol Learn Mem 78:610–624, 2002

Volkow ND, Fowler JS, Wang GJ: The addicted human brain: insights from imaging studies. J Clin Invest 111:1444–1451, 2003

Volkow ND, Fowler JS, Wang GJ, et al: Dopamine in drug abuse and addiction: results from imaging studies and treatment implications. Mol Psychiatry 9:557–569, 2004

Wang GJ, Volkow ND, Fowler JS, et al: Regional brain metabolic activation during craving elicited by recall of previous drug experiences. Life Sci 64:775–784, 1999

Wilens TE, Faraone SV, Biederman J, et al: Does stimulant therapy of attention-deficit/ hyperactivity disorder beget later substance abuse? A meta-analytic review of the literature. Pediatrics 111:179–185, 2003

Yu Q, Larson DF, Watson RR: Heart disease, methamphetamine and AIDS. Life Sci 73:129–140, 2003

Yuferov V, Kroslak T, Laforge KS, et al: Differential gene expression in the rat caudate putamen after "binge" cocaine administration: advantage of triplicate microarray analysis. Synapse 48:157–169, 2003

Zhang D, Zhang L, Lou DW, et al: The dopamine D1 receptor is a critical mediator for cocaine-induced gene expression. J Neurochem 82:1453–1464, 2002

Zhang D, Zhang L, Tang Y, et al: Repeated cocaine administration induces gene expression changes through the dopamine D1 receptors. Neuropsychopharmacology 30: 1443–1454, 2005

Zhu LX, Sharma S, Stolina M, et al: Delta-9 tetrahydrocannabinol inhibits antitumor immunity by a CB2 receptor-mediated, cytokine-dependent pathway. J Immunol 165:373–380, 2000

12

Alcoholism

Developmental Patterns of Drinking and Prevention of Alcohol Use Disorders

Ting-Kai Li, M.D.
Ellen Witt, Ph.D.
Brenda G. Hewitt, B.A.

The production and use of alcoholic beverages in many cultures predate written history, and the majority of adults who drink alcohol experience few if any adverse consequences from these practices. However, an estimated 28% of U.S. adults 18 years and older engage in high-risk drinking patterns—drinking too much too fast and too much too often—that significantly increase their odds of developing drinking-related problems, including alcohol abuse and dependence. Furthermore, although use by individuals younger than 21 years is illegal, a troubling number of adolescents and young adults not only drink but engage in high-risk drinking patterns that can lead to serious and often fatal consequences for them both acutely and over the course of their lives. Animal and human studies have begun to shed light on the complex interplay of hormonal and neuronal systems with such behavioral patterns common to adolescence (e.g., risk-taking behavior) that makes adolescent alcohol use so much more deadly than the traditionally viewed "rite of passage." Recent research also reveals that alcohol use disorders are highly comorbid with drug use disorders and major psychiatric illnesses. Identification of similarities in the age of onset of alcohol dependence and that of many co-occurring illnesses—between 18 and 25 years—coupled with our increasing understanding of the differences between the adolescent and the adult brain, is leading to a shift in paradigm of alcohol prevention and intervention which considers adolescence and early adulthood critical windows of opportunity for preventing the early onset of alcohol use disorders and/or beginning early treatment. Continued progress in understanding the mechanisms involved in periadolescent development, how alcohol affects them, and their relationship to co-occurring problems in adolescents will link biology and psychology and provide evidence-based approaches for effective prevention and intervention. Finally, evidence-based screening based on quantity/frequency measures and brief intervention in adult primary health care populations have been shown to help patients who engage in high-risk drinking to reduce consumption. Correlating these measures with screening tools for adolescent populations remains to be done. An important next step in preventing alcohol use disorders (AUDs) and their many complications for both adults and adolescents is to develop models of dimensional severity in alcohol use disorders (as has been done in other disorders, such as diabetes, and hypertension).

ALCOHOL CONSUMPTION, ABUSE, AND DEPENDENCE IN THE UNITED STATES

In the United States, 67% of the population age 18 years and older are drinkers (individuals who have reported drinking at least one drink in the past 12 months); more men are drinkers than women (76% vs. 24%); and a majority of the alcohol consumed (61%) is used by a relatively small population (10%) of very heavy drinkers (Greenfield and Rogers 1999). It is this heavy-drinking population that is largely responsible for the considerable impact of alcohol use disorders on our nation's health, society, and economy.

Individual Variations in Responses to Alcohol

A U.S. standard drink contains about 14 grams (about 0.6 fluid ounces) of pure alcohol. Thus, 12 oz. of beer or cooler, 8.5 oz. of malt liquor, 5.0 oz. of table wine, 3.5 oz. of fortified wine, 2.5 oz. of a cordial, liqueur, or aperitif, 1.5 oz. of distilled spirits (e.g., vodka, bourbon) are all equivalent measures. However, whereas *drinks* are standardized, *drinkers* are not. There is a three- to fourfold variation among individuals in the pharmacokinetics of alcohol absorption, distribution, and metabolism and a two- to threefold difference among individuals in the pharmacodynamic or subjective and objective responses to alcohol. About one-half of these differences is due to genetics. These individual variations determine, in part, why individuals can experience the effects of alcohol, such as feeling intoxicated ("high") or impaired motor coordination, from different amounts of alcohol consumed.

GENETIC AND ENVIRONMENTAL FACTORS IN THE DEVELOPMENT OF ALCOHOL DEPENDENCE

Alcohol dependence is a common complex disorder/disease involving the interactions of different sets of genes in different people exposed to different environments. As noted previously, approximately 50% of the risk for developing alcohol dependence is genetic. This level of genetic risk is similar to that for other common, serious health disorders, such as adult-onset diabetes, hypertension, asthma, and manic-depressive illness. Genetic factors are both nonspecific and specific. Nonspecific factors include personality/temperament and externalizing/internalizing disorders (e.g., antisocial personality disorder, mood and anxiety disorders). Specific factors include those that influence the absorption and metabolism of alcohol and those that influence the objective and subjective responses to alcohol. Environmental influences (e.g., childhood abuse and trauma and nonfamilial influences such as peer relationships, stress, and substance availability) account for the remaining 50% of the risk for developing alcohol dependence. These influences are mostly nonshared (Kendler et al. 2003) and change over the life span (Knopik et al. 2004). Environmental risks predominate in adolescence; genetic factors become more and more important with age and experience in drinking and in the quantity and frequency of drinking.

ALCOHOL USE DISORDERS

Alcohol abuse, defined as recurring personal, interpersonal, and societal problems, and alcohol dependence, which includes loss of control over drinking, a preoccupation with drinking, compulsive drinking, and physical dependence, together constitute AUDs. The cost of AUDs is significant. For example, 18 million Americans, or 8.5% of the U.S. population age 18 years and older, suffer from alcohol abuse or alcohol dependence (B. F. Grant et al. 2004). In addition, AUDs are associated with an estimated 85,000 deaths annually and are the third leading cause of preventable death in the United States (Mokdad et al. 2004). Alcohol-related problems are estimated to cost the U.S. economy $185 billion annually (Harwood et al. 1999).

Developmental Patterns of Drinking

Historically, alcoholism has been characterized as a chronic relapsing disease of mid-to-late adulthood, because the disease becomes readily apparent to health professionals only after patients have manifested its multiple adverse consequences over many years. By then, the disease is usually in its late, severe, chronic form. Recent findings from epidemiological research concerning the age at onset of AUDs and other co-occurring conditions have radically changed the way in which we must think about the onset of AUDs and how to prevent them. These findings are converging with findings from the biological and behavioral neurosciences to reveal that not only are adolescents at risk for the early onset of AUDs, but a part of their vulnerability stems from the nature of adolescence (i.e., the influence of hormones and genetics on brain development and behavior in adolescence, and the impact of alcohol use on both).

Underage Drinking: Prevalence and Problems

Data from the National Epidemiological Survey on Alcohol and Related Conditions (NESARC), a national survey directed by the National Institute on Alcohol Abuse and Alcoholism (NIAAA) of the National Institutes of Health, contain a wealth of clues about alcohol use disorders and who is at risk for them. The NESARC, conducted in 2001–2002, was a representative survey of the U.S. civilian noninstitutionalized population age 18 years and older on alcohol and substance use and disorders and major psychiatric conditions based on DSM-IV (American Psychiatric Association 1994) diagnostic criteria (B. F. Grant et al. 2003). More than 43,000 American adults participated in the survey, which had a response rate of 81%. Among its purposes, the NESARC is intended to identify prevalence, onset, and remissions over the life course of alcohol and co-occurring mental and substance use disorders and is designed to be longitudinal with data collected in successive studies.

Analysis of data from the NESARC and from the NIAAA's 1991–1992 National Longitudinal Alcohol Epidemiological Survey (NLAES) has provided an eye-opening view on adolescent vulnerability to alcohol use and co-occurring conditions. For example, the NESARC reveals that alcohol, nicotine, and cannabis are used by youth as young as 10–12 years of age, use of all three substances rise steeply by age 15 years, and alcohol is clearly the substance of choice for many underage youth (Figure 12–1). Even more striking is the age of onset of alcohol, nicotine, and cannabis use disorders. Each of these disorders displays a similar steep developmental trajectory in prevalence up through age 15–16 years which declines steeply after age 25 years for both alcohol dependence and cannabis use disorders. The ages of first use and onset of illness become even more important when viewed in terms of the age of onset of brain disorders that are comorbid with alcohol and drug use disorders. Obsessive-compulsive disorders and eating disorders typically have their onsets between 10 and 13 years of age, and bipolar disorder, panic disorder, and social phobia typically have onsets between the ages of 13 and 20 years, all corresponding with the age of first use of alcohol. The NESARC data on age at first substance use and age at onset of illness are further substantiated by an analysis of the survey's prevalence data by age. The highest 12-month prevalence of DSM-IV alcohol dependence was among individuals ages 18–29 years (9%), versus a prevalence of 6% for *all other ages combined* (B.F. Grant et al. 2004). These youth and young adults whose lives and careers are just beginning are not only developing alcohol dependence early in their lives, but they are more likely to also develop a co-occurring psychiatric condition. Alcohol-dependent individuals are 2½ times more likely to develop an anxiety disorder, 7 times more likely to develop antisocial personality disorder, and 37 times more likely to develop drug dependence than individuals who are not alcohol dependent (B.F. Grant et al. 2005a, 2005b).

Consequences of Underage Drinking

Alcohol is the most commonly used drug by children and adolescents. In 2003, 17.7% of young people ages 12–17 years reported past-month use of alcohol, versus 11.2% for any illicit drug (including nonmedical use of psychotherapeutic medications) and 14.4% for any tobacco product (Substance Abuse and Mental Health Services Administration 2003). The consequences of underage drinking are significant during adolescence, a period of rapid and profound physical and mental development, and continue throughout the individual's life. For example, teenagers who begin drinking before age 15 years have four times the risk of developing alcohol dependence later in life (B.F. Grant and Dawson 1997). In addition, adolescents with histories of extensive alcohol use have noticeable changes in brain function that impair learning, memory, and problem solving (Caldwell et al. 2005) and smaller hippocampal volume (De Bellis et al. 2000) compared with adoles-

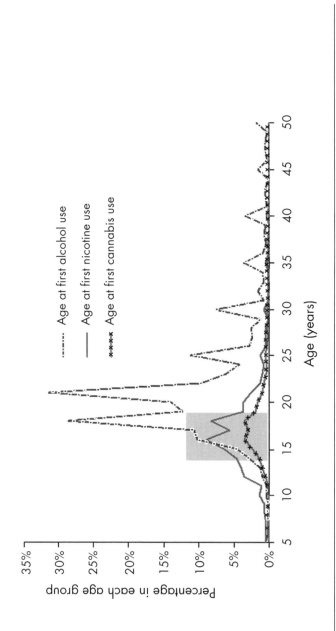

FIGURE 12–1.   Age at first use of alcohol, nicotine, and cannabis.

Source.   National Institute on Alcohol Abuse and Alcoholism (NIAAA) National Epidemiologic Survey on Alcohol and Related Conditions, 2003. Available at: http://niaaa.census.gov.

cents who do not have such histories. Finally, teens who use alcohol and drugs are more likely to be involved in violent behaviors (Swahn et al. 2004).

Adolescent Drinking Patterns

The drinking patterns of adolescents differ from those of adults. Youth ages 12–17 years drink less frequently but more per occasion than do adults, in a pattern frequently referred to as binge drinking (Substance Abuse and Mental Health Services Administration 2003). Individuals who start to drink before age 13 years are 9 times more likely to binge-drink frequently (5+ drinks on an occasion at least 6 times per month) as high school students than those who begin drinking later. Compared with nondrinkers, a greater proportion of frequent binge drinkers engage in other risky behaviors, including carrying a gun (24% vs. 2%), using marijuana (71% vs. 6%), using cocaine (22% vs. 4%), and having sex with 6 or more partners (32% vs. 3%) (Hingson 2004). This pattern of drinking is harmful at any age, but adolescents are particularly vulnerable because they are in the process of making the rapid biological and behavioral changes that will usher in adulthood.

There are significant consequences of drinking for college students, many of whom are also underage drinkers. For instance, in 2001 more than 1,700 college students ages 18–24 years died from alcohol-related unintentional injuries, including motor vehicle crashes; 2.8 million of the 8.9 million college students in the U.S. drove under the influence of alcohol; and more than 600,000 were hit or assaulted by another student who had been drinking (Hingson et al. 2005).

Underage Drinking: Biology and Behavior

Research indicates that the human brain continues to develop into a person's mid-20s. The number and kinds of nerve cells in the brain are changing, and connections between brain cells are reforming. During this time, adolescents face not only major physiological changes but also changes in their social roles, and decision-making competes strongly with emotions for control of behavior. Evidence from both animal and human studies strongly suggests that people who suffer from alcohol dependence (and major depression, cannabis dependence, and tobacco addiction) are influenced by this developmental process.

Although early alcohol use alone is a significant risk factor for developing lifetime alcohol dependence, genetics also plays a part. Nearly 60% of youngsters with a positive family history of alcohol dependence who begin drinking by the age of 15 years will develop alcohol dependence at some point during their life course. This compares with less than 30% of those who have a negative family history who begin drinking by the same age. Early adolescent problem behavior identifies a subset of youth who are at especially high risk for developing adult psychopathology, including AUDs, suggesting general, rather than specific, mechanisms of risk (McGue and Iacono 2005). Early abuse of alcohol is familial, heritable in males, and caused in part by genetic risk for disinhibitory psychopathology in males and to shared environmental factors in females (McGue et al. 2001). There is further evidence from electrophysiological studies that identifies disinhibited or externalizing psychopathology as a nonspecific (non-alcohol-related) risk factor for developing alcohol dependence (Carlson et al. 2004).

Adolescent Motivation

Understanding adolescent motivation is critical for understanding why so many young people drink alcohol and engage in associated behaviors such as drinking and driving and sexual risk-taking. In one recent study (Bjork et al. 2004), adolescents showed less activity than adults in brain regions that motivate behavior to obtain rewards. For both age groups, the researchers found that the anticipation of potential gain activated portions of the ventral striatum, right insula, dorsal thalamus, and dorsal midbrain, with the magnitude of ventral striatum activation sensitive to magnitude of the anticipated gain. In adolescents, however, there was lower activation of the right ventral striatum centered in the nucleus accumbens, a region at the base of the brain that is a key component of the reward system.

Animal models have also demonstrated a difference in initial tolerance and sensitivity to alcohol by adolescents compared with adults. For example, adolescent rats consume higher absolute levels of alcohol than older animals due to a combination of factors. These include less sensitivity than adult animals to the aversive effects of acute intoxication (sedation, ataxia, social impairment, and acute withdrawal/hangover effects), greater sensitivity to alcohol-induced social facilitation and stimulation of alcohol intake by social experiences (Spear and Varlinskaya 2005). The neural basis for these developmental differences in initial response to alcohol remains speculative. However, recent evidence suggests that the relative resistance of adolescents to the sedative effects of alcohol is related in part to both accelerated development of acute tolerance (Silveri and Spear 1998) and developmental immaturity of the gamma-aminobutyric acid (GABA) and/or N-methyl-D-aspartate (NMDA) receptor systems (Silveri and Spear 2004a). The available data on the consequences of longer-term adaptations (i.e., rapid and chronic tolerance) to alcohol's effects in adolescents are inconsistent, with studies indicating more tolerance in adolescents than adults, similar levels of tolerance, or the appearance of sensitization rather than tolerance after repeated adolescent exposures.

PUBERTY, HORMONES, AND SEX DIFFERENCES IN ALCOHOL ABUSE AND DEPENDENCE

Converging evidence from the National Survey on Drug Use and Health (Substance Abuse and Mental Health Services Administration 2003), an in-person survey of individuals ages 12 years and older, and from a study of 4,010 Australian twin pairs (Knopik et al. 2004) shows that adolescent males and females between the ages of 12 and 17 years have similar patterns of alcohol use (frequency and quantity) as well as prevalence of DSM-IV alcohol abuse and dependence. By about age 17 years, however, the gender-specific patterns and prevalence begin to diverge and remain disparate across the ages surveyed (12–65+ years), with females reporting fewer drinking days in the past month, fewer days of drinking 5 or more drinks in the past month, and lower prevalence of alcohol abuse and dependence. Recent cross-sectional survey data of 10- and 15-year-old subjects in the United States and Australia (Patton et al. 2004) found that pubertal stage is associated with higher rates of substance use and abuse, including alcohol. In this study, adolescents in later pubertal stages were found to be two to three times more likely to report lifetime and recent substance use than were those at an early pubertal stage, independent of age and school grade level. A few studies, which focused on adolescent girls, found that earlier puberty is associated with younger age at onset of drinking and smoking (Dick et al. 2000). The usual interpretation for this finding is that social factors and environmental stressors mediate the relationship between maturational changes during puberty and the onset of alcohol or substance use. However, the biologically based mechanisms that could explain the progression of gender differences in alcohol drinking patterns during puberty, such as changes in reproductive hormones and stress responses and their effects on developmental neurobiological processes, remain relatively unexplored.

Puberty and the Onset of Substance Use and Abuse

Puberty ushers in a phase of heightened risk for alcohol and substance use. The strongest social factor associated with pubertal stage and substance use was peer associations (Patton et al. 2004). Questions remain about whether, and if so, to what extent, socialization changes during pubertal stage of development and subsequent gender differences in alcohol dependence are biologically driven by sex hormones and by ontogenetic changes in ethanol-elicited corticosterone response in the HPA (Silveri and Spear 2004b).

Hormonal Changes Associated With the Onset of Puberty

Puberty is a gradual physiological process that occurs between the ages of 6 and 12 years and results in the attainment of sexual maturation. The two main stages of pubertal development are the adrenarche and gonadarche. During the adrenarche period (between 6 and 9 years of age), there is a rise in levels of a variety of androgens, including adrenal androgens. The second stage of pubertal development, the gonadarche, brings about the production of gonadal steroids that are critical for "activating" sex differences in specific behaviors. At puberty, the primary activating role of gonadal steroids is to support the development of sex differences in reproductive physiology and behavior. In both males and females, puberty is a period of reawakening of the hypothalamic-pituitary-gonadal (HPG) axis, which is dormant during early to mid-childhood. This reactivation is followed by marked increases in gonadal sex steroid output (estrogen and testosterone).

Sex differences in alcohol self-administration have been observed in adult nonhuman primates, with males consuming approximately 1.5-fold more alcohol than females (Vivian et al. 2001). In contrast to humans and nonhuman primates, female rodents tend to drink more alcohol than do males (Lancaster and Spiegel 1992), although these differences may be influenced by environmental variables (Middaugh et al. 1999), body weight differences, and stress (K. Eriksson and Pikkarainen 1968). Of greater interest is that increased voluntary ethanol intake in female rats relative to males occurs at around the time of puberty, suggesting a hormonal basis for this difference (Lancaster et al. 1996). Other rodent studies have shown sex differences in behavioral responses to intoxication, such as locomotor activation, and loss of the righting reflex (Jones and Whitfield 1995), which may also be affected by species or age (Webb et al. 2002). Finally, one study examined a potential neural mechanism for sex differences in alcohol consumption and found that female rats show greater extracellular release of dopamine in the nucleus accumbens relative to males, as well as greater consumption of alcohol (Blanchard et al. 1993). These sex differences in alcohol consumption and behavioral response to alcohol could be due to hormonal changes that modulate neural sensitivity to alcohol. However, sex and ontogenetic differences in the pharmacokinetics of ethanol, which affects the amount of alcohol that reaches the brain, could also explain the gender differences in these behaviors during development (Brasser and Spear 2002). To date, most of the research on sex differences in alcohol drinking and response to alcohol has been conducted in adult subjects. Only one study (Lancaster et al. 1996) has focused on the emergence of differential drinking patterns during the early postpubertal period, although others suggest that age may be an important factor in the expression of sex differences (Collins et al. 1975; Middaugh et al. 1992). Clearly, more research is needed to characterize the evolution of sex differences in alcohol consumption and response to alcohol during the pubertal period.

Alcohol, Hormones, and Adolescents

Researchers have used a number of approaches to investigate the role of gonadal hormones in the observed sex differences in patterns of alcohol consumption and response to alcohol. For example, correlational studies have found evidence that gonadal hormones are associated with drinking behavior and other responses to alcohol, such as aggression. A positive relationship was also found between alcohol intake, testosterone levels, and aggressive responding in adult male human and nonhuman primates (von der Pahlen 2005). Two self-report studies, in male and female college students (La Grange et al. 1995) and in female adolescents (Martin et al. 1999), found a positive correlation of testosterone with alcohol consumption in male and female college students, but the correlation was stronger in males. In female adolescents, current alcohol use (within the past month) was associated with higher levels of testosterone and estradiol (suggesting involvement of gonadal and adrenal steroids with alcohol use in these women). A recent study on the relationship between testosterone and alcohol use among male twins found significant relationships between higher levels of testosterone and ever drinking, frequent intoxication, greater number of drinks within 24 hours, more alcohol symptoms and DSM-III-R (American Psychiatric Association 1987) diagnoses of alcohol dependency (C.J. Eriksson et al. 2005). The authors note the interesting hypothesis that underlying testosterone elevations may be related to the promotion of alcohol consumption through a hypothalamic opiate mechanism. Finally, a single study in male hamsters on the relationship between puberty, drinking, and testosterone found that adolescent animals that voluntarily drank large quantities of ethanol had twice the blood levels of testosterone of controls (Ferris et al. 1998). However, this difference disappeared by adulthood. Nevertheless, the authors suggest that elevated exposure to testosterone during puberty may have permanently altered the HPG axis, because these same animals showed augmented aggression in adulthood.

At present, inconsistent findings within and between species, as well as the lack of controls in human studies, make it difficult to establish a clear association between changes in endogenous hormone levels during the menstrual cycle of females and alterations in drinking patterns.

Effects of Reproductive Hormone Changes on Neural Circuits Associated With Alcohol-Seeking Behavior

It is well known that gonadal steroids play an "organizational" role during brief periods of early brain development to permanently establish differences between males and females in brain structures and functions. During later development and throughout adulthood, gonadal steroids are critical for "activating" gender-related differences in specific behaviors. Although puberty is primarily linked with hormonal activation of sexual reproductive behaviors, gonadal steroids are also responsible for sex differences in brain structure and function unrelated to reproduction via effects on their respective receptors distributed throughout the brain (Cameron 2004; Rubinow and Schmidt 1996). In humans and/or animals, actions of gonadal steroids have been implicated in gender-related differences in nonreproductive behaviors, such as aggression, motor activity, learning, memory, and affect regulation, as well as responses to alcohol and other drugs (Cameron 2004).

Alcohol, Hormones, and Adolescents—Neurosteroids

The term *neuroactive steroids* refers to steroids synthesized in the brain, adrenals. and gonads that affect neuronal excitability by acting in a rapid nongenomic manner at the membrane surface of certain neurotransmitter receptors (Barbaccia 2004; Paul and Purdy 1992; Rupprecht 2003). There is now considerable evidence that neuroactive steroids, particularly the progesterone metabolite allopregnanolone (3-hydroxy-5-pregnan-20-one), interact with alcohol at the GABA type A ($GABA_A$) receptor to produce electrophysiological, pharmacological, and behavioral effects (Devaud et al. 2003; Morrow et al. 1999, 2001). Allopregnanolone and ethanol are both positive modulators of GABAA receptors and share similar pharmacological properties, the most prominent being their anxiolytic and anticonvulsant effects.

A few studies have investigated the role of allopregnanolone in modulating sex differences in susceptibility to alcohol abuse. Pretreatment with allopregnanolone was found to increase voluntary ethanol intake in male mice (Sinnott et al. 2002). Furthermore, consumption of ethanol increased brain allopregnanolone levels in male, but not female mice (Finn et al. 2004; K. A. Grant et al. 1997). Because brain and plasma baseline levels of allopregnanolone are greater in female than in male rats, even at puberty, and fluctuate during the estrus and menstrual cycle in rodents and nonhuman primates, sex differences in basal levels of allopregnanolone or changes in circulating levels of allopregnanolone across the menstrual cycle could account for differences in sensitivity to exogenously administered ethanol (Finn et al. 2004; K. A. Grant et al. 1997) and/or development of physical dependence (Morrow et al. 1995). However, the ability of allopregnanolone to differentially modulate the effects of ethanol in males and females has not been examined from a developmental perspective, particularly at the onset of puberty.

Interaction of Stress and Gonadal Hormones at Puberty and Gender Differences in Alcohol-Seeking Behavior

The interrelationship between the stress response of the hypothalamic-pituitary-adrenal (HPA) axis and alcohol consumption is complex. Although humans and animals often consume alcohol in response to stress, the conditions under which this occurs are extremely variable and depend on many factors such as genetic vulnerability; early life stress experiences; individual drinking patterns; the intensity and type of the stressor and control over it; individual coping ability; and the availability of social support (Fahlke et al. 2000). There are both gender and age differences in the types of psychological and social stressors that precipitate drinking (Fillmore et al. 1995; King et al. 2003; Spear 2000), and there are individual physiological differences in response to alcohol as a stressor (Silveri and Spear 2004a). In addition, even though alcohol is usually consumed to diminish stress and anxiety, alcohol can also stimulate a stress response by activating the HPA axis (Rivier 1996). In general, it has been found that corticosterone response increases during adolescence in response to alcohol and that sex differences in adulthood are more pronounced than the sex differences in adolescence. Thus, studying the interaction between stress hormones, gonadal hormones, and alcohol consumption at puberty could further our understanding of gender differences in drinking behavior that begin to emerge during that developmental period.

PREVENTION: CONNECTING DRINKING PATTERNS TO SEVERITY OF ALCOHOL-RELATED DISORDERS

Screening and Interventions for Alcohol Use Disorders

As noted in the beginning of this chapter, both adults and adolescents in the United States engage in high-risk drinking patterns—drinking too much too fast and too much too often—that significantly increase their odds of developing drinking-related problems, including alcohol abuse and dependence. A growing body of research shows that clinicians, particularly those in primary care settings, can significantly reduce both problem drinking and its medical consequences—especially for patients who are not alcohol-dependent—by screening to identify those who are at risk for developing or who have already developed alcohol abuse and dependence and by conducting brief interventions with individuals who are engaging in risky drinking patterns but have not yet met the DSM-IV criteria for alcohol dependence (Ballesteros et al. 2004; D'Onofrio and Degutis 2002).

The recognition that alcohol-related problems are not limited to alcohol-dependent individuals has important implications for our nation's health care system. It suggests that health care professionals need to switch from an exclusive focus on identifying and treating persons who are alcohol-dependent to the inclusion of persons who are "at risk" and problem drinkers. The screening process allows health care professionals to do just this. Once a problem—or a level of increased risk—is found, steps can be taken to help the patient minimize or prevent future problems. Often this intervention takes the form of advice or counseling to encourage the patient to alter behaviors that are contributing to the problem. Such an intervention may be brief—taking only a few minutes— or may require more time to convey a number of health messages. Screening for alcohol-related problems can involve structured interviews or self-report questionnaires. It may also involve laboratory tests to detect abnormalities associated with excessive alcohol consumption. Recent research has identified an individual's pattern of alcohol consumption (that may include frequent regular drinking of small amounts, or infrequent episodes of consuming very large quantities all at one time), is an important determinant of risk for problems. For example, one of the alcohol consumption questions from the Alcohol Use Disorders Identification Test (AUDIT-C)—How often do you have 6 or more drinks on an occasion?—has been shown to screen a primary care population with 79% sensitivity and 81% specificity for individuals who are engaging in drinking patterns that place them at high risk for AUDs (Bush et al. 1998). When alcohol-related problems are identified, more detailed assessments can be undertaken to specify the nature and extent of the problems so that appropriate treatment can be undertaken. If the screening and assessment results indicate that a patient is an at-risk or problem drinker but not alcohol dependent, a brief intervention on the part of the health care provider can significantly reduce alcohol use and associated problems (Bien et al. 1993; Fleming et al. 1997; Wilk et al. 1997). Although used most often with patients who are not alcohol dependent, brief interventions may also hold promise as part of a "stepped care" approach that involves specialized treatment settings (Drummond 1997).

U.S. Adult Drinking Patterns and Risks

About 72% of the U.S. adult population age 18 years and older who drink alcohol do not exceed weekly alcohol screening limits (B. F. Grant et al. 2004). These limits are 14 drinks in a typical week and 4 on any day for men, and 7 drinks in a typical week and 3 on any day for women. Yet nearly 3 in 10 adults engage in risky drinking, and more than 1 in 4 of these risky drinkers already meet DSM-IV diagnostic criteria for alcohol abuse or dependence (National Institute on Alcohol Abuse and Alcoholism: "Unpublished analysis of data from the 2001–2002 National Epidemiologic Survey on Alcohol and Related Conditions [NESARC], a nationwide survey of 43,093 U.S. adults aged 18 or older," 2004). A significant proportion of problems related to alcohol use, including motor vehicle crashes, other injuries, health problems, and family difficulties, occur in persons who are risky drinkers. The more alcohol consumed and the more frequently it is consumed dramatically increases an individual's odds of developing an AUD. For example, adults who exceed only the daily limit once a week or more are 31 times as likely to develop alcohol abuse and 82 times as likely to develop alcohol dependence than adults who never exceed the weekly or daily screening limits (National Institute on Alcohol Abuse and Alcoholism: "Unpublished analysis of data from the 2001–2002 National Epidemiologic Survey on Alcohol and Related Conditions [NESARC], a nationwide survey of 43,093 U.S. adults aged 18 or older," 2004).

Treatment for AUDs involves a mix of behavioral and pharmacological therapies. Behavioral therapies include brief intervention, motivational enhancement therapy, cognitive-behavioral therapy, couples (marital) and family therapies, and community reinforcement. Current medications approved for treating alcohol dependence are disulfiram, naltrexone, and acamprosate. The amount of alcohol an individual drinks (quantity) over what period of time (frequency) can be used to determine whether an individual requires intervention for drinking and the level of intervention required. As a common complex disease, alcohol dependence has relapse rates comparable to those of hypertension, diabetes, and asthma (McLellan et al. 2000).

CONCLUSION

There is a critical window of opportunity for preventing the onset of alcohol-related problems in adolescence. Continued progress in understanding the mechanisms involved in periadolescent development, how alcohol affects these mechanisms, and their relationship to co-occurring problems in adolescents will link biology and psychology and provide evidence-based approaches for effective prevention and intervention. Screening for high-risk drinking in primary care settings is an important and effective tool in identifying individuals who have or who are at risk for alcohol-related problems. Brief intervention has been found to be effective in helping nondependent high-risk drinkers reduce or moderate their drinking to lower their risk for developing abuse and/or dependence. An important next step in preventing AUDs and their many complications is to develop models of dimensional severity in alcohol use disorders (as has been done in other disorders, such as diabetes and hypertension).

CLINICAL IMPLICATIONS

Many adults and adolescents demonstrate drinking patterns that increase the probability of developing drinking-related problems. Clinicians may significantly reduce both problem drinking and subsequent consequences by screening to identify those who are at risk and administering brief interventions. Alcohol-related problems also occur in individuals without alcohol dependence. Clinicians need to switch from an exclusive focus on identifying and treating persons who are alcohol dependent to the inclusion of persons who are "at risk" and problem drinkers. If clinicians utilize effective screening, they will be able to use brief interventions that provide advice and counseling. These brief interventions can be very effective.

REFERENCES

American Psychiatric Association: Diagnostic and Statistical Manual of Mental Disorders, 3rd Edition, Revised. Washington, DC, American Psychiatric Association, 1987

American Psychiatric Association: Diagnostic and Statistical Manual of Mental Disorders, Fourth Edition. Washington, DC, American Psychiatric Association, 1994

Ballesteros J, Duffy JC, Querejeta I, et al: Efficacy of brief interventions for hazardous drinkers in primary care: systematic review and meta-analyses. Addiction 9:103–108, 2004

Barbaccia ML: Neurosteroidogenesis: relevance to neurosteroid actions in brain and modulation by psychotropic drugs. Crit Rev Neurobiol 16:67–74, 2004

Bien TH, Miller WR, Tonigan JS: Brief interventions for alcohol problems: a review. Addiction 88:315–335,1993

Bjork JM, Hommer DW, Grant SJ, et al: Impulsivity in abstinent alcohol-dependent patients: relation to control subjects and type 1-/type 2-like traits. Alcohol 34:133–150, 2004

Blanchard BA, Steindorf S, Wang S, et al: Sex differences in ethanol-induced dopamine release in nucleus accumbens and in ethanol consumption in rats. Alcohol Clin Exp Res 17:968–973, 1993

Brasser SM, Spear NE: Physiological and behavioral effects of acute ethanol hangover in juvenile, adolescent, and adult rats. Behav Neurosci 116:305–320, 2002

Bush K, Kivlahan DR, McDonell MB, et al: The AUDIT Alcohol Consumption Questions (AUDIT-C): an effective brief screening test for problem drinking. Ambulatory Care Quality Improvement Project (ACQUIP). Alcohol Use Disorders Identification Test. Arch Intern Med 158:1789–1795, 1998

Caldwell LC, Schweinsburg AD, Nagel BJ, et al: Sex and adolescent alcohol use disorders on bold blood oxygen level dependent response to spatial working memory. Alcohol Alcoholism 40:194–200, 2005

Cameron JL: Interrelationships between hormones, behavior, and affect during adolescence: understanding hormonal, physical, and brain changes occurring in association with pubertal activation of the reproductive axis. Introduction to part III. Ann N Y Acad Sci 1021:110–123, 2004

Carlson SR, Iacono WG, McGue M: P300 amplitude in nonalcoholic adolescent twin pairs who become discordant for alcoholism as adults. Psychophysiology 41:841–844, 2004

Collins AC, Yeager TN, Lebsack ME, et al: Variations in alcohol metabolism: influence of sex and age. Pharmacol Biochem Behav 3:973–978, 1975

De Bellis MD, Clark DB, Beers SR, et al: Hippocampal volume in adolescent-onset alcohol use disorders. Am J Psychiatry 157:737–744, 2000

Devaud LL, Alele P, Chadda R: Sex differences in the central nervous system actions of ethanol. Crit Rev Neurobiol 15:41–59, 2003

Dick DM, Rose RJ, Viken RJ, et al: Pubertal timing and substance use: associations between and within families across late adolescence. Developmental Psychology 36:180–189, 2000

D'Onofrio G, Degutis LC: Preventive care in the emergency department: screening and brief intervention for alcohol problems in the emergency department: a systematic review. Acad Emerg Med 9:627–638, 2002

Drummond DC: Alcohol interventions: do the best things come in small packages? Addiction 92:375–380, 1997

Eriksson CJ, Kaprio J, Pulkkinen L, et al: Testosterone and alcohol use among adolescent male twins: testing between-family associations in within-family comparisons. Behav Genet 35:359–368, 2005

Eriksson K, Pikkarainen PH: Differences between the sexes in voluntary alcohol consumption and liver ADH-activity in inbred strains of mice. Metabolism 17:1037–1042, 1968

Fahlke C, Lorenz JG, Long J, et al: Rearing experiences and stress-induced plasma cortisol as early risk factors for excessive alcohol consumption in nonhuman primates. Alcohol Clin Exp Res 24:644–650, 2000

Ferris CF, Shtiegman K, King JA: Voluntary ethanol consumption in male adolescent hamsters increases testosterone and aggression. Physiol Behav 63:739–744, 1998

Fillmore KM, Golding JM, Kniep S, et al: Gender differences for the risk of alcohol-related problems in multiple national contexts. Recent Dev Alcohol 12:409–439, 1995

Finn DA, Sinnott RS, Ford MM, et al: Sex differences in the effect of ethanol injection on consumption on brain allopregnanolone levels in C57BL/6 mice. Neuroscience 123:813–819, 2004

Fleming MF, Barry KL, Manwell LB, et al: Brief physician advice for problem alcohol drinkers. A randomized controlled trial in community-based primary care practices. JAMA 277:1039–1045, 1997

Grant BF, Dawson DA: Age of onset of drug use and its association with DSM-IV drug abuse and dependence: results from the National Longitudinal Alcohol Epidemiologic Survey. J Subst Abuse 9:103–110, 1997

Grant BF, Moore TC, Kaplan K: Source and Accuracy Statement: Wave 1 National Epidemiologic Survey on Alcohol and Related Conditions (NESARC), 2003. Available at: http://niaaa.census.gov/pdfs/source_and_accuracy_statement.pdf. Accessed September 16, 2006.

Grant BF, Dawson DA, Stinson FS, et al: The 12-month prevalence and trends in DSM-IV alcohol abuse and dependence: United States, 1991–1992 and 2001–2002. Drug Alcohol Depend 74:223–234, 2004

Grant BF, Stinson FS, Dawson DA, et al: Co-occurrence of DSM-IV personality disorders in the United States: results from the National Epidemiologic Survey on Alcohol and Related Conditions. Compr Psychiatry 46:1–5, 2005a

Grant BF, Hasin DS, Stinson FS, et al: Co-occurrence of 12-month mood and anxiety disorders and personality disorders in the US: results from the National Epidemiologic Survey on Alcohol and Related Conditions. J Psychiatr Res 39:1–9, 2005b

Grant KA, Azarov A, Shively CA, et al: Discriminative stimulus effects of ethanol and 3-hydroxy-5-pregnan-20-one in relation to the menstrual cycle phase in cynomolgus monkeys (Macaca fascicularis). Psychopharmacology 130:59–68, 1997

Greenfield TK, Rogers JD: Who drinks most of the alcohol in the US? The policy implications. J Stud Alcohol 60:78–89, 1999

Harwood HJ, Fountain D, Fountain G: Economic cost of alcohol and drug abuse in the United States, 1992: a report. Addiction 94:631–635, 1999

Hingson R: Advances in measurement and intervention for excessive drinking. Am J Prev Med 27:261–263, 2004

Hingson R, Heeren T, Winter M, et al: Magnitude of alcohol-related mortality and morbidity among U.S. college students ages 18–24: changes from 1998 to 2001. Annu Rev Public Health 26:1–24, 2005

Jones BC, Whitfield KE: Sex differences in ethanol-related behaviors in genetically defined murine stock, in Recent Developments in Alcoholism, Vol 12: Women and Alcoholism. Edited by Galanter M. New York, Plenum, 1995, pp 223–230

Kendler KC, Prescott C, Myers J, et al: The structure of genetic and environmental risk factors for common psychiatric and substance use disorders in men and women. Arch Gen Psychiatry 60:929–937, 2003

King AC, Bernardy NC, Hauner K: Stressful events, personality, and mood disturbance: gender differences in alcoholics and problem drinkers. Addict Behav 28:171–187, 2003

Knopik VS, Heath AC, Madden PA, et al: Genetic effects on alcohol dependence risk: reevaluating the importance of psychiatric and other heritable risk factors. Psychol Med 34:1519–1530, 2004

La Grange L, Jones TD, Erb L, et al: Alcohol consumption: biochemical and personality correlates in a college student population. Addictive Behavior 20:93–103, 1995

Lancaster FE, Spiegel KS: Sex differences in patterns of drinking. Alcohol 9:415–420, 1992

Lancaster FE, Brown TD, Coker KL, et al: Sex differences in alcohol preference and drinking patterns emerge during the early postpubertal period in Sprague-Dawley rats. Alcohol Clin Exp Res 20:1043–1049, 1996

Martin CA, Mainous AG, Curry T, et al: Alcohol use in adolescent females: correlates with estradiol and testosterone. Am J Addictions 8:9–14, 1999

McLellan AT, Lewis DC, O'Brien CP, et al: Drug dependence, a chronic medical illness: implications for treatment, insurance, and outcomes evaluation. JAMA 284:1689–1695, 2000

McGue M, Iacono WG, Legrand LN, et al: Origins and consequences of age at first drink, II: familial risk and heritability. Alcohol Clin Exp Res 25:1166–1732, 2001

McGue M, Iacono WG: The association of early adolescent problem behavior with adult psychopathology. Am J Psychiatry 162:1118–1124, 2005

Middaugh LD, Frackelton WF, Boggan WO, et al: Gender differences in the effects of ethanol on C57BL/6 mice. Alcohol Clin Exp Res 9:257–260, 1992

Middaugh LD, Kelley BM, Bandy AE, et al: Ethanol consumption by C57BL/6 mice: influence of gender and procedural variables. Alcohol 17:175–183, 1999

Mokdad AH, Marks JS, Stroup DF, et al: Actual causes of death in the United States, 2000. JAMA 29:1238–1245, 2004

Morrow AL, Devaud LL, Purdy RH, et al: Neuroactive steroid modulators of the stress response. Ann N Y Acad Sci 771:257–272, 1995

Morrow AL, Janis GC, VanDoren MJ, et al: Neurosteroids mediate pharmacological effects of ethanol: a new mechanism of ethanol action: Alcoholism Clin Exp Res 23:1933–1940, 1999

Morrow AL, VanDoren MJ, Penland SN, et al: The role of GABAergic neuroactive steroids in ethanol action, tolerance, and dependence. Brain Res Rev 37:98–109, 2001

Patton GC, McMorris BJ, Toumbourou JW, et al: Puberty and the onset of substance use and abuse. Pediatrics 114:300–306, 2004

Paul SM, Purdy RH: Neuroactive steroids. FASEB J 6:2311–2322, 1992

Rivier C: Alcohol stimulates ACTH secretion in the rat: mechanisms of action and interactions with other stimuli. Alcohol Clin Exp Res 20:240–254, 1996

Rubinow DR, Schmidt PJ: Androgens, brain, and behavior. Am J Psychiatry 153:974–984, 1996

Rupprecht R: Neuroactive steroids: mechanisms of action and neuropharmacological properties. Psychoneuroendocrinol 28:139–168, 2003

Silveri MM, Spear LP: Decreased sensitivity to the hypnotic effects of ethanol early in ontogeny. Alcohol Clin Exp Res 22:670–676, 1998

Silveri MM, Spear LP: The effects of NMDA and GABAA pharmacological manipulations on acute and rapid tolerance to ethanol during ontogeny. Alcohol Clin Exp Res 28:884–894, 2004a

Silveri MM, Spear LP: Characterizing the ontogeny of ethanol-associated increases in corticosterone. Alcohol 32:145–155, 2004b

Sinnott RS, Phillips TJ, Finn DA: Alteration of voluntary ethanol and saccharin consumption by the neurosteroid allopregnanolone in mice. Psychopharmacology (Berl) 162:438–447, 2002

Spear L: The adolescent brain and age-related behavioral manifestations. Neurosci Biobehav Rev 24:417–463, 2000

Spear LP, Varlinskaya EI: Adolescence. Alcohol sensitivity, tolerance, and intake. Recent Dev Alcohol 17:143–159, 2005

Substance Abuse and Mental Health Services Administration: National Survey on Drug Use and Health, 2003. Available at: http://www.oas.samhsa.gov. Accessed July 22, 2005.

Swahn MH, Simon TR, Hammig BJ, et al: Alcohol-consumption behaviors and risk for physical fighting and injuries among adolescent drinkers. Addict Behav 29:959–963, 2004

Vivian JA, Green HL, Young JE, et al: Induction and maintenance of ethanol self-administration in cynomolgus monkeys (*Macaca fascicularis*): long-term characterization of sex and individual differences. Alcohol Clin Exp Res 25:1087–1097, 2001

von der Pahlen B: The role of alcohol and steroid hormones in human aggression. Vitam Horm 70:415–437, 2005

Webb B, Burnett PW, Walker DW: Sex differences in ethanol induced hypnosis and hypothermia in young Long-Evans rats. Alcohol Clin Exp Res 26:695–704, 2002

Wilk AI, Jensen NM, Havighurst TC: Meta-analysis of randomized control trials addressing brief interventions in heavy alcohol drinkers. J Gen Intern Med 12:274–283, 1997

Part V

Challenges for the
Near Future

13

Prevention of Alzheimer's Disease

Principles and Prospects

John C.S. Breitner, M.D., M.P.H.

This chapter describes several lessons learned in the long process of seeking a method of preventing Alzheimer's disease. While the work deals specifically with Alzheimer's disease, it seems probable that some of these lessons could be usefully applied in the search for prevention of other neuropsychiatric diseases.

PRINCIPLE 1

Alzheimer's disease is not only a dementia of old age but also a chronic disease that evolves over decades.

The familiar dementia of Alzheimer's disease is indeed the most common form of dementia, and there is no doubt that this dementia poses an enormous public health challenge worldwide as populations age. But there is much evidence to suggest that this dementia is an end stage of a much lengthier disease process.

It is now clear that individuals with a family history of Alzheimer's disease who also bear at least one copy of the epsilon 4 allele at the apolipoprotein E (*APOE*) locus (which encodes the cholesterol transport protein apolipoprotein E) will have already acquired suggestive neurocognitive changes by the fifth and sixth decade of life. *APOEε4* is a prominent genetic risk factor for Alzheimer's disease, and the presumption is that most of these ε4-positive individuals with a family history of Alzheimer's disease will eventually develop Alzheimer's dementia. On neuroimaging (Reiman et al. 1996), they also have a characteristic pattern of temporoparietal hypometabolism that is relatively specific to Alzheimer's disease (Phelps et al. 1983). Furthermore, neuropsychological changes are detectable over time in *APOEε4*-positive individuals who are decades away from developing Alzheimer's dementia (Flory et al. 2000).

The time therefore seems ripe for a change in nomenclature, with the term *Alzheimer's neuropathology* reserved for the identification of the underlying pathological or pathogenetic processes of the condition, while the term *Alzheimer's dementia* may be used more specifically to denote the familiar, fully evolved symptomatic stages of the illness. The term *Alzheimer's disease* would then generically encompass both of the above.

The chronic disease model of Alzheimer's disease, attributable originally to Robert Katzman, suggests three identifiable stages in the progression of Alzheimer's disease. The foregoing evidence suggests at least two decades of disease evolution, and perhaps more, during which the pathogenetic process is undetectable without invasive or high-resolution techniques. I use the term *latent stage* for this period, because, from a symptoms perspective at least, the disease is unapparent. As the process continues, there is sufficient destruction of the neural substrate of cognition that early symptoms appear. When these are sufficiently notable that an individual (or family or physician) recognizes that the patient is not his or her "old self," there is also typically a demonstrable cognitive deficit that is not (yet) severe enough to meet criteria for dementia. From the perspective of symptomatic Alzheimer's dementia, at least, one may think of this as a *prodromal stage*. The Alzheimer's disease prodrome, which is easy to conceive but harder to identify, is frequently described nowadays as "mild cognitive impairment" (Winblad et al. 2004). Finally, of course, there is the familiar dementia syndrome itself, or *symptomatic stage*, which is well known to be progressive and increasingly disabling over time.

Of course, these three identifiable stages of the Alzheimer's pathogenetic process are not distinct; they merge imperceptibly into one another. But in concept at least they offer three distinct opportunities for therapeutic or preventive interventions. The basic notions of this argument are summarized in Figure 13–1.

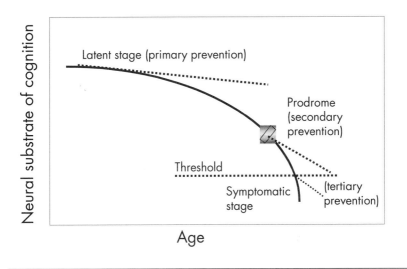

FIGURE 13–1. Several potential targets for preventive interventions.

Currently available treatments (cholinesterase inhibitors, memantine) provide symptomatic improvement for some patients with Alzheimer's dementia, but they are not known to attenuate the further progression of the underlying disease process. There is opportunity, therefore, for better interventions at this stage which offer what the U.S. Food and Drug Administration (FDA) terms a "disease-modifying" effect (I would suggest that this term might well apply to earlier stages also). Here the hope is that by slowing the further progression of the underlying disease process, one may also slow the progression of symptomatic severity.

In theory, at least, one may also intervene in the prodromal stage. Here again, the aim would be to find an intervention that slows the progression of the underlying disease process. The result would not be restitution of lost cognitive abilities, but rather a delay in the expected progression of symptom severity, first to a more severe prodromal state and eventually to fully symptomatic dementia. A number of randomized trials have attempted intervention at this stage, with the intended outcome being reduction in the rate of "conversion" from "mild cognitive impairment" to dementia (Petersen et al. 2005; Reines et al. 2005).

Finally, we consider the possibility of intervention in the latent stage. Now the intent would be to prevent or delay the progression of the disease process so that symptomatic stages (including prodromal illness) may be avoided altogether. From a symptomatic perspective, at least, this last form of intervention may be termed "primary prevention." In the same framework, one may think of intervention at the prodromal stage as "secondary prevention" (i.e., prevention of the full syndrome when early or suggestive symptoms are apparent), and of "disease modifying" interventions in the fully symptomatic stage as "tertiary prevention" (prevention of worsening in symptoms or of complications). In fact, I would argue that the use of these three terms—primary, secondary, and tertiary prevention—would help avoid confusion and serve as a helpful reminder of the true nature of the condition referred to as Alzheimer's disease.

How may we identify strategies for primary, secondary, and tertiary prevention? This brings us to Principle 2.

PRINCIPLE 2

Trials data should be used, when possible, to identify strategies for prevention, but data from carefully conducted observational studies should not be dismissed without further exploration.

A corollary is, if trials data do not confirm observational results, do not assume a priori that the observational data are "wrong" or are simply a result of "bias" or "confounding." That may be so, but unless the conditions of the observational study were congruent with those of the trial(s), the observational data may tell us something that is true and yet different from the conclusions of the trial. It is imprudent simply to discard observational data! Many studies now show that the overwhelming majority of carefully gathered observational study findings are confirmed (not refuted) when results of trials become available (Concato and Horwitz 2004). Rather than simply dismissing them, we should explore them to discover the reasons why they differ from the trial results. It has long been thought foolish to discard observations simply because they are not in accord with our preconceptions of reality. Here we may recall Thomas Hunt Morgan's maxim, "Treasure your exceptions." They may contain the kernel of important discovery. I suggest that it is similarly foolish to dismiss observational study results as "wrong" without offering (or better yet, demonstrating) a reason why the studies may disagree.

One important reason why trials data and observational study data may differ is the *timing* of the exposure in relation to the outcome. In the remainder of this chapter, I shall draw several examples to highlight the importance of timing of intervention (i.e., distinctions among primary, secondary, and tertiary prevention). Furthermore, I will attempt to demonstrate the potential importance of contrasting results from trials and observational studies.

Hormone Therapy and Alzheimer's Disease

Consider first the example of the relation of postmenopausal hormone therapy and Alzheimer's disease. There is more than a decade's worth of accumulated observational data that examine this relationship. Among six adequate case–control studies (reviewed by Zandi et al. 2002b), the results are decidedly mixed or equivocal, with some suggestion of protection over all. However, particular note may be paid to one very carefully conducted study conducted among enrollees in the Group Health Cooperative health maintenance organization in the Puget Sound area (Brenner et al. 1994). This study ascertained women from this population who had developed dementia over a 10-year interval. The research also capitalized on the extraordinary resource of the computerized pharmacy database of Group Health, enabling the investigators to identify with accuracy the exposure status of each case and of a set of age-matched control women *over the same 10-year interval*. Application of the case–control method then yielded adjusted odds ratios that were indistinguishable from the null value of 1.0.

Yet three out of four prospective studies that have examined this same relationship suggested a moderately strong "protective" effect of hormones (Kawas et al. 1997; Mayeux and Tang 1996; Zandi et al. 2002b). The most recent prospective study was reported from the very large Cache County (Utah) cohort (Zandi et al. 2002b) and suggested an inverse relation of prior hormone use and subsequent onset of Alzheimer's disease. The result appeared to be strengthened by a clear increase in the apparent effect with longer duration of treatment. Again, however, it is worth a moment's consideration to the "outlier" that failed to show protection (Seshadri et al. 2001). That study was conducted using the resources of the U.K. general practice database, which supplied both exposure information and outcomes results *over a specified 10-year interval*. The adjusted hazard ratios were again very close to 1.0.

Within a year of the publication from Cache County came the first report of the Women's Health Initiative Memory Study (WHIMS), an ancillary study to the well-known Women's Health Initiative (Shumaker et al. 2003). This randomized controlled trial of hormone therapy (conjugated equine estrogens and medroxyprogesterone acetate) showed an unequivocal increase in the risk of dementia and Alzheimer's dementia over the 3–6 years the women were exposed to the treatments. Later reports from the same group are reported to have shown equivocal but suggestive increases in dementia risks among a different group of women exposed to estrogens alone (Shumaker et al. 2004). How can this be?

A reanalysis of the Cache County data, together with a reconsideration of the variations in methods from the other observational studies, may suggest the answer. The original Cache County report included separate analyses of dementia risks in women who were current users of hormones at the study's baseline assessment versus those who reported variable durations of use earlier in their lives. While the apparent effects in former users were strong and dependent on duration of treatment, there was no apparent effect in the current users, with a possible exception among those who reported more than 10 years of lifetime use. In fact, the paper reported trend-level increases in dementia incidence among current users who reported either 0–3 or 3–10 years of exposure. Following the first WHIMS results, we performed the simple expedient of combining these two groups of "recent users" (Breitner and Zandi 2003), now observing an adjusted hazard ratio of 2.22 (95% confidence interval [CI] = 1.05–4.34). This estimate agrees remarkably with the original WHIMS relative risk of 2.05 (95% CI = 1.21–3.48).

Now consider the other observational studies. Note that the one case–control and one prospective study showing null results counted as "exposed" only those women who had used hormones within the same 10-year interval as the occurrence of dementia onset. A parsimonious and attractive interpretation of all this information is shown in Figure 13–2.

The figure suggests that hormones may protect against Alzheimer's disease when they are taken during the perimenopausal or early menopausal period or more than a decade before the risk period for dementia. Later, the situation seems to reverse itself, and exposure within less than a decade of dementia onset seems to increase risk. The stippled bar in the upper right of the figure shows the approximate timing of exposure (relative to dementia onset) in WHIMS. The other portion of this same bar shows that the results of a randomized controlled treatment trial (i.e., a tertiary prevention trial) with hormones also suggested *increased* risks with treatment (Mulnard et al. 2000). Although this trial was reported as having "null" results, the data were at least suggestive of a negative outcome (i.e., an increase in risk).

A point to ponder is that exposure within a few years of dementia onset may be equivalent to exposure during the Alzheimer's disease prodrome. I therefore suggest that patients and families be advised to *avoid* use of hormones when there is a suggestion of early cognitive impairment.

NSAIDs and Alzheimer's Disease

We now turn to the other well known strategy for primary prevention of Alzheimer's disease, long-term administration of nonsteroidal anti-inflammatory treat-

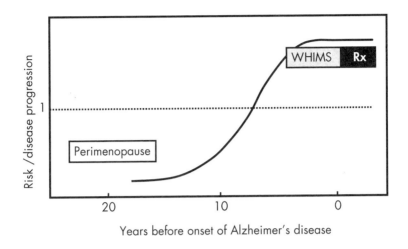

FIGURE 13–2. What the observational and trials data suggest about hormone therapy's effects on dementia risks.

Rx = treatment; WHIMS = Women's Health Initiative Memory Study.

ments (NSAIDs). The potential for anti-inflammatory interventions in Alzheimer's disease was first suggested by observations from Patrick McGeer and colleagues (McGeer et al. 1990) and was first demonstrated formally in the Duke Twin Studies of Alzheimer's disease (Breitner et al. 1994). Since those publications, more than 25 observational studies have suggested that long-term use of NSAIDs may prevent the onset of Alzheimer's disease. This topic was recently reviewed by Szekely et al. (2004), who considered seven strong case–control studies that appeared consistent in their findings and produced a meta-analytic summary odds ratio estimate of 0.51 (95% CI = 0.40–0.66). This review also cited four population-based prospective studies, three of which disclosed durations of treatment among the "exposed" groups (in 't Veld et al. 2001; Stewart et al. 1997; Zandi et al. 2002a). Considering the individuals from these three studies who reported 2 or more years of NSAID use, the results were again consistent and suggested a meta-analytic hazard ratio of 0.42 (95% CI = 0.26–0.66) (Szekely et al. 2004).

These promising results contrast with results from three well conducted randomized controlled trials of NSAIDs or other anti-inflammatory interventions for tertiary prevention of dementia progression (Aisen et al. 2000, 2003; Van Gool et al. 2001). None of those trials produced relative risk estimates that appeared to deviate meaningfully from the null value of 1.0. Again, how can this be?

Again, a review of the observational data may hold the answer. Of note, the highly regarded Rotterdam Study (in 't Veld et al. 2001), which showed very strong "protection" against Alzheimer's disease with more than 2 years of exposure to NSAIDs, found no evidence for protection when NSAIDs were used within 2 years of dementia onset. Only with exposures before this time did the effect increase with duration of exposure. A similar result was suggested, if less elegantly, in the Cache County study (Zandi et al. 2002a). The Cache County investigators reported no "protective" effect in current users of NSAIDs at baseline unless these individuals reported 2 or more years of earlier use. By contrast, prior users showed relatively impressive "protective" hazard ratios, and the strongest effects were suggested among prior users with longer durations of exposure.

Taken together, these studies suggest not only that NSAIDs are not helpful to those who have already developed the dementia of Alzheimer's disease, but also that NSAIDs may not be useful for those who are a few years away from dementia onset. Again, a parsimonious interpretation would state that NSAIDs should be ineffective among those with prodromal "mild cognitive impairment." We predicted this in the Cache County report (Zandi et al. 2002a). Sadly, it is now evident from randomized controlled trial results that at least one NSAID, the selective COX-2 inhibitor rofecoxib (no longer marketed), does not prevent conversion of mild cognitive impairment to dementia (Reines et al. 2005). In fact, the results of that trial are even more sobering, because they show a *negative* result, with a hazard ratio near 1.5, which differs from the null with a P value smaller than 0.05. One may wonder whether the increase in risk could be a reflection of the recently reported thrombogenic effects of rofecoxib. It is important, however, to consider that this may not be the case, and that the administration of other NSAIDs to those with prodromal Alzheimer's disease may produce adverse results. Caution is urged here particularly because by this time there is considerable public hope and expectation that NSAIDs may prevent Alzheimer's disease. Indeed they may, but it is at least possible that they have opposite effects when individuals' disease has advanced to the point of prodromal symptoms.

CLINICAL IMPLICATIONS

The prospects for the prevention of Alzheimer's disease appear cloudy. Much may depend on the timing of intervention during a long process of disease pathogenesis that appears to include a "latent" stage in middle life. Interventions that appear to be protective when given several years before the onset of Alzheimer's dementia may lose this effect as the disease process progresses, and may even become harmful. As Richard Nixon once said, "Timing is everything." This maxim may well hold for the prevention of Alzheimer's dementia. If so, the pursuit of preventative strategies becomes substantially more complex. It is not immediately apparent how one can test this idea experimentally, but at least we should be cautious about the interpretation of the data available.

From a clinical as well as a research perspective, it is probably very useful to think of a continuum of Alzheimer's disease, ranging from a latent stage, through a prodromal stage, and finally to a symptomatic stage. Evidence indicates that various interventions (e.g., hormones, NSAIDs) may be effective at different stages. Indeed, interventions may have opposite effects, depending on the stage during which they are administered.

REFERENCES

Aisen PS, Davis KL, Berg JD, et al: A randomized controlled trial of prednisone in Alzheimer's disease. Alzheimer's Disease Cooperative Study. Neurology 54:588–593, 2000

Aisen PS, Schafer KA, Grundman M, et al: Effects of rofecoxib or naproxen vs placebo on Alzheimer disease progression: a randomized controlled trial. JAMA 289:2819–2826, 2003

Breitner JC, Gau BA, Welsh KA, et al: Inverse association of anti-inflammatory treatments and Alzheimer's disease: initial results of a co-twin control study. Neurology 44:227–232, 1994

Breitner JC, Zandi PP: Effects of estrogen plus progestin on risk of dementia. JAMA 290:1706–1708, 2003

Brenner DE, Kukull WA, Stergachis A, et al: Postmenopausal estrogen replacement therapy and the risk of Alzheimer's disease: a population-based case-control study. Am J Epidemiol 140:262–267, 1994

Concato J, Horwitz RI: Beyond randomized versus observational studies. Lancet 363:1660–1661, 2004

Flory JD, Manuck SB, Ferrell RE, et al: Memory performance and the apolipoprotein E polymorphism in a community sample of middle-aged adults. Am J Med Genet 96:707–711, 2000

in 't Veld B, Ruitenberg A, Hofman A, et al: Nonsteroidal antiinflammatory drugs and the risk of Alzheimer's disease. N Engl J Med 345:1515–1521, 2001

Kawas C, Resnick S, Morrison A, et al: A prospective study of estrogen replacement therapy and the risk of developing Alzheimer's disease: the Baltimore Longitudinal Study of Aging. Neurology 48:1517–1521, 1997

Mayeux R, Tang M-X: Oestrogen and Alzheimer's disease. Lancet 348:1029–1030, 1996

McGeer PL, McGeer E, Rogers J, et al: Anti-inflammatory drugs and Alzheimer disease. Lancet 335:1037, 1990

Mulnard RA, Cotman CW, Kawas C, et al: Estrogen replacement therapy for treatment of mild to moderate Alzheimer disease: a randomized controlled trial. Alzheimer's Disease Cooperative Study. JAMA 283:1007–1015, 2000

Petersen RC, Thomas RG, Grundman M, et al: Vitamin E and donepezil for the treatment of mild cognitive impairment. N Engl J Med 352:2379–2388, 2005

Phelps ME, Schelbert HR, Mazziotta JC: Positron computed tomography for studies of myocardial and cerebral function. Ann Intern Med 98:339–359, 1983

Reiman EM, Caselli RJ, Yun LS, et al: Preclinical evidence of Alzheimer's disease in persons homozygous for the epsilon 4 allele for apolipoprotein E. N Engl J Med 334:752–758, 1996

Reines S, Thal LJ, Ferris S: A randomized, double-blind, study of rofecoxib in patients with mild cognitive impairment. Neuropsychopharmacology 30:1204–1215, 2005

Seshadri S, Zornberg GL, Derby LE, et al: Postmenopausal estrogen replacement therapy and the risk of Alzheimer disease. Arch Neurol 58:435–440, 2001

Shumaker SA, Legault C, Rapp SR, et al, WHIMS investigators: Estrogen plus progestin and the incidence of dementia and mild cognitive impairment in postmenopausal women: the Women's Health Initiative Memory Study: a randomized controlled trial. JAMA 289:2651–2662, 2003

Shumaker SA, Legault C, Kuller L, et al: Conjugated equine estrogens and incidence of probable dementia and mild cognitive impairment in postmenopausal women: Women's Health Initiative Memory Study. JAMA 291:2947–2958, 2004

Stewart WF, Kawas C, Corrada M, et al: Risk of Alzheimer's disease and duration of NSAID use. Neurology 48:626–632, 1997

Szekely C, Thorne J, Zandi PP, et al: Nonsteroidal anti-inflammatory drugs for the prevention of Alzheimer's disease: a systematic review. Neuroepidemiology 23:159–169, 2004

Van Gool W, Weinstein H, Scheltens P, et al: Effect of hydroxychloroquine on progression of dementia in early Alzheimer's disease: an 18-month randomised, double-blind, placebo-controlled study. Lancet 358:455–460, 2001

Winblad B, Palmer K, Kivipelto M, et al: Mild cognitive impairment—beyond controversies, towards a consensus: report of the International Working Group on Mild Cognitive Impairment. J Intern Med 256:240–246, 2004

Zandi PP, Anthony J, Hayden K, et al: Reduced incidence of AD with NSAID but not H2 receptor antagonists: the Cache County Study. Neurology 59:880–886, 2002a

Zandi PP, Carlson MC, Plassman BL, et al: Hormone replacement therapy and incidence of Alzheimer disease in older women—the Cache County Study. JAMA 288:2123–2129, 2002b

14

Five Facts About Preventing Drug Dependence

James C. Anthony, Ph.D.

By the end of this chapter, the reader will know five facts about preventing drug dependence. Before turning to these facts, I must provide an orientation to some basic but sometimes bewildering issues of drug dependence as a phenomenon or object of study in psychopathology.

This chapter is a revised and shortened version of an invited lecture presented at the 95th Annual Scientific Meeting of the American Psychopathological Association in New York City on Saturday, 5 March 2005. Some of the material presented in the lecture could not be included in the chapter; it is still undergoing peer review for primary publication in scientific journals.

The preparation of this chapter was supported primarily by a National Institutes of Health National Institute on Drug Abuse Senior Scientist Award (5K05DA015799) and institutional research support from Michigan State University. Sara Vasilenko provided helpful bibliographical research assistance.

DRUG DEPENDENCE AS A PHENOMENON

What's in a Name?

In public health outreach and early intervention activity, we learn that much stigma is attached to the terms *drug addiction* and *drug addict*, and even more to *drug abuse* and *drug abuser*. There is less stigma attached to the term *drug dependence*. For this reason, we adopt the term *drug dependence* in our epidemiological research and public health–oriented outreach and early intervention work.

This change in terminology was recommended more than 40 years ago by the World Health Organization (WHO) Expert Committee on Addiction-Producing Drugs (World Health Organization 1964), which subsequently became the WHO Expert Committee on Drug Dependence. There is widespread belief that public health outreach and early intervention efforts will be more successful if we abandon terms with stigma attached to them. Indeed, during my experience with public health outreach and early intervention over more than 30 years, if I insist that insight should meet the pithy requirements of Sir Aubrey Lewis' definition ("correct attitude to a morbid change in oneself"; Lewis 1934), a good many individuals with treated drug dependence have insight and call themselves by the names *drug addict* or *drug abuser*; among the never-treated cases, this characteristic is quite uncommon.

Table 14–1 presents the WHO Expert Committee's initial descriptions of drug dependence, as communicated through the *Bulletin of the World Health Organization* (Isbell and Chrusciel 1970). Here we see a clear display of Cartesian dualism in relation to definitions for "psychic dependence" and "physical dependence." Origins of this concept of psychic dependence can be traced back to early primate studies of cocaine pharmacology. During these studies, cocaine hydrochloride powder (hereinafter referred to as *cocaine*) was administered repeatedly, but abrupt cessation of this sustained cocaine dosing was not followed by any clearly recognizable abstinence syndrome of the type seen when heroin, morphine, or other opioids were studied using the same protocols (e.g., see Tatum and Seevers 1929). Some 35–40 years after this work by Tatum and Seevers, the term *behavioral dependence* entered the vocabulary of behavioral pharmacology and was joined by the terms *psychic* (or *psychological*) *dependence* and *physical dependence*: "Behavioral dependence always accompanies physical dependence, in that discontinuation of chronic drug treatment produces behavioral as well as physiological disruptions" (Schuster and Thompson 1969, p. 498).

Roughly concurrently, Edwards and Gross (1976) started to develop a somewhat different concept of an "alcohol dependence syndrome" that has be-

Table 14–1. WHO Expert Committee definitions for drug dependence

Drug dependence: "A state, psychic and sometimes also physical, resulting from the interaction between a living organism and a drug, characterized by behavioral and other responses that always include a compulsion to take the drug on a continuous or periodic basis in order to experience its psychic effects, and sometimes to avoid the discomfort of its absence. Tolerance may or may not be present. A person may be dependent on more than one drug."

Psychic dependence: "A compulsion that requires periodic or continuous administration of a drug to produce pleasure or avoid discomfort. This compulsion is the most powerful factor in chronic intoxication with psychotropic drugs.... Psychic dependence, therefore, is the universal characteristic of drug dependence. Operationally, it is recognized by the fact that the dependent continues to take the drug in spite of conscious admission that it is causing harm to his health and to his social and familial adjustment, and that he takes great risks to obtain and maintain his supply of the drug."

Physical dependence: "A pathological state brought about by repeated administration of a drug and that leads to the appearance of a characteristic and specific group of symptoms, termed an abstinence [or withdrawal] syndrome, when the administration of the drug is discontinued or—in the case of certain drugs—significantly reduced. In order to prevent the appearance of an abstinence syndrome the continuous taking of the drug is required. Physical dependence is a powerful factor in reinforcing psychic dependence upon continuing drug use or in relapse to drug use after withdrawal."

Source. Isbell and Chrusciel 1970.

come quite influential in conceptualization of dependence on drugs other than alcohol. The Edwards-Gross description of the alcohol dependence syndrome includes the following features: 1) tolerance, 2) withdrawal, 3) drinking to relieve or avoid withdrawal symptoms, 4) subjective awareness of the compulsion to drink, 5) drink-seeking behavior, 6) return to drinking after a period of abstinence, and 7) narrowing of the drinking repertoire. Here, *tolerance* refers to decreased drug effect after repeated administration, as in the nicotine tolerance model (e.g., see Csajka and Verotta 2006). *Withdrawal* refers to an abstinence syndrome that appears upon abrupt discontinuation of sustained use, sometimes with reductions in daily doses, and in some instances when precipitated by an effective antagonist drug, as described below in the prevention section of this chapter.

Mindful that my trainees and colleagues sometimes have difficulty remembering seven items in a list, I have tried to simplify the Edwards-Gross list, grouping the features under three main subheadings, as shown in Table 14–2. It is noteworthy that "Drug use to relieve or avoid withdrawal" appears under two headings (i.e., both "Observable manifestations of neuroadaptation" and "Observable obsession-like clinical features" in Table 14–2). This circumstance is a manifestation of an observed interdependency between these two clinical features. That is, drug use to relieve or avoid withdrawal is one of the manifestations of the obsession-like character of drug dependence, but this feature cannot be present unless withdrawal symptoms have been experienced in the process of neuroadaptation.

Regrettably, expert panels assembled to develop the third edition of the American Psychiatric Association's *Diagnostic and Statistical Manual of Mental Disorders* (DSM-III; American Psychiatric Association 1980) were not markedly influenced by these generalizable Edwards-Gross concepts when they formulated their own case definitions and diagnostic criteria for drug dependence. Instead, they wrote a separate set of diagnostic criteria for each general class of drug compounds (e.g., cannabis, opioids), which made it impossible to hold the diagnostic criteria constant while estimating the occurrence of drug-specific dependence syndromes. That is, each drug class had its own definition and diagnostic criteria. This approach retarded the development of a "comparative epidemiology" of drug dependence (i.e., comparisons of the occurrence of drug dependence syndromes across drug classes) because, for example, the DSM-III "apples" of alcohol dependence were not strictly comparable to the DSM-III "oranges" of cannabis dependence. In specific, the diagnostic criteria for cannabis dependence did not admit to the existence of a cannabis abstinence or withdrawal syndrome; tolerance alone sufficed as evidence of neuroadaptation. By contrast, DSM-III diagnostic criteria for alcohol dependence offered substitutability of tolerance or the alcohol withdrawal syndrome. This deficiency of DSM-III was remedied in DSM-III-R (American Psychiatric Association 1987), DSM-IV (American Psychiatric Association 1994), and ICD-10 (Isaac et al. 1994; World Health Organization 1992), which made possible comparative studies in which the case definition for drug dependence can be held constant (e.g., see Anthony et al. 1994), in contrast to prior comparisons (e.g., see Anthony and Helzer 1991).

A second defect in DSM-III was mixing the issue of drug-related social and occupational impairment with the issue of defining the drug dependence phenomenon under study. This defect is not present in ICD-10 and (for the most part) was removed in DSM-III-R and DSM-IV, which demonstrate the influence of the Edwards-Gross construct (e.g., see Rounsaville 2002). Nonetheless, many researchers maintain an erroneous belief that all cases of drug dependence necessar-

---

Table 14–2.   Three main subgroups for clinical features of drug dependence

1. Observable manifestations of neuroadaptation

    Subjectively felt or demonstrated tolerance (a)

    Characteristic withdrawal/abstinence syndrome (b)

    Drug use to relieve or avoid withdrawal/abstinence (c)

2. Observable obsession-like clinical features

    Subjective awareness of compulsion to use the drug (d)

    Drug-seeking behavior (e)

    Drug use to relieve or avoid withdrawal/abstinence (c)

3. Observable compulsion-like clinical features

    Return to drug use after withdrawal/abstinence (f)

    Narrowing of the drug-using behavior (g)

Note.   Letters within parentheses refer to text-item listings for the Edwards-Gross criteria (Edwards and Gross 1976).

ily have some degree of drug-related social or occupational impairment. This belief has led to regrettable mistakes in the scripting of drug-dependence assessments (e.g., interview branching patterns that do not ask about clinical features of drug dependence unless drug-related impairment or social maladaptation has been reported). As a consequence, in the resulting study data, it is impossible to find drug-dependence cases that lack these impairments or maladaptation.

A third defect in DSM-III, corrected in ICD-10 but not in DSM-III-R or DSM-IV, was an interpenetration of politics with psychopathology when the "drug abuse" and "nondependent abuse" categories were formed. In ICD-10, there is a category of "harmful drug use," but the stigmatizing and political implications of the term *drug abuse* have been jettisoned. By contrast, DSM-III, DSM-III-R, and DSM-IV declare that legal difficulties are evidence of social maladaptation (or impairment) due to drug taking. In consequence, a U.S. citizen who smokes cannabis once a week will qualify for the DSM psychiatric diagnosis of nondependent cannabis abuse after just two arrests for violation of cannabis possession laws, unless cannabis dependence is present, in which case nondependent abuse is ruled out (via a formal exclusion). The same U.S. citizen who moves to Amsterdam after the first cannabis arrest will not qualify for the diagnosis of cannabis abuse (unless he or she moves back to the U.S. and is arrested for cannabis possession yet again). This is a peculiar interpenetration of politics and psychopathology, no matter which drug is under consideration. Moreover, stigma attached to the term *drug abuse* gives good reason to abandon this term in the medical and psychiatric nomenclature and classifications such as DSM-V, as has been done in ICD-10, in hope that the victims might be more responsive to public health outreach and early intervention efforts.

Should Drug Dependence Be Grouped With the Obsessional Disorders?

From Table 14–2 and topics covered in the previous section, the reader will see that the phenomenon of drug dependence can be understood in relation to neuroadaptational changes (e.g., tolerance, abstinence/withdrawal), observable obsession-like clinical features (e.g., subjective awareness of a compulsion to use the drug, sometimes described as a "craving"), and observable compulsion-like clinical features (e.g., return to drug use even after bouts of abstinence, and when the user self-describes a failed strenuous effort to thwart reinstatement). In this context of psychopathological analysis, it might be useful to ask whether drug dependence is simply a subtype of obsession.

Here again, as in our definition of "insight," we can turn to Sir Aubrey Lewis, this time in two essays, one titled "Problems of Obsessional Illness" (Lewis 1936) and another titled "Obsessional Illness" (Lewis 1957). In this pair of essays, Lewis implicitly (not explicitly) gave us reasons to group drug dependence with the obsessions. To begin, there is a similarity. As noted by Edwards and Gross (1976), alcohol dependence includes a subjective awareness of the compulsion to use the drug, as do the dependence syndromes secondary to the use of other nonalcohol drugs (e.g., see Table 14–1). This type of subjective awareness is central to the experience of obsessions, elucidated by Lewis in relation to a definition provided by Schneider: obsessions are "contents of consciousness which, when they occur, are accompanied by the experience of subjective compulsion, and which cannot be got rid of, though on quiet reflection they are recognized as senseless" (Lewis 1936, p. 326). Lewis claims that "senselessness" is not a necessary condition of obsessions. Instead, he argues that there should be some feeling that one should resist the obsession: "This resistance is experienced as that of one's free will" (Lewis 1936, p. 326). As made clear by Edwards and Gross (1976), the experience of subjective compulsion is quite prominent during the drug dependence process. If it is not present beforehand, early intervention and effective treatment induce the resistance, as described.

Lewis also noted the secondary phenomena in obsessions, namely, behaviors that develop "in order to obtain relief from the primary disturbance" (Lewis 1957,

p. 324)—that is, the subjectively felt compulsions to act. Here, we can map the concept of this type of secondary behavior onto what Edwards and Gross call "drug use to relieve or avoid withdrawal" as well as "drug-seeking behavior" (see Table 14–2), each of which develop as efforts to obtain relief from the primary disturbances in drug dependence.

The narrowing of the drinking repertoire (e.g., less diversity among types and number of alcoholic beverage drinks consumed per occasion) may have the character of the secondary rituals seen in cases of the obsessions. This type of narrowed and ritualized behavior also has been observed in relation to dependence on other drugs (e.g., rituals associated with rolling of cigarettes, "smoking the dragon" preparations when heroin is inhaled, cooker rituals when heroin is injected).

This form of narrowed behavior sometimes is confused with a separable secondary complication of the drug dependence process, which involves a narrowing of the nondrug behavioral repertoire. This phenomenon is seen when drug dependence and accompanying behaviors (e.g., drug seeking) expand to fill the hours of the victim, with concomitant giving up of other activities that previously served reinforcing functions (e.g., music, sports).

Nevertheless, despite superficial resemblances to obsessions, it seems that the best we can do in psychopathology is to avoid forced confluence of drug dependencies with obsessional disorders (as we apply the Cartesian advice to "divide up every difficulty into as many parts as are possible"). Instead, we note that some of the features of drug dependence are obsession-like in nature and form, without claiming that drug dependence should be classified as an obsession or grouped with the obsessional disorders.

Some psychopathologists have been quite strident on this point. For example, Kraupl-Taylor (1983, p. 83) has insisted that "patients with self-damaging addictions are the victims of compulsions which are not obsessional because they are more self-indulgent than distressing and because resistance against them either is absent or weak-willed." In a direct contradiction of Edwards and Gross, Kraupl-Taylor argued that "the compulsion of alcohol dependence is not obsessional; it is not sufficiently distressing and anxiety-dominated to oust the lure of the addiction and the craving of self-indulgence. There is also the difference that alcohol dependence does not give rise to secondary obsessional phenomena in the form of superstitious and compulsive rituals to combat the craving that is in due course more desired than dreaded" (Kraupl-Taylor 1983, p. 83). Regrettably, Kraupl-Taylor tars all cases of alcohol and drug dependence with the same brush. Nonetheless, even so, there is no need to group all alcohol or other drug dependence syndromes among the obsessions or obsessional disorders. It is enough to say that at least one of the clinical features of these syndromes is obsession-like in its character.

Natural Histories and Clinical Courses of Drug Dependence

Many research groups have contributed evidence about the natural history of drug dependence, and one of the lessons is that there is no single "natural history" of this condition; rather, there are many "natural histories." Some of the diversity is due to the many different types of pharmacological compounds that can give rise to a drug dependence syndrome. This diversity prompted the WHO Expert Committee to recommend distinctions: "Therefore, better understanding should be attained by substitution of the term drug dependence of this or that type, according to the agent or class of agents involved, in discussions of these conditions, especially interdisciplinary [discussions]" (World Health Organization 1965, p. 44). Accordingly, our research group has produced evidence on drug dependence of the cannabis type (e.g., Chen et al. 2005), drug dependence of the cocaine type (O'Brien and Anthony 2005), and so on.

A quite distinct source of diversity is the social context. In this regard, drug dependence is not really very different from other conditions. As noted by Carstairs (1962, pp. 125–126):

> In one sense, every follow-up study in the literature is a contribution to this field of inquiry; but one has to remember that the phrase "natural history of the illness" can be misleading. The course of a disease cannot be studied without reference to the social context in which it occurs, and this context contains factors—such as new drugs, new developments in treatment facilities, changes in public attitude toward the illness—which can radically alter its outcomes. In the writer's own professional lifetime new chemotherapies and antibiotics have radically changed the picture of organic disease in pneumonias, venereal diseases and tuberculosis.

It is difficult to challenge Professor Carstairs' claim that the social context helps produce multiple natural histories of the same condition; public attitudes certainly play a role. Nevertheless, it is possible to distinguish "natural history" from "clinical course," and there may be good reason to think of the natural history of cannabis dependence as a progression through linked states and processes in the absence of effective clinical intervention. Once we can introduce effective interventions, we no longer have a "natural" history in its original sense. Rather, we have the "clinical course" of the condition, subject to manipulation by effective clinical intervention. Indeed, during the mid-1980s, I was part of a research group led by the late Frank

Polk and his protégé, David Vlahov, which set out to investigate the natural history of HIV infection and AIDS among injecting drug users. Midway through the study, effective antiretroviral drugs became more widely available, and we had to change our specific aims for focus on the possibility that clinical course of HIV infection and AIDS were being changed by these medicines. Our study of "natural history" became a study of "clinical course," except for those HIV-infected injecting drug users who did not take the recommended regimens.

In some of our natural history research on drug dependence, we have worked forward through the first weeks and months after first drug self-administration (e.g., O'Brien and Anthony 2005). Nevertheless, much can be learned by working backward toward earlier predrug segments of life history, along the lines recommended by Lee N. Robins. As noted elsewhere, Professor Robins encouraged a *staging* concept in natural-history research on drug dependence, beginning with antecedents of the first chance to try a drug (i.e., before the start of drug use). Naming this concept "drug exposure opportunity," our research group sought to pay homage also to Wade Hampton Frost, first professor of epidemiology at Johns Hopkins University, whose early twentieth-century work in infectious disease epidemiology drew careful distinctions between effective contact with an infective agent and the "exposure opportunity" for such contact, noting that there is no risk of infection or disease where there is no exposure opportunity. Just as we have worked our way from the first weeks and months of drug use to observe rapid transitions and onset of drug dependence in the articles just cited, we also have worked our way from the first weeks and months of drug exposure opportunity to observe the first occurrence of drug use. To illustrate, with respect to cocaine in the United States during the early 1990s, an estimated 20%–25% of the U.S. population reported having had at least one chance to try cocaine (median age at onset: 19–20 years). Among those presented with a first chance to try cocaine, about one-third tried the drug within 1 year after the first cocaine exposure opportunity (Van Etten and Anthony 1999). Based on estimates from the first National Comorbidity Survey in the U.S., with data gathered about the same time as data on drug exposure opportunities, we learned that among individuals who tried cocaine, the risk of developing a cocaine dependence syndrome during the first year after first cocaine use was about 5%–6%; more than 80% who tried cocaine never developed cocaine dependence during 10 or more years after onset of cocaine use (Wagner and Anthony 2002). More recent epidemiological survey estimates have confirmed the 5%–6% value (i.e., little change in risk to develop cocaine dependence in the first year after onset of cocaine use, over the span from the early 1990s to 2000–2001; O'Brien and Anthony 2005).

Corresponding values for cannabis have been estimated as follows: in the general population, roughly 50% reported having experienced at least one chance to try cannabis (median age at onset: 16 years). Once the first cannabis exposure opportunity occurred, an estimated 40%–45% made a rapid transition from cannabis exposure opportunity to cannabis use (within 1 year of first opportunity; Van Etten and Anthony 1999). Based on data from the early 1990s, an estimated 2%–5% made the rapid transition to a cannabis dependence syndrome within 1 year of first cannabis use (Wagner and Anthony 2002). The corresponding estimate from 2000–2001 epidemiological survey data was 3.9% (Chen et al. 2005).

Drug Dependence Phenotype as Developmental Trajectory

Before leaving the topic of drug dependence as a phenomenon, it might be worthwhile to note a growing tendency to reorient our concept of phenotypes in the direction of developmental trajectories. That is, in the earlier sections of this chapter, we have assumed a state-like character of drug dependence, but it is possible to conceive of drug dependence as a process that unfolds in a trajectory. More definitive evidence might be gained, particularly in research on the genetic epidemiology of drug dependence, if we were to reconceptualize the phenotype as a developmental trajectory or as a vector of sequentially experienced developmental trajectories, one for each discrete stage of drug involvement—from the first drug exposure opportunity, to the first actual use of the drug, and onward toward the onset of drug dependence syndromes and their aftermath. This topic is worthy of more detailed coverage, given its resonance with related developments in trajectory studies of paleobiological processes, tree and plant growth, cockroach development, honeybees, human hypertension, and swordtail fish; interested readers will find more on this topic in articles now under review.

PREVENTION OF DRUG DEPENDENCE: FIVE FACTS

In this section of the chapter, I offer five facts or observations about preventing drug dependence. All five facts are based on recommendations made by the National Academy of Sciences/National Research Council (NAS/NRC) Committee on Data and Research for Policy on Illegal Drugs (Manski et al. 2001), of which I was a member. My intent is to explain these observations in more detail.

Fact 1—Most Psychopathologists Do Not Appreciate the Billions Spent on Prevention and Control of Drug Dependence

In the United States during 1999, federal expenditures on prevention and control of illegal drugs exceeded $17 billion. When annual expenditures are combined across federal, state, and local government allocations, the value is more than $30 billion. In relation to expenditures during the 5 years before 1999 and the 5 years after 1999, these values from 1999 are normative. For the most part, whether this massive annual expenditure actually prevents drug dependence or other drug-related hazards is almost completely unknown. It is difficult to imagine what might be accomplished if these funds were to be reallocated to prevention of other psychiatric disturbances and related behaviors such as suicide. One suspects that modest transfers would not increase the risk of becoming drug dependent, and might reduce the risk of drug dependence, to the extent that occurrence of drug dependence can be caused by preexisting psychiatric disturbances (O'Brien et al. 2004).

Most of these dollars are spent on macro-level programs, with no consideration of possibilities for randomization or controlled comparisons. Even when there are possibilities for between-jurisdiction or over-time nonexperimental contrasts, the evidence generally has been disregarded. For example, one investigation produced evidence that federal drug-scheduling decisions had little or no impact on occurrence of drug-related hazards, unless the decision was to take a previously unscheduled prescription medicine and to move it into the same scheduled category with cocaine, morphine, and other medically prescribed controlled substances; incremental rescheduling of a controlled drug from one low level of federal scheduling to the next highest level of scheduling seemed to yield no discernible impact (Anthony 1979). Evidence from nonexperimental studies of cannabis decriminalization is balanced on both sides of the decriminalization debate, with some studies suggesting no decriminalization impact in terms of cannabis use or problems, and with other studies suggesting adverse impact (e.g., see Joffe and Yancy 2004). In research on the recent National Youth Anti-Drug Media Campaign, most of the evidence either is being neglected (i.e., not published in the scientific literature) or is being actively suppressed, perhaps because early reports suggested a "boomerang" effect—for example, with young adolescents showing less rejection of cannabis use the more they were exposed to the campaign's anti-cannabis public service announcements. Notwithstanding negative or mixed evidence of this type, the nation continues to regard incremental rescheduling of already scheduled medicines as an effective maneuver in prevention of drug dependence; there is active federal resistance to state- and substate-level innovation in relation to the legal status of cannabis; the antidrug media campaign rolls on.

One of the most heavily financed drug prevention programs in U.S. schools is called Drug Abuse Resistance Education (DARE). After more than 15 years of repeated evaluations of DARE's impact on youthful drug involvement, the evidence is balanced toward the null—that is, at best no impact. Rather than change course and urge a different approach, the response of DARE leaders has been to renovate DARE and to reinitiate the cycle of evaluation. Given its momentum, one suspects that DARE will receive massive support for another 15–20 years before yet another reevaluation and renovation. In this field, perhaps more than in other fields, prevention efforts seem to take on lives of their own, thriving despite evidence that they are having no effect or perhaps even a negative effect.

Fact 2—Most Evidence About Drug Dependence Prevention Concerns the Low-Hanging Fruit

Our NAS/NRC committee noted that available evidence is not about effects of the entire spectrum of plausible approaches to prevention proposed or in use. Rather, the available evidence mainly is about the interventions that are most readily evaluated. To illustrate, a large fraction of the annual billions spent in the name of prevention and control of drug dependence is allocated to drug law enforcement and supply reduction, both overseas and domestically (e.g., crop eradication, crop substitution, border control, controlled purchases to set up prosecution of illegal drug traffickers). These prevention and control activities have never been scrutinized in serious evaluation research. Instead, the focus has been on what might well be the least expensive of the drug prevention and control initiatives—namely, the drug education curriculum initiatives and innovative drug prevention programs developed with support from the National Institute on Drug Abuse (NIDA).

It is quite likely that one of the most effective drug dependence prevention techniques has been to combine a dependence-causing drug compound with an antagonist for that compound, as was done by combining naloxone (an opioid antagonist) with pentazocine (Talwin) more than 20 years ago (e.g., see Senay 1985). This type of combination has resurfaced recently in efforts to reduce hazards associated with buprenorphine use (i.e., harm reduction via a buprenorphine-naloxone combination). These combination drug products exploit the capacity of the antagonist to counteract the influence of the agonist opioid. As described in the first sections of this chapter, antagonists can be used to precipitate abstinence/withdrawal syndromes when opioid dependence is present; they also can be used to dampen the reinforcing functions served by opioid drugs when they are administered in relatively small doses in these combination products.

During recent months, despite evidence of the value of the buprenorphine–naloxone combination in relation to successful opioid dependence treatment experiences (e.g., see Ling et al. 2005), there is pressure on the International Narcotics Control Board to reassign buprenorphine to the highest levels of controlled substance scheduling. One consequence of this board action, if it occurs, will be to dampen efforts to place effective drug dependence treatment regimens in the hands of specially trained and certified primary care practitioners who are visited by patients suffering from opioid dependence. Evaluation research on drug policy shifts of this type is more difficult than completion of evaluation research in the school setting (which has serious challenges of its own). Nonetheless, most of our evaluations of drug dependence prevention initiatives are in the domain of research on the school drug education curriculum; little work has been done on the high-cost macro-level interventions.

Fact 3—We Know Little About Drug Prevention Program Effects Under Conditions of Normal Practice

Here, our NAS/NRC committee asked for renewed attention to the difference between efficacy studies of prevention impact versus effectiveness studies. Drawing from our own experience, we have implemented a "Good-Behavior Game" (GBG) curriculum during the first 2 years of schooling, in an effort to assess whether teachers might exert a lasting influence on risk of drug use initiation during these years, after training to organize the primary school curriculum so as to clarify standard social task demands that must be learned when students first enter primary school (e.g., paying attention to the rules) (see Brown et al., Chapter 15, this volume). Studied to mid-adolescence, the effects of the GBG intervention seem quite remarkable—for example, with roughly a 50% reduction in the incidence of tobacco smoking initiation by age 14 years among boys (e.g., see Kellam and Anthony 1998, and later studies). Nonetheless, in the just-cited trial and the replication that followed, evaluation research was conducted under fairly tightly controlled conditions of NIDA-funded research (i.e., as efficacy research) and not under the conditions of normal practice (i.e., not as effectiveness research). As such, we have not yet assessed the impact of the GBG intervention on tobacco smoking or other forms of drug involvement or drug dependence under the conditions of normal practice. We are in the same position with respect to other more recently developed and evaluated drug prevention programs (e.g., see Spoth et al. 2005).

Fact 4—We Know Little About the Effects of Combined Drug Prevention Programs

For most children in the U.S., the schooling experience includes a succession of drug prevention programs, each with a different developmental orientation, each with a somewhat related message. Do these sequential prevention initiatives combine well? Do they complement one another? Do they detract from one another? These are fairly basic questions, but we do not yet have good evidence to answer them, except to say that programs might be more effective when they include booster sessions (i.e., postintervention follow-up to seek enhanced effects), as discussed by Manski and colleagues (2001, Chapter 7).

Fact 5—Experimentally Induced Delays in Drug-Use Onset Might Not Yield Reduced Risk of Drug Dependence

Progress in epidemiology and prevention research over the past 40 years points toward a plausible mechanism linking the effects of early prevention initiatives with later effects in the form of reduced risks of drug dependence. In specific, there is evidence to suggest delays in onset of smoking and other drug-taking behaviors following the GBG intervention in primary school (mentioned above), and following other more generic interventions intended to increase resistance to peer pressure toward drug use (e.g., social skills resistance training). A concurrently developing line of research tends to support the observation that onset of drug-taking in early adolescence (or before) is more malignant, in the sense that earlier-onset drug users are more likely to develop problems associated with drug dependence (e.g., see Anthony and Petronis 1995; Robins and Przybeck 1985). These two lines of research offer hope that experimentally induced delays in onset of drug use might yield later reduced risk of drug dependence. Nonetheless, this is a crucially important gap in knowledge that cannot be filled by additional observational studies, which leave great uncertainty about whether the vulnerabilities that give rise to early-onset drug use happen to be strongly associated with the vulnerabilities that give rise to later heightened risk of drug dependence. That is, early-onset drug use might be no more than a marker of increased vulnerability to later drug dependence, as opposed to a causal determinant of a later increased risk of drug dependence.

PAST RESEARCH AND FUTURE DIRECTIONS

Quantitative research in psychiatric epidemiology has a 200-year history and dates back to formal population surveys of mental disorders conducted in the early nineteenth century. In contrast, not counting alcohol studies, the traditions of epidemiological research on problems related to drug dependence started no more than about 100 years ago, with surveys of pharmacists who might know of chronic drug-seeking cases in their home communities (e.g., see Anthony and Van Etten 1998). Fortunately, with increased support for drug-dependence studies over the past 30 years, the field of epidemiology and prevention research on drug dependence has begun to make up for lost time.

This is not the place for a summary of the rapidly developing body of evidence on genetic polymorphisms that appear to influence the risk of drug dependence once drug-taking starts. Nor is it an appropriate place to summarize recent developments in "vaccines" to help protect drug users from the effects of psychoactive drugs once they have been administered. Nevertheless, one might forecast a time when parents living in high-risk neighborhoods, knowing of their own family histories of drug dependence, might choose to buy some time for their children, in the hope that a "vaccine induced" delay in onset and repetition of drug self-administration might lead to a markedly reduced risk of drug dependence in later years. One also might forecast a time when a government executive decides that the youth of a community need to be "vaccinated" or quarantined in order to avert an impending epidemic of drug dependence, possibly with attention focused on youths who carry risk-enhancing genetic traits. Advances in drug dependence genetics research and medications development might lead us to these circumstances sooner rather than later. The result will be challenges on multiple fronts, not only in relation to public health action and public health research, but also in relation to ethics, choice, and governance in a free society challenged by external threats and internal vulnerabilities.

CLINICAL IMPLICATIONS

Clinicians should be aware that not all cases of drug dependence necessarily involve some degree of drug-related social or occupational impairment. Stigma attached to the term *drug abuse* gives good reason to abandon this term in medical and psychiatric classifications such as DSM-V, in hope that the victims might be more responsive to public health outreach and early clinical interventions. Although at least one of the clinical features of substance dependence syndromes is obsession-like in its character, there is no need to group all alcohol or other drug dependence syndromes among the obsessions or obsessional disorders. There is no single "natural history" of substance dependence; rather, there are many "natural histories." There is a growing tendency to reorient our concept of phenotypes in the direction of developmental trajectories. It is worth noting that there is some evidence that prominent efforts at the prevention of substance abuse may produce a "boomerang" effect—for example, young adolescents may show less rejection of cannabis use the more they are exposed to anti-cannabis public service announcements.

One promising clinical approach for preventing drug dependence may be to combine a dependence-causing drug compound with an antagonist for that compound. It has been observed that onset of drug-taking in early adolescence (or before) is more malignant in the sense that such earlier-onset drug users are more likely to develop problems associated with drug dependence. However, there is uncertainty about whether the vulnerabilities that give rise to early-onset drug use are strongly associated with the vulnerabilities that give rise to later heightened risk of drug dependence. That is, early-onset drug use might be no more than a marker of increased vulnerability to later drug dependence, as opposed to a causal determinant of a later increased risk of drug dependence.

REFERENCES

American Psychiatric Association: Diagnostic and Statistical Manual of Mental Disorders, 3rd Edition. Washington, DC, American Psychiatric Association, 1980

American Psychiatric Association: Diagnostic and Statistical Manual of Mental Disorders, 3rd Edition, Revised. Washington, DC, American Psychiatric Association, 1987

American Psychiatric Association: Diagnostic and Statistical Manual of Mental Disorders, 4th Edition. Washington, DC, American Psychiatric Association, 1994

Anthony JC: The effect of federal drug law on the incidence of drug abuse. J Health Polit Policy Law 4:87–108, 1979

Anthony JC, Helzer JE: Syndromes of drug abuse and dependence, in Psychiatric Disorders in America: The Epidemiologic Catchment Study. Edited by Robins LN, Regier DA. New York, Free Press, 1991, pp 116–154

Anthony JC, Petronis KR: Early onset drug use and risk of later drug problems. Drug Alcohol Depend 40:9–15, 1995

Anthony JC, Warner LA, Kessler RC, et al: Comparative epidemiology of dependence on tobacco, alcohol, controlled substances and inhalants: basic findings from the National Comorbidity Survey. Exp Clin Psychopharmacol 2:244–268, 1994

Anthony JC, Van Etten ML: Epidemiology and its rubrics, in Comprehensive Clinical Psychology. Edited by Bellack A, Hersen M. Oxford, UK, Elsevier Science Publications, 1998, pp. 355–390

Carstairs GM: Some targets for future epidemiological research, in The Burden on the Community: The Epidemiology of Mental Illness: A Symposium. London, Oxford University Press, 1962

Chen CY, O'Brien MS, Anthony JC: Who becomes cannabis dependent soon after onset of use? Epidemiological evidence from the United States: 2000–2001. Drug Alcohol Depend 79:11–22, 2005

Csajka C, Verotta D: Pharmacokinetic-pharmacodynamic modelling: history and perspectives. J Pharmacokinet Pharmacodyn (epub Jan 11):1–53, 2006

Edwards G, Gross MM: Alcohol dependence: provisional description of a clinical syndrome. BMJ 1:1058–1061, 1976

Isaac M, Janca A, Sartorius N: ICD-10 Symptom Glossary for Mental Disorders. Geneva, Switzerland, World Health Organization Division of Mental Health, 1994

Isbell H, Chrusciel TL: Dependence liability of "non-narcotic" drugs. Bull World Health Organ 43:1–111, 1970

Joffe A, Yancy WS: Legalization of marijuana: potential impact on youth. Pediatrics 113:e632–e638, 2004

Kellam SG, Anthony JC: Targeting early antecedents to prevent tobacco smoking: findings from an epidemiologically based randomized field trial. Am J Public Health 88:1490–1495, 1998

Kraupl-Taylor F: Descriptive and developmental phenomena, in Handbook of Psychiatry, Vol 1: General Psychopathology. Edited by Shepherd M, Zangwill OL. New York, Cambridge University Press, 1983, pp 59–94

Lewis A: The psychopathology of insight. Br J Med Psychol 14:332–328, 1934

Lewis A: Problems of obsessional illness. Proc Royal Soc Med 29:325–336, 1936

Lewis A: Obsessional illness. Acta Neuropsiqiatrica Argentina 3:323–335, 1957

Ling W, Amass L, Shoptaw S, et al: A multi-center randomized trial of buprenorphine-naloxone versus clonidine for opioid detoxification: findings from the National Institute on Drug Abuse Clinical Trials Network. Addiction 100:1090–1100, 2005

Manski CF, Pepper JV, Petrie CV: Informing America's Policy on Illegal Drugs: What We Don't Know Keeps Hurting Us. Washington, DC, National Academy Press, 2001

O'Brien CP, Charney DS, Lewis L, et al: Priority actions to improve the care of persons with co-occurring substance abuse and other mental disorders: a call to action. Biol Psychiatry 56:703–713, 2004

O'Brien MS, Anthony JC: Risk of becoming cocaine dependent: epidemiological estimates for the United States, 2000–2001. Neuropsychopharmacology 30:1006–1018, 2005

Robins LN, Przybeck TR: Age at onset of drug use as a factor in drug and other disorders, in Etiology of Drug Abuse: Implications for Prevention (DHHS Pub. No. ADM 85 1335). Edited by Jones CL, Battjes RJ. Washington, DC, NIDA Research Monograph 56, 1985

Rounsaville BJ: Experience with ICD-10/DSM-IV substance use disorders. Psychopathology 35:82–88, 2002

Schuster CR, Thompson T: Self administration of and behavioral dependence on drugs. Annu Rev Pharmacol 9:483–502, 1969

Senay EC: Clinical experience with T's and B's. Drug Alcohol Depend 14:305–312, 1985

Spoth R, Randall GK, Shin C, et al: Randomized study of combined universal family and school preventive interventions: patterns of long-term effects on initiation, regular use, and weekly drunkenness. Psychol Addict Behav 19:372–381, 2005

Tatum AL, Seevers MH: Experimental cocaine addiction. Journal of Pharmacology and Experimental Therapeutics 36:401–410, 1929

Van Etten ML, Anthony JC: Comparative epidemiology of initial drug opportunities and transitions to first use: marijuana, cocaine, hallucinogens and heroin. Drug Alcohol Depend 54:117–125, 1999

Wagner FA, Anthony JC: From first drug use to drug dependence; developmental periods of risk for dependence upon marijuana, cocaine, and alcohol. Neuropsychopharmacology 26:479–488, 2002

World Health Organization: WHO Expert Committee on Addiction-Producing Drugs: Thirteenth Report (Technical Report Series 273). Geneva, Switzerland, World Health Organization, 1964

World Health Organization: WHO Expert Committee on Dependence-Producing Drugs: Fourteenth Report (Technical Report Series 312). Geneva, Switzerland, World Health Organization, 1965

World Health Organization: International Statistical Classification of Diseases and Related Health Problems, 10th Revision (ICD-10). Geneva, Switzerland, World Health Organization, 1992

15

Prevention of Aggressive Behavior Through Middle School Using a First-Grade Classroom-Based Intervention

C. Hendricks Brown, Ph.D.

Sheppard G. Kellam, M.D.

Nick Ialongo, Ph.D.

Jeanne Poduska, Sc.D.

Carla Ford, Ph.D.

This work was supported by grants from the National Institute of Mental Health (MH38725, MH42968, and MH40859). Principal collaborators have included the above authors and James C. Anthony, Lawrence Dolan, and Lisa Werthamer.

This work would not have been possible without the support and collaboration of the Baltimore City Public School System and the parents, children, teachers, and principals who participated. We would also like to thank our collaborators in the Prevention Science and Methodology Group for their many helpful comments and suggestions.

Population-based epidemiological studies have identified a number of robust risk factors in childhood that predict conduct disorder, delinquency and criminal behavior, unprotected sexual behavior, and substance use during adolescence. One common antecedent to all of these externalizing behaviors in adolescence is early aggressive behavior. Ratings of aggression by first-grade teachers, for example, are associated with 1.5 to 2.0 times the risk of being a regular cigarette or marijuana user 10 years later (Fleming et al. 1982; Kellam et al. 1982a, 1982b, 1982c, 1983); similar relative risks occur for exhibiting high delinquency or being arrested, as well as completing high school (Ensminger and Slusarcick 1992). The continuity of early aggressive behavior continues well into adulthood, with elevated lifetime cocaine use found among individuals who were aggressive in first grade (Ensminger et al. 2002). Children who are aggressive often have other concurrent risk factors. For example, we have reported that virtually all children who were rated by teachers as aggressive were also nominated by peers as being among the most aggressive and least-liked children in the classroom, and these children almost always had serious learning problems as well (Kellam et al. 1991). When a teacher rates a child as aggressive, the child's mother is much more likely to rate the child as aggressive, although mothers' ratings of aggression have lower predictability of aggressive behavior than do teachers' ratings (Kellam et al. 1982a). Furthermore, a subset of children who exhibit aggressive behavior also exhibit shy–withdrawn behavior. This combination of shy-aggressiveness, or what DSM-III-R (American Psychiatric Association 1987) called *undersocialized aggression*, is associated with an extremely high risk of adolescent externalizing behavior, because these children are rejected by prosocial-behaving peers and more readily join deviant peer groups at an early age (Kellam et al. 1982a, 1982b, 1982c).

In response to a number of national committees and the priorities of the National Institute of Mental Health's establishment of its prevention branch that first began targeting the prevention of conduct disorder and other externalizing behaviors, the Baltimore Prevention Program at the Johns Hopkins University Department of Mental Hygiene began a series of randomized field trials designed to modify aggressive behavior, as well as other specific risk factors, among first-graders so as to reduce their long-term risk of developing externalizing behaviors in adolescence. The National Institute on Drug Abuse also provided funding for this program. This trial is continuing to be evaluated, with the original two cohorts of first-graders being followed into adolescence and young adulthood. It is directed by Dr. Sheppard Kellam and his colleagues at the American Institutes for Research, with collaboration from the Johns Hopkins Prevention Research Center, the Baltimore City Public School System, and the Prevention Science and Methodology Group (PSMG) centered at the University of South Florida.

THEORETICAL FRAMEWORK

Much of our work in prevention has been guided by a three-tiered frame that we have termed *developmental epidemiology* (Kellam and Van Horn 1997; Kellam et al. 1982a, 1991, 1994a, 1994b, 1999), which comfortably coexists with more specific biopsychosocial theories for the etiology and prevention of conduct disorder (Reid et al. 1999, 2002), drug use (Botvin and Griffin 2003; Botvin et al. 1995), and major mental disorders. The first frame in developmental epidemiology is *community epidemiology*, which provides a population-based approach to prevention and early intervention. It is central to our public health perspective on reducing the burden of mental disorder and drug abuse. Our community epidemiological perspective relies on understanding the distribution over time of person-level and environmental risk factors and service utilization within the community.

Our work also grows out of a *life-course developmental* perspective—the second frame in developmental epidemiology—that is grounded in both developmental and environmental influences and is increasingly being informed by biology. This life-course development incorporates both person-level and environmental influences and their interaction on behavior and psychopathology across different stages of life. The integration of life-course development with community epidemiology allows the study of variation in developmental antecedents and paths in a defined population in defined ecological contexts. Because entire populations are studied, subject selection bias can be minimized, which is a major advantage over many clinic and treatment trials. This allows antecedents along developmental paths to be precisely targeted, their frequencies determined, and the variation in their function assessed with marked precision. An important focus of this approach is on the variation in the frequency and function of risk factors within and across subgroups in the population, rather than merely on the central tendencies or averages of risk factors for the population as a whole. This is only possible by controlling selection bias through examination of the entire study population or a representative sample.

The third frame in developmental epidemiology has involved the fundamental role of *randomized field trials* to test and refine our theories, particularly as we examine their impact on hypothesized mediators and their differential effect on subgroups characterized by different person and environment factors. Since we are interested in measuring the effects of these interventions on defined populations, we rely on field trials, or carefully designed intervention trials conducted under natural community settings, to examine program effectiveness, sustainability, scalability, and dissemination (Kellam and Langevan 2003). This developmental epidemiology perspective allows us to map the effects of an intervention within a population across different individuals, across different contexts, and across time and stage of life.

LIFE COURSE AND SOCIAL FIELD THEORY

The life-course development theory underlying the trials in Baltimore make use of life course/social field theory (Kellam and Rebok 1992; Kellam et al. 1975). This theory provides a framework within which to consider the interactions between children and others in their lives. At its center, life course/social field theory posits that as they develop, individuals move through different stages of life, each involving a set of relevant social fields with specific task demands. For example, the two main social fields for first-grade children are the family of origin and the classroom. As children grow up, other social fields become important, such as the peer group, the family of procreation, and the workplace. Within each of the social fields, "natural raters" define the social task demands and rate individuals' performance on these task demands. Thus, the teacher and the child's classmates are natural raters in the classroom; parents are natural raters in the family of origin. Kellam et al. (1975) named this process of social task demand and behavioral response *social adaptation*. The rating of an individual's adequacy on task demands by the natural rater is termed *social adaptational status* (SAS). For example, elementary teachers consistently identify three major social adaptational dimensions related to success in school:

1. Children must be able to sit still, obey rules, and not be disruptive or aggressive.
2. Children must be able to interact socially with their peers.
3. Children must be able to learn to read and achieve mastery in subject matter.

Often, SAS is assessed formally, as with grades and standardized achievement tests in the classroom. Where no such formal SAS dimensions exist, they may be assessed through direct interviews with the teacher (Werthamer-Larsson et al. 1991), as well as by direct observation of, say, aggressive/disruptive behavior in the classroom.

Each measure of SAS is a socially relevant construction influenced by the interaction of the individual, the natural rater, and the context. For example, there are a number of individual-level behavioral interventions that can successfully reduce a child's actual level of aggressive behavior, but often teachers and peers continue to rate the child as aggressive, perhaps remembering all too well their past conflictual encounters with the child. If the child recognizes that teacher and peer responses are not contingent on his or her current behavior, then there is little to reinforce better behavior in the long term. Thus, the child's actual level of aggressive behavior in the classroom, obtained through direct observation of the child by an independent assessor, is conceptually distinct from and potentially quantitatively different from the teacher's and peers' ratings of that child on classroom aggression and also distinct from the parent's rating of aggressiveness for the child. We would therefore expect that the predictability of long-term conduct disorder in children may differ across these different measures of SAS. In fact, we and others have noted that teacher ratings of aggressive behavior are more predictive of long-term outcomes than are similar aggressive ratings by mothers (Kellam et al. 1982a, 1982b, 1982c).

In keeping with Cicchetti and Schneider-Rosen (1984), we hypothesize that success in mastering social task demands specific to one stage of development and social field leads to an increase in later successes across developmental stages and across social fields. For example, if an individual learns the social skill of working with others early in life within the classroom social field, that individual has an increased likelihood of success later in life working with co-workers in the work social field. Competencies in early stages of life can also be activated and used during times of stress, crisis, novelty, or creativity. It follows that early successful social adaptation in the face of prominent developmental challenges tends to promote later adaptation as the individual encounters new and different social task demands across social fields. This key developmental principle, along with a growing empirical literature, forms the basis for our focus on successful adaptation to first grade as a means of improving social adaptational status over the life course.

Our conceptualization of the pathway from SAS to psychological measures and psychiatric conditions is grounded in social learning theory, with the additional recognition that there are also genetic factors that interact with environmental exposures. From a social learning point of view, the more successful individuals are in meeting the demands of their natural raters, the more likely they are to be reinforced for success and experience positive psychological well-being. Alternatively, failure to meet the natural raters' demands will be associated with reductions in reinforcement and increases in punishment, which may then lead to decrements in psychological well-being.

We also hypothesize that the salience of adaptation in certain social fields and at different times is more relevant than others. For example, failure to accept authority in a first-grade classroom setting, which involves a major life transition into a structured setting, compared to similar ratings by parents, should be more predictive of conduct disorder in adolescence. Specific key transition periods that require new social task demands, such as first grade and entry into middle school, should be more predictive of later outcomes and therefore important places to conduct preventive trials.

Life course/social field theory postulates that social maladaptation is often reciprocally related to *psychological well-being* (PWB). PWB is an internal assessment reflecting the psychological status of the individual in regard to such constructs as self-esteem, psychiatric symptoms or disorders, and neurobiological or neuropsychological conditions. Thus, measurement of attention through the Continuous Performance Task is a PWB measure. By contrast, an assessment by the teacher of the child's ability to stay on task within a classroom setting is a SAS measure. PWB, which can be assessed by symptom reports, standardized neuropsychological tests, or clinical observation, may be an antecedent and/or a consequence of social maladaptation. For example, if a child manifests neuropsychological deficits in attention, these psychological characteristics, if untreated, may lead to poor performance in school, a SAS measure. We have reported in our work that directing interventions at SAS during the key transition point of first grade shows promise of improving both later SAS and PWB, particularly among children already having SAS and/or PWB problems (Dolan et al. 1993; Ialongo et al. 1999). In terms of the pathway from PWB to SAS, we hypothesize that the concentration problems and feelings of helplessness and low self-efficacy frequently associated with decrements in PWB (Kovacs and Goldston 1991) reduce the likelihood that the individual will succeed in meeting social task demands such as academic achievement. This hypothesized link between SAS and PWB provides an additional rationale for targeting early SAS as a means of reducing the risk for decrements in PWB, which, in reciprocal fashion, should further reduce the likelihood of social adaptational failure.

Directionality and malleability in these relationships have been tested in our preventive field trial by specifically targeting single or combinations of risk factors (Dolan et al. 1993; Ialongo et al. 1999; Kellam et al. 1994a, 1994b, 1998a, 1998b).

AGGRESSION, CONDUCT DISORDER, AND ANTISOCIAL BEHAVIOR

Our framework for understanding the etiology and course of antisocial behavior relies heavily on the integration of our developmental epidemiological perspective with the developmental model of antisocial behavior described by Patterson et al. (1992) and, more recently, by Capaldi and Patterson (1994). A basic tenet of the Patterson et al. (1992) model is that family interactions, both early in the child's life and through adolescence, are the prime determinants of antisocial and delinquent behavior. However, family processes are seen as embedded within and transacting across the larger contextual fields of the community, neighborhood, and school. According to Patterson et al. (1992), one of the major pathways to delinquency and antisocial behavior in adolescence and adulthood begins in the toddler years. Parents' failure to effectively punish aggressive behavior and to teach reasonable levels of compliance becomes the first step in an escalating spiral of coercive behaviors among family members, which serve to "train" the child to become progressively more antisocial. Upon the transition to school, such children can prove difficult for either teachers or peer groups to teach, due to their coercive and noncompliant stance. Over the course of elementary school, Patterson and colleagues postulate that these children's coercive style ultimately leads to rejection by teachers and well-adjusted peers. Coercive, noncompliant children are likely to have difficulty engaging fully in academic tasks and may fall behind in school as well. Thus, rejection and failure at home and at school lead to deficits in academic, social, and occupational skills, as parents and teachers fail to adequately monitor the child and reinforce prosocial behavior and academic achievement. The failure of parents to adequately monitor their children is seen as particularly critical during adolescence, when children are seeking greater independence and are spending more time outside of their parents' direct supervision. Ultimately, the lack of adequate monitoring by parents in early adolescence, combined with rejection by parents and mainstream peers, precipitates "drift" into a deviant peer group, where reinforcement is provided for a wide array of antisocial and delinquent behavior, including alcohol and drug use (Dishion et al. 1996; Sampson and Groves 1989). This, in turn, results in an increase in these behaviors and their maintenance over time.

THEORY OF THE GOOD-BEHAVIOR GAME INTERVENTION

In 1985 we conducted a randomized trial of two first-grade classroom interventions, the Good-Behavior Game (GBG) and the Mastery Learning (ML) curriculum for reading. The GBG was chosen because it had a successful track record for reducing aggressive behavior in classroom settings. ML was chosen to improve learning in first and second grade, a protective factor for adolescent depression and other psychiatric symptoms (Dolan et al. 1993). Although we have reported on beneficial impact from both of these interventions, it is clear that the effects of the GBG are broader than those of ML, continuing throughout adolescence and into adulthood. We therefore limit the discussion in this chapter to the GBG intervention.

The GBG was developed more than 35 years ago (Barrish et al. 1969) by a teacher (Saunders in the reference cited above), who used group contingencies to reinforce positive behavior in a chaotic classroom. The GBG intervention tested in the Baltimore City Public School System is a highly articulated behavioral intervention that begins with the teacher clearly specifying four classroom rules for the students to follow: 1) working quietly; 2) being polite to others; 3) getting out of one's seat only with permission; and 4) following directions. These rules are defined and categorized into four clearly measurable behaviors. For example, "talking or verbal disruption" is defined as "talking without being permitted by the teacher, whistling, singing, yelling, or making other sounds." The associated rule is "We will work quietly." Similarly, "aggression or physical disruption" means "physical contacts, such as hitting, kicking, pushing, making someone stumble, hair pulling, pinching, throwing objects, pencil fighting, intentional pencil breaking, taking or destroying property of others." The associated rule is "We will be polite to others." These rules and behaviors are repeatedly stated with specifications, such as no talking allowed during reading period.

The game is played in the classroom by first dividing the class into heterogeneous teams of 4–7 students, establishing a set time and duration in which the game will be played, setting a standard for number of violations (i.e., four or fewer occurrences of rule breaking), and then counting rule infractions for each team. Whenever a misbehavior occurs, the teacher immediately names the behavior, identifies the child, and praises the other teams for behaving appropriately. Teachers do not punish individual children for their misbehavior; rather, they record behaviors for each team on a scoreboard. At the end of the game, each team that has fewer than a set number of rule infractions receives an appropriate reward. Although teams do not compete against one another, they naturally use the peer group to shape their own team member's behavior. With supervision from a GBG coach, the teacher continues to use the game throughout the school year, extending the time the game is played, lessening the rewards as well, and making sure that the teams remain relatively even. As children become socialized to the role of student, they develop their own intrinsic rewards for good behavior. As implemented in Baltimore schools, the GBG was continued throughout all of first and second grade. Teachers were provided with 40 hours of GBG training and continued to receive supervision during the first year they delivered the intervention.

The GBG has several benefits over other behavioral interventions aimed at reducing aggressive behavior. Most important, because individual children are not removed from the classroom for correction of bad behavior, there is no labeling of children. Such labeling conflicts with the long-term strategy of having children reintegrated with prosocial peers. A second benefit is that the GBG provides teachers with a general tool for organizing classroom behavior, something that unfortunately is almost exclusively taught only to special education teachers. In our baseline studies, nearly half of the first-grade teachers were unable to manage aggressive classroom behavior at baseline (Kellam et al. 1998a). In such chaotic environments, many children have reduced chances of learning.

Specific Hypotheses About the Good-Behavior Game

We have hypothesized that the GBG reduces conduct problems and eventually antisocial behavior and substance use in the following manner. First, the game is designed to reduce aggressive and coercive behavior in the first and second grade. This, in turn, reduces rejection of problem children by teachers and peers. Consequently, teachers and peers are able to "teach" these children key social survival skills—academic as well as interpersonal. As a result, these children are less likely to drift into deviant peer groups or be assigned to poor-achieving, aggressive-behaving classes or tracks, where reinforcement of antisocial and delinquent behavior is provided. Ultimately, these youths will be less likely to engage in antisocial behavior and substance use and abuse. Moreover, these individuals will be less likely to fail in the fields of work and intimate social relations and to develop antisocial and substance abuse and dependence disorders as young adults.

We anticipate that the GBG may vary in impact by level of aggressiveness at baseline. Specifically, we would not anticipate that the GBG would have much effect among minimally aggressive children; as a group, such children are already at low risk for later externalizing behavior. When we began our study, we anticipated that the GBG intervention could improve outcomes among children who were moderately aggressive, but we conjectured that for children with the highest levels of aggressive behavior they would be the hardest to change and therefore would receive a more moderate level of impact from GBG. These predictions have implications for analytical strategies as well. For example, even though the average rate of aggressive behavior in GBG classrooms could decrease compared to control classrooms, this overall decrease may be relatively small, because the benefit would be seen mostly in the more at-risk group of children. In terms of analyses, we anticipated the need to examine not only GBG's main effects but also its potential interactions with baseline levels of aggressive behavior. Furthermore, since there was a possibility that the intervention effect could be highest among the middle level of aggressive behavior, we would need to use statistical methods for examining this treatment-by-baseline interaction that would allow detection of such nonlinear patterns. In the analytic method below, we describe several methods that we have used.

Measures

Teacher Observation of Classroom Adaptation—Revised

The Teacher Observation of Classroom Adaptation—Revised (TOCA-R; Werthamer-Larsson et al. 1991) is a brief measure of each child's adequacy of performance on the core tasks in the classroom as defined by the teacher. We have used this instrument to collect key SAS measures repeatedly on the study children twice in first and second grade when the intervention was going on, and then yearly thereafter until the eighth grade. It is a structured interview administered by a trained member of the assessment staff. The interviewer records the teacher's ratings of the adequacy of each child's performance on six basic tasks: accepting authority (aggressive behavior), social participation (shy or withdrawn behavior), self-regulation (impulsivity), motor control (hyperactivity), concentration (inattention), and peer likeability (rejection). These ratings are recorded for each child in the classroom. Werthamer-Larsson et al. (1991) reported test–retest correlations over a 4-month interval with different interviewers of 0.60 or higher and coefficient alphas of 0.80 and higher for each of these subscales. With respect to concurrent validity, scores on the Attention/Concentration subscale correlated 0.62 with the reading total score on the California Achievement Test in first grade. In addition, a correlation of 0.67 was found between the Authority Acceptance subscale and peer nominations for "gets into trouble." The TOCA-R Likeability/Rejection subscale correlated 0.44 with peer nominations for likeability/rejection.

Direct Observation of Classroom Behavior

We developed a behavior coding system based on observation by independent classroom observers, who rated children's social interactions, aggression, and off-task behavior. Each item was defined by accepted behavioral definitions (R.N. Kent, G. Miner, W. Kay, and K.D. O'Leary, "Stonybrook Observer Manual" [unpublished manuscript], 1974; K.D. O'Leary, R.G. Ronamczyk, R.E. Kass,

A. Dietz, and D. Santograssi, "Procedures for Classroom Observation of Teachers and Children" [unpublished manuscript], 1971). Additionally, we coded what activity the target child was engaged in at that instant; this ranged from the teacher working with the target child in a small group, to group instruction, to unsupervised seat work or no assignment. To collect sufficient behavior observation data, we did time sampling of six consecutive 10-second time intervals of observation for each child in the classroom, coding all relevant behaviors for that child during each 10-second time interval. By repeating this microbehavior coding, we obtained 10 minutes of observation on each child per day of observation. For both the first and second cohorts of first graders, we obtained measures just before and after TOCA-R administration in the fall, and just before and after TOCA-R administration in the late spring. Forty minutes of observation were done per child during the year.

Peer Assessment Inventory

The Peer Assessment Inventory (PAI) is a modified version of the Revised Pupil Evaluation Inventory (R-PEI; Pekarik et al. 1976) and is designed to assess the child's adaptation to the demands of the classroom peer group. Ten items were selected from the original R-PEI on the basis of their relevance to three key constructs: authority acceptance/aggressive behavior (e.g., "Which of the children starts fights?"), social participation/shy behavior (e.g., "Which of the children plays alone a lot?"), and likeability/rejection ("Which children don't you like?"). In terms of administration, a question is read aloud to the class, and the children are then instructed to circle the pictures of all children in their classroom described by the question. Thus, children are able to make unlimited nominations of classmates for each question. Raw scores on each of the above dimensions are converted to standard scores based on the distribution of nominations within a child's classroom. As indicated above, a correlation of 0.67 was found between the Authority Acceptance subscale and peer nominations for "gets into trouble." The TOCA-R Likeability/Rejection subscale had a correlation of 0.44 with peer nominations for likeability/rejection.

Analytic Models

It has been our view that the designs and analytic models used to evaluate prevention programs need to be directly tuned to the questions driving the research. Our perspectives have included the development of new methodologies to examine intervention impact over long periods of time, leading to a number of growth modeling techniques for examining intervention impact over time. Because we are concerned with examining variation in impact over time, we have developed new tools that allow for examining how growth depends on intervention by baseline interactions (Curran and Muthén 1999; Muthén and Curran 1997; Muthén et al. 2002), for examining nonlinear impact with additive models (Brown 1993a, 1993b; Ialongo et al. 1999), and for examining impact on different classes of growth trajectories (Carlin et al. 2002; Muthén et al. 2002). We have also been concerned with examining how intervention impact on the most proximal targets of the intervention affect the longer-term distal outcomes, a strategy we call proximal-distal modeling. General growth mixture models (Muthén et al. 2002) provide an important way to determine impact on growth as well as distal diagnoses, syndromes, or time-to-event measures. All of these analytic models require careful handling of missing data, and we have provided several approaches for both ignorably missing and nonignorably missing data (Brown 1990; Brown et al. 2000).

Randomized Trial Design

All of these analytical techniques would be of relatively little value in the absence of a carefully designed randomized trial that allows one to infer causality about the intervention's impact from the statistical analyses. The inferential advantages of a well-conducted randomized trial over other designs have been described in philosophical and statistical terms involving a *counterfactual* (Brown 1993a, 2004; Rubin 1974). A counterfactual considers two potential outcomes for each subject, one under each intervention condition. It is the conceptualized difference in response for each individual that corresponds to that individual's intervention impact. Of course, a realized experiment provides information on only one of these outcomes—either under intervention or control condition—and thus one cannot obtain a direct estimate of intervention impact for any individual (Brown 2004). However, when those who are assigned to the intervention condition have outcomes that have the same distribution as that for the entire population if given the intervention, and similarly those in the control condition have outcomes that have the same distribution as that of the entire population if not given the intervention, then the difference in average responses for those assigned to the intervention and those assigned to the control condition provides an unbiased estimate of the average intervention effect over the entire population. In randomized trials, these two conditions, which are known as strongly ignorable treatment assignment, can be realized, provided assessors are blind to intervention condition and there is no attrition bias. This counterfactual argument allows one to define theoretically what is meant by intervention effect at the individual and group level and to specify what must occur for an unbiased estimate of this effect (Brown 1993a, 2003).

Unit of Intervention Assignment

In the Baltimore trial, some classes received the GBG intervention, others received an enhanced ML intervention, and still others received a standard setting. Depending on the teacher's school, teachers were randomly assigned to GBG or ML or to one of three control conditions (described later). Our rationale for examining each of these conditions separately was that we wanted to test the salience of each of the two correlated risk factors of aggressive behavior and learning problems through interventions targeting each separately. We could then determine whether crossover effects occurred (e.g., Did achievement improve among classes who received the GBG intervention to reduce aggression and disruption?). In two follow-up trials, we have combined intervention components in systematic evaluations that allow us to examine their combined effects (Ialongo et al. 1999).

In the trials we have conducted in Baltimore, whole classrooms are randomized as a group to the intervention condition. (We used other levels of randomization as well, as described below.) *Unit of assignment* refers to which units in a design—for example, children, families, classroom, schools, neighborhoods, or regions—are assigned as a unit to the intervention condition. In most pharmacological trials, individuals are typically assigned to the intervention. In many drug prevention trials, whole schools are assigned to the intervention condition (see, e.g., similar school-based randomized trials conducted by Reid et al. 1999, 2002), and there are examples of public housing, clinics, and villages being randomized as well. Although a number of considerations determine which unit of assignment should be used, the most important of these is what has been called the *unit of intervention*. *Unit of intervention* refers to the level at which an intervention is theoretically intended to function. The GBG, for example, is an intervention delivered by a teacher to an entire class; here, the classroom is the unit of intervention. Clearly, one cannot randomize at a lower level than the unit of intervention—for example, randomly assigning a subset of the class to the intervention—since this will dissipate the strength of the intervention. It is possible to randomize at a level higher than the unit of intervention—for example, randomizing at the school level means that all classes in the school at the same grade level receive the same intervention condition. Randomizing at a higher level reduces the risk of intervention leakage. However, this randomization at a higher level generally comes at a very large cost in statistical power. We have noted, for example, that randomization at the level of the classroom (after ensuring that classrooms were balanced across classes) reduced the sample size by a factor of 3 in our first Baltimore Prevention Program trial, compared with a design that used school-level random assignment (Brown and Liao 1999).

In addition to assigning intervention conditions at the individual or group level, one can also assign intervention conditions at different times. For example, in the Linking the Interests of Families and Teachers (LIFT) trial, all schools began as controls, and each year a random subset of schools were randomized to the intervention condition (Reid et al. 1999, 2002; see also Brown et al. 2006). In the first trial of the Baltimore Prevention Program, we kept each first-grade classroom-teacher in the same intervention condition for 2 consecutive years. Our rationale for this fixed two-cohort design was to increase power through increased sample size. Unfortunately, we found that the overall impact of the GBG intervention was much smaller in the second cohort than in the first cohort, a point we will come back to later.

GBG Trial Design

In order to select elementary schools, classroom, teachers, and children, we began by selecting five sociodemographically distinct school regions in eastern Baltimore. These five contiguous regions represented diversity in terms of socioeconomic status, ranging from very poor to moderate income, and variation in ethnicity, ranging from mostly African American, mixed, and mostly white. The areas, each of which was relatively homogeneous, were required to serve as catchment areas for four or five somewhat similar elementary schools, so that the random assignment of schools within each region would bring about a balanced design at the school level. We randomized schools within each of these regions to one of three types. One school within each region was designated to be a school where GBG was being implemented in randomly selected classrooms. In one of the other schools in each region, we designated that school to be one where our enhanced ML was being implemented in randomly selected classrooms. All other schools served as "external control schools" where only standard practice was taking place. It is important to note that the entire school system was implementing ML as a reading curriculum at that time. Our enhanced ML condition provided substantially more structure, training, and supervision than the ML curriculum received by the remaining classrooms. Children in the external control schools were used to evaluate each intervention against this standard setting. Although we knew that these external controls would not be contaminated by either of the interventions, we did realize that school-to-school variation would likely add variability to the GBG versus external control comparison relative to that achievable with comparison classrooms within the same school (Brown and Liao 1999).

During the summer before the interventions were to begin, we completed random assignment of classes. In those schools where GBG was to take place, we first excluded the few first-grade special education classes and then randomly selected one classroom/teacher to serve as an internal control classroom for GBG. The other one or two classrooms were then assigned to the GBG condition. Likewise, for schools where the enhanced ML intervention was to be implemented, we randomly selected one classroom/teacher to serve as an internal control classroom for enhanced ML and then assigned the other one or two classes to receive the enhanced ML. We further realized that comparisons within school would succeed only if the classes themselves were quite similar. Thus, during the summer before school started, we had principals assign all students sequentially to the different classes. Classes within school were checked for balance on kindergarten experience and academic and behavioral performance, and where there was imbalance the children were reassigned. Children who moved into any of these school districts during the year were assigned to classrooms in a balanced fashion as well, except that some provision was made to keep the class sizes comparable. These procedures produced very balanced classrooms within schools. (In our two succeeding trials in Baltimore, our research staff has prepared random assignment lists so that true random allocation occurs for all children in the study. Although full randomization did not occur in the first trial that we describe here, we have no indication that the randomization of schools and randomization of classes within schools, coupled with balanced assignment of children, causes any threat to our inferences about intervention impact.)

Both interventions were delivered over the course of 2 years in two successive cohorts. In the second year, the first cohort of first graders moved en masse as a class to second grade, remaining in the same intervention condition. Thus, children receiving GBG in first grade also received GBG during second grade. Also in the second year, a second cohort of first graders was assigned in a balanced fashion to classroom, and the same teacher stayed in the same intervention condition. In this manner, two separate cohorts received the same intervention over the first 2 years of elementary school.

Beginning in 1985, two successive cohorts (NI = 1,196; NII = 1,115) of urban first-graders were recruited from a total of 43 classrooms in 19 elementary schools located in 5 sociodemographically distinct areas in eastern Baltimore. In each school, 8 classrooms were assigned to the GBG intervention, 6 classrooms served as internal controls, and 12 classrooms served as external controls.

In regard to gender, ethnicity, and age of the subject population at entrance into the study, in cohort 1, 49.1% were male, 65.6% were African American, 31.6% were European American, 0.3% Asian, 1.0% Native American, 0.3% Hispanic, and for 1.2% of the children, ethnicity was either missing or refused. For first graders, the mean age was 6.55 years (SD ± 0.48). In cohort 2, these summary statistics were quite similar.

Of the 1,196 cohort 1 students, 1,084 (91%) were available for data collection at baseline in the fall of 1985. Of these 1,084, 871 (80%) remained enrolled in project schools through grade 1; 96% of the 871 completed the second year of their assigned intervention or control condition. Of the 835 receiving the entire 2-year intervention, 71% (593) remained enrolled in the Baltimore City Public School System (BCPSS) through grade 9. Of the 1,115 cohort 2 students, 910 (82%) were available for data collection at baseline. Of these 910, 878 (96%) completed the second year of their assigned intervention or control condition. Of the 878 receiving the entire 2-year intervention, 579 (70%) remained enrolled in the BCPSS through the 1993–1994 academic year. Departure from the BCPSS or transfer from a project to a nonproject school was unrelated to assigned condition initially and from grade 1 through the 1993–1994 academic year. Of the 2,311 children originally enrolled in cohorts 1 and 2, 1,431 remained enrolled in the BCPSS at the end of the 1993–1994 year.

Effects of the GBG Intervention on Aggressive Behavior

We report here on the published results on the first cohort. We limit this to analyses on the first cohort because we found overall smaller GBG effects in the second cohort compared to the first. These results appear most likely to be the result of lower sustainability of the GBG in the second year compared with the first. It appears that while GBG designated teachers received extensive training and supervision the first year, the supervision they received the second year did not provide sufficient structure for them to continue its implementation at the level they had used the previous year. The fact that sustaining such interventions requires a concerted structure has been integrated into our current trial designs.

We also point out that for the analyses described below, we do not provide full details about their effects and standard errors, particularly those dealing with adjustments for randomization at the classroom and higher levels (see Brown 1993a).

The earliest time for evaluating impact of GBG is with the end of first grade measures. Using the fall of first grade measures as covariates, we found for cohort 1 that there were significant reductions in aggressive behavior for GBG boys and girls compared with controls and that these differences were most pronounced for children with higher aggressive ratings at baseline (Dolan et al. 1993). We start by describing results on teacher ratings of aggressive behavior. GBG boys had a significantly lower level of teacher ratings of aggression (TOCA-R authority acceptance) compared with external controls, and the difference with internal controls was nonsignificant but in the same direction. We also found that GBG benefit for boys was highest when concentration problems were present at baseline (Rebok et al. 1996). For girls, there was a significant reduction in teacher ratings of aggressive behavior for GBG compared with internal controls and a nonsignificant but similar pattern of higher aggression for the external controls. Thus, both boys and girls showed important gains due to GBG, and even though the patterns of effects were identical, the significance levels varied somewhat, depending on whether we used the internal or external controls as comparisons.

For boys, results for peer nominations of aggressive behavior were identical to results for teacher ratings of aggression. GBG boys had significantly lower rates of aggression compared with internal controls and nonsignificantly lower levels compared with external controls (Dolan et al. 1993). The largest intervention impact again was among the high-aggression males (Brown 1993a). For girls' ratings of peer nominations, there were no significant differences, although again GBG girls had lower levels of aggressive nominations. One reason that we did not find a significant effect on peer nominations for girls is that the nomination rate for girls was much lower than that for boys (Dolan et al. 1993).

Although both teacher and peer ratings of aggression were found to be reduced in GBG children, it is possible that GBG could have changed the rating behavior of these natural raters alone without actually changing the behaviors themselves. To examine behaviors directly, we used classroom observation of off-task behavior to assess the impact of the intervention on observable behaviors. We found a strong and consistent reduction in off-task behavior among the GBG children compared with the controls. Overall, the rate of off-task behavior decreased more than threefold by the end of first grade in GBG children compared with internal controls, and here detailed adjustments for the various levels of randomization still showed a highly significant reduction (Brown 1993a). We also found that this GBG effect was highest when the child was engaged in seat work and not being directly supervised by the teacher, something that we would expect since GBG focuses on self-regulation. Additionally, we found that observations of aggressive/disruptive behavior were also reduced in GBG children compared with controls. Thus, taken together, GBG had beneficial effects across both teacher and peer ratings of aggressive behavior as well as reductions in observed off-task and aggressive/disruptive behavior.

We have also conducted a number of evaluations of the patterns in growth trajectories for teacher ratings of aggressive behavior from first through eighth grades. Growth mixture models (Muthén et al. 2002; Schaeffer et al. 2003; Wang et al. 2005) and general growth mixture models (Muthén et al. 2002) were used as statistical modeling techniques to characterize these multiple trajectories across time. These models are similar to the growth modeling techniques of Nagin and colleagues (Nagin and Tremblay 1999; Shaw et al. 2003), except that these allow for within-cluster variation, something that we have found to be useful in explaining autocorrelation in the data (Wang et al. 2005).

As Moffitt (1993) concluded earlier, children differed in their patterns of aggression through elementary and middle school. About 10% of the boys had high levels of aggressive behavior throughout the study; these continuing high-aggression children were much more likely to have concentration problems and be rejected by their peers compared with the other classes (Muthén et al. 2002; Schaeffer et al. 2003). These continuing high-aggression males closely resembled Moffitt's (1993) and Loeber et al.'s (1998) life-course-persistent groups. About half of the boys had more moderate levels of aggressive behavior throughout. They began with fewer conduct problems and were more liked by their peers than were those in the continuing high-aggression group (Schaeffer et al. 2003). About a third of the boys maintained a very low level of aggressive behavior throughout elementary and middle school. They had less concentration problems and were more liked by their peers. Finally, we found a limited amount of evidence for the existence of a small number of males who showed substantial increase in aggressive behavior, and very few in the control group showed a marked decrease over time. These last two groups were too small to examine intervention impact and for most analyses have been subsumed into the other classes.

Our growth models have been able to determine how the GBG intervention differentially affects different subgroups. Our analyses indicate that significant reduction in aggression occurs among the continued high aggressive group (the group most at risk), with other growth trajectory groups being little affected by GBG (Muthén et al. 2002). That is, the GBG appears to have a long-term beneficial impact among the highest-risk males.

CONCLUSION

This chapter gives an overview of GBG impact on aggressive behavior through middle school. The data suggest that GBG has its major impact on those at highest risk, that is, those who begin with high levels of aggression (and who in the absence of intervention would likely remain aggressive). The strength of the randomized trial design adds credibility that the observed differences can be attributed causally to GBG and are not artifacts of selection or assignment bias (Brown 2003).

The GBG is a universal intervention—that is, it is designed to be used for the full classroom. Nevertheless, the GBG's impact on aggression is primarily in the high-risk group, a fact that increases its utility and its appeal. Indeed, the prevention field is finding a number of universal preventive interventions that have their largest impact among the highest-risk group (Brown and Liao 1999). Thus, it appears feasible to have population-based interventions that improve those at highest risk and also avoid labeling problems when at-risk children are removed from their natural environments.

This first-generation trial demonstrated that a portion of aggressive behavior or conduct disorder is preventable through adequate structuring of a child's environment in early elementary school. It is far more difficult to treat seriously conduct disordered adolescents. Thus, the GBG by itself can be a beginning of a strategy to reduce aggressive behavior, especially in males. We have found that GBG is well accepted by schools and communities. Part of its appeal is that it not only helps the teacher organize the classroom and reduce aggression, but also aids the higher-risk children in becoming more liked as it shapes their behavior. We note that the GBG by itself is likely not to be as powerful as more integrated prevention programs that target multiple risk factors. Such integrated interventions are now being tested by our team.

The intervention impact appeared most prominent in the first cohort, and we have been forced to conclude that the most probable explanation is that the already-trained teachers did not implement GBG with the same level of precision in the second year as they did in the first. Now that we have had more experience with effectiveness trials, in which an intervention such as the GBG is designed to be implemented by teachers in their own settings and they may vary in their level of implementation, we recognize the need to provide some technical support for maintaining the degree of implementation that is required to produce beneficial effects. This is not very different from medical settings, however; maintaining good practice standards for treatment of attention-deficit/hyperactivity disorder in the community would also likely require continued reinforcement to many practitioners.

Note also that many of the SAS risk factors studied here, including poor peer relations, off-task behavior, shy/withdrawn behavior, and learning problems and poor achievement, have parallels later on in life with negative symptoms that have prominence in the progression toward psychosis. All of these SAS measures can be rated reliably and measured in natural environments. We have demonstrated that the GBG, an early environmental intervention that can be delivered by teachers, helps improve a number of these outcomes early on in life. This early malleability may have relevance to population-based strategies for prevention of psychosis and related conditions as well. To date, no one has attempted to design a trial to evaluate how modification of these early risk factors can affect the risk for psychosis or other major psychopathologies (Brown and Faraone 2004; Faraone et al. 2002).

CLINICAL IMPLICATIONS

It is important that clinicians be aware that there are reliable early predictors of later conduct disorder and substance use disorders. It is possible to intervene, and interventions that provide structure and feedback are the most effective, particularly for high-risk groups.

REFERENCES

American Psychiatric Association: Diagnostic and Statistical Manual of Mental Disorders, 3rd Edition, Revised. Washington, DC, American Psychiatric Association, 1987

Barrish HH, Saunders MW, Wolf MM: Good behavior game: effects of individual contingencies for group consequences on disruptive behavior in a classroom. J Appl Behav Analysis 2:119–124, 1969

Botvin GJ, Baker E, Dusenbury L, et al: Long-term follow-up results of a randomized drug abuse prevention trial in a white middle-class population. JAMA 273:1106–1112, 1995

Botvin GJ, Griffin KW: Drug abuse prevention curriculum in schools, in Handbook of Drug Abuse Prevention: Theory, Science, and Practice. Edited by Bukoski WJ, Sloboda Z. New York, Kluwer Academic/Plenum, 2003, pp 45–69

Brown CH: Protecting against nonrandomly missing data in longitudinal studies. Biometrics 46:143–155, 1990

Brown CH: Statistical methods for preventive trials in mental health. Stat Med 12(3–4): 289–300, 1993a

Brown CH: Analyzing preventive trials with generalized additive models. Am J Community Psychol 21:635–664, 1993b

Brown CH: Design principles and their application in preventive field trials, in Handbook of Drug Abuse Prevention: Theory, Science, and Practice. Edited by Bukoski WJ, Sloboda Z. New York, Kluwer Academic/Plenum, 2003, pp 523–540

Brown CH, Faraone SV: Prevention of schizophrenia and psychotic behavior: definitions and methodological issues, in Early Clinical Intervention and Prevention in Schizophrenia. Edited by Stone WS, Faraone SV, Tsuang MT. Totowa, NJ, Humana, 2004, pp 255–284

Brown CH, Liao J: Principles for designing randomized preventive trials in mental health. Am J Community Psychol 27:673–710, 1999

Brown CH, Indurkhya A, Kellam SG: Power calculations for data missing by design: application to a follow-up study of lead exposure and attention. J Am Stat Assoc 95:383–395, 2000

Brown CH, Wyman PA, Guo J, et al: Dynamic wait-listed designs for randomized trials: new designs for prevention of youth suicide. Clin Trials 3:259–271, 2006

Capaldi DM, Patterson GR: Interrelated influences of contextual factors on antisocial behavior in childhood and adolescence for males, in Psychopathy and Antisocial Personality: A Developmental Perspective. Edited by Fowles D, Sutker P, Goodman S. New York, Springer, 1994, pp 165–198

Carlin JB, Wolfe R, Brown CH, et al: A case study on the choice, interpretation, and checking of multilevel models for longitudinal, binary outcomes. Biostatistics 2:397–416, 2002

Cicchetti D, Schneider-Rosen K: Toward a transactional model of childhood depression. New Directions for Child Development 26:5–27, 1984

Curran P, Muthén B: The application of latent curve analysis to testing developmental theories in intervention research. Am J Community Psychol 27:567–595, 1999

Dishion TJ, Spracklen KM, Andrews DW, et al: Deviancy training in male adolescent friendships. Behav Ther 27:373–390, 1996

Dolan LJ, Kellam SG, Brown CH, et al: The short-term impact of two classroom-based preventive interventions on aggressive and shy behaviors and poor achievement. J Appl Developmental Psychology 14:317–345, 1993

Ensminger ME, Slusarcick AL: Paths to high school graduation or dropout: a longitudinal study of a first grade cohort. Sociology of Education 65:95–113, 1992

Ensminger ME, Juon HS, Fothergill KE: Childhood and adolescent antecedents of substance use in adulthood. Addiction 97:833–844, 2002

Faraone SV, Brown CH, Glatt SJ, et al: Preventing schizophrenia and psychotic behaviour: definitions and methodological issues. Can J Psychiatry 47:527–537, 2002

Fleming JP, Kellam SG, Brown CH: Early predictors of age at first use of alcohol, marijuana, and cigarettes. Drug Alcohol Depend 9:285–303, 1982

Ialongo N, Werthamer L, Brown CH, et al: The proximal impact of two first grade preventive interventions on the early risk behaviors for later substance abuse, depression and antisocial behavior. Am J Community Psychol 27:599–642, 1999

Kellam SG, Langevin DJ: A framework for understanding "evidence" in prevention research and programs. Prev Sci 4:137–153, 2003

Kellam SG, Van Horn Y: Life course development, community epidemiology, and preventive trials: a scientific structure for prevention research. Am J Community Psychol 25:177–187, 1997

Kellam SG, Branch JD, Agrawal KC, et al: Mental Health and Going to School: The Woodlawn Program of Assessment, Early Intervention, and Evaluation. Chicago, IL, University of Chicago Press, 1975

Kellam SG, Brown CH, Fleming JP: Social adaptation to first grade and teenage drug, alcohol and cigarette use. J Sch Health 52:301–306, 1982a

Kellam SG, Brown CH, Fleming JP: The prevention of teenage substance abuse: longitudinal research and strategy, in Promoting Adolescent Health: A Dialog on Research and Practice. Edited by Coates TJ, Petersen AC, Perry C. New York, Academic Press, 1982b, pp 171–200

Kellam SG, Brown CH, Fleming JP: Developmental epidemiological studies of substance use in Woodlawn: implications for prevention research strategy. NIDA Res Monogr 41:21–33, 1982c

Kellam SG, Brown CH, Rubin B, et al: Paths leading to psychiatric symptoms and substance use: developmental epidemiologic studies in Woodlawn, in Childhood Psychopathology and Development. Edited by Guze SB, Earls F, Barrett JE. New York, Raven, 1983, pp 17–51

Kellam SG, Werthamer-Larsson L, Dolan LJ, et al: Developmental epidemiologically based preventive trials: Baseline modeling of early target behaviors and depressive symptoms. Am J Community Psychol 19:563–584, 1991

Kellam SG, Rebok GW, Ialongo N, et al: The course and malleability of aggressive behavior from early first grade into middle school: results of a developmental epidemiologically based preventive trial. J Child Psychol Psychiatry 35:359–382, 1994a

Kellam SG, Rebok GW, Mayer LS, et al: Depressive symptoms over first grade and their response to a developmental epidemiologically based preventive trial aimed at improving achievement. Dev Psychopathol 6:463–481, 1994b

Kellam S, Ling X, Merisca R, et al: The effects of the level of aggression in the first grade classroom on the course and malleability of aggressive behavior into middle school. Dev Psychopathol 10:165–185, 1998a

Kellam SG, Mayer LS, Rebok GW, et al: Effects of improving achievement on aggressive behavior and of improving aggressive behavior on achievement through two preventive interventions: an investigation of causal paths, in Adversity, Stress, and Psychopathology. Edited by Dohrenwend BP. New York, Oxford, 1998b, pp. 486–505

Kellam S, Koretz D, Moscicki E: Core elements of developmental epidemiologically based prevention research. Am J Community Psychol 27:463–482, 1999

Kovacs M, Goldston D: Cognitive and social cognitive development of depressed children and adolescents. J Am Acad Child Adolesc Psychiatry 30:388–392, 1991

Loeber R, Farrington DP, Stouthamer-Loeber M, et al: The development of male offending: key findings from the first decade of the Pittsburgh Youth Study. Studies on Crime and Crime Prevention 7:141–171, 1998

Moffitt TE: Adolescence-limited and life-course-persistent antisocial behavior: a developmental taxonomy. Psychol Rev 100:674–701, 1993

Muthén B, Curran P: General growth modeling in experimental designs: a latent variable framework for analysis and power estimation. Psychological Methods 2:371–402, 1997

Muthén BO, Brown CH, Masyn K, et al: General growth mixture modeling for randomized preventive interventions. Biostatistics 3:459–475, 2002

Nagin D, Tremblay RE: Trajectories of boys' physical aggression, opposition, and hyperactivity on the path to physically violent and nonviolent juvenile delinquency. Child Dev 70:1181–1196, 1999

Patterson GR, Reid JB, Dishion TJ: A Social Learning Approach, Vol 4: Antisocial Boys. Eugene, OR, Castalia, 1992

Pekarik E, Prinz R, Leibert C, et al: The Pupil Evaluation Inventory: a sociometric technique for assessing children's social behavior. J Abnorm Child Psychology 4:83–97, 1976

Rebok GW, Hawkins WE, Krener P, et al: The effect of concentration problems on the malleability of aggressive and shy behaviors in an epidemiologically based preventive trial. J Am Acad Child Adolesc Psychiatry 35:193–203, 1996

Reid JB, Eddy JM, Fetrow RA, et al: Description and immediate impacts of a preventive intervention for conduct problems. Am J Community Psychol 27:483–517, 1999

Reid JB, Patterson GR, Snyder JJ (eds): Antisocial Behavior in Children and Adolescents: A Developmental Analysis and Model for Intervention. Washington, DC, American Psychological Association, 2002

Rubin DB: Estimating causal effects of treatments in randomized and nonrandomized studies. Journal of Educational Psychology 66:688–701, 1974

Sampson RJ, Groves WB: Community structure and crime: testing social-disorganization theory. Am J Sociology 94:774–802, 1989

Schaeffer CM, Petras H, Ialongo N, et al: Modelling growth in boys' aggressive behavior across elementary school: links to later criminal involvement, conduct disorder, and antisocial personality disorder. Dev Psychol 39:1020–1035, 2003

Shaw DS, Gilliom M, Ingoldsby EM, et al: Trajectories leading to school-age conduct problems. Dev Psychol 39:189–200, 2003

Wang CP, Brown CH, Bandeen-Roche K: Residual diagnostics for growth mixture models: examing the impact of a preventive intervention on multiple trajectories of aggressive behavior. J Am Stat Assoc 100:1054–1076, 2005

Werthamer-Larsson L, Kellam SG, Wheeler L: Effect of first-grade classroom environment on child shy behavior, aggressive behavior, and concentration problems. Am J Community Psychol 19:585–602, 1991

16

Conceptually Driven Pharmacological Approaches to Acute Trauma

Roger K. Pitman, M.D.

Douglas L. Delahanty, Ph.D.

Posttraumatic stress disorder (PTSD) is a serious public health problem. The National Comorbidity Survey (Kessler et al. 1995) estimated the lifetime prevalence of PTSD in the United States at 7.8%. The lifetime prevalence among Vietnam veterans was estimated at 31% (Kulka et al. 1990). Research has shown

This chapter was previously published in the journal *CNS Spectrums* (Volume 10, Issue 2, pages 99–106, February 2005).

Dr. Pitman received support from the National Institutes of Health (grants MH58671 and MH68603). Dr. Delahanty received support from the National Institute of Mental Health (grant MH062042).

Disclosure: Because there are no drugs with a U.S. Food and Drug Administration indication for the prevention of posttraumatic stress disorder, all potential clinical applications of currently marketed drugs in the U.S. discussed in this chapter are "off label."

that approximately 69% of nonmilitary respondents reported experiencing a traumatic event in their lifetimes (Norris 1992; Resnick et al. 1993). Motor vehicle accidents alone accounted for over 3 million injurious accidents in the U.S. in 1999 (National Highway Traffic Safety Administration 1998). Incidence rates of PTSD after motor vehicle accidents range from 19% to 47% (Blanchard et al. 1995, 1996).

Although they come to medical attention less frequently than do motor vehicle accidents, interpersonal traumas (rape, assault) often result in even higher rates of PTSD (Norris 1992; Resnick et al. 1993). Little is available in the way of prophylaxis (i.e., prevention) for this potentially disabling mental disorder. *Primary prevention* of PTSD involves the prevention of traumatic events. *Secondary prevention* involves intervening in the aftermath of a traumatic event to forestall the development of PTSD. *Tertiary prevention* involves interventions designed to reduce symptomatology and disability after PTSD has developed. The current state of PTSD mental hygiene consists largely of tertiary prevention, which is often of limited benefit. Until recently, the most popular secondary preventive intervention for PTSD was psychological debriefing. However, recent reviews (Rose et al. 2003; Suzanna et al. 2002) of controlled studies have failed to confirm its efficacy, and at least one study (Mayou et al. 2000) reported adverse long-term effects from this intervention. These developments led the United Kingdom Department of Health to go on record with the statement that "Routine debriefing following traumatic events is not recommended" (Parry 2001).

The collapse of the empirical basis for debriefing underscores the need to find other secondary preventions for PTSD. Treating acute stress disorder with cognitive-behavioral therapy (CBT) has been reported to have preventive value for subsequent PTSD (Bryant et al. 1998). Secondary pharmacological prevention of PTSD has received little research attention but is a topic of increasing medical interest (Larkin 1999). Medical and surgical house officers carry emergency care manuals that list many preventive actions. Examples include prescribing anticoagulants to prevent pulmonary embolism from venous thrombophlebitis and antibiotics to prevent secondary infection in burn victims. In these manuals, it is difficult to find any mention of preventive mental health interventions, including any targeted toward acutely traumatized persons.

SIGNIFICANCE FACILITATES REMEMBRANCE

As McGaugh (1990) noted, "Significance facilitates remembrance." Most everyone is likely to remember in fair detail where they were and what they were doing on the morning of September 11, 2001. By contrast, few are likely to remember in any detail, if at all, where they were and what they were doing on the morning of September 10, 2001. We are more likely to remember significant life events than trivial ones, and this is surely the result of natural selection. Suppose a hypothetical primitive hominid decided to take a new route to a watering hole, and on her way she encountered a crocodile. Should she fail to remember in the future that a crocodile inhabited that route, she would be more likely to take the same route again and be eliminated from the gene pool.

Influence of Stress Hormones on Memory Consolidation

Evolution appears to have enabled significance to facilitate remembrance by means of modulatory effects exerted by neurohormones on the consolidation of memory traces—or alternately stated, on the acquisition of conditioned emotional responses. Because emotionally arousing events mobilize neurohormones, facilitation of learning by these hormones amounts to a mechanism whereby the intensity of the unconditioned emotional response to an arousing event regulates the strength of the resultant conditioned response. Evolution favors parsimony; if it can achieve two adaptations through one mechanism, it often will. In the above hypothetical example, the same adrenaline (or epinephrine) that enabled the primitive hominid to run away from the crocodile acted in her brain to strengthen her memory of the frightful encounter. Stress hormones that have been shown to facilitate memory and conditioning in experimental animals include not only epinephrine, but also corticotropin-releasing hormone, adrenocorticotropin (ACTH), arginine vasopressin (AVP), and cortisol (Croiset et al. 2000; McGaugh and Roozendaal 2002). Exogenous administration or endogenous activation of these substances shortly following a learning trial leads to the formation of a conditioned response that is particularly strong and resistant to extinction. Pharmacological blockade of stress hormones produces the opposite effect. This body of findings (McGaugh 2003) represents one of the most exciting discoveries in the history of physiological psychology. In rats trained in a passive avoidance task, retention was enhanced by systemic posttraining injections of epinephrine (Gold and Buskirk 1975). This finding has been replicated in numerous independent experiments. The memory-enhancing effect of epinephrine is counteracted by the pretraining administration of the beta-adrenergic receptor blocker propranolol (Sternberg et al. 1985). Posttraining administration of systemic propranolol to rats also impairs subsequent memory for a stressful spatial water maze task (Cahill et al. 2000). Cahill et al. (1994) found that oral propranolol abolished the memory-enhancing effect of negative emotional arousal in humans. Although propranolol interferes with sympathetic α-adrenergic transmission both peripherally and centrally, evidence suggests that its central action is responsible for blocking memory enhancement. The beta-adrenergic blocker nadolol, which does not cross the blood–brain barrier, does not share this effect of systemic propranolol (van Stegeren et al. 1998).

Role of the Amygdala

The basolateral nucleus of the amygdala (BLA) appears to be the critical brain structure involved in both fear conditioning (Davis 1990; LeDoux 1996) and the memory-enhancing effects of emotional arousal (McIntyre et al. 2003). Post-training intra-BLA microinjections of norepinephrine enhance conditioning, and this effect is blocked by simultaneous intra-BLA administration of propranolol (Liang et al. 1986). Beta-adrenergic neurotransmission in the BLA is a final common pathway for the influence of most stress hormones on memory, and propranolol acts to block this pathway (McGaugh et al. 2002).

A Translational Model of Posttraumatic Disorder Pathogenesis

In 1989, Pitman advanced a novel theory of the pathogenesis of PTSD based on the above-described animal research on the memory-enhancing effects of stress hormones. Specifically, he postulated that in trauma victims who subsequently develop PTSD, the traumatic event (unconditioned stimulus) stimulates an excessive release of stress hormones (unconditioned response), resulting in overconsolidated memories of the event (Figure 16–1, Loop A), which subsequently manifest themselves in the intrusive recollections and reexperiencing symptoms found in PTSD. Pitman (1989) further hypothesized that reminders of the traumatic event (conditioned stimuli) lead to retrieval of the traumatic memories, with the additional release of stress hormones (conditioned response). These further enhance the strength of the traumatic memory, thereby creating a positive feedback cycle (Figure 16–1, Loop B). This model regards PTSD as a quantitative overshoot of a normally adaptive mechanism, in which too much significance leads to too much remembrance. There are several lines of evidence in humans that support the hypothesized pathogenesis of PTSD depicted in Figure 16–1, Loop A. The current diagnostic criteria for PTSD require an acute response to the traumatic event of intense fear, helplessness, or horror. Such a response is highly likely to mobilize stress hormones such as epinephrine. Elevated heart rate in the aftermath of a traumatic event, indicative of a hyperadrenergic state, was found to predict subsequent PTSD in three (Bryant et al. 2000; Shalev et al. 1998; Zatzick et al. 2005) of four (Blanchard et al. 2002) published studies. The paradoxical finding that quadriplegic injury is less often associated with PTSD than is paraplegic injury (Radnitz et al. 1998) is potentially explained by the severing of the connection between the brain and the adrenal glands in the former but not the latter condition. However, challenges to the pathogenic model of PTSD presented here are posed by the viewpoints that PTSD may not be properly regarded as a maladaptive process that occurs immediately following a trauma, but rather as a process involving the lack of resolution of an acute stress reaction; also that PTSD may not involve a normative response to an extreme trauma event, but rather an endocrinologically atypical response (McFarlane and Yehuda 2000). The hypothetical capacity of conditioned responses to reinforce—rather than extinguish—conditioned responding has been termed "paradoxical enhancement" or "incubation." Eysenck (1968) postulated that incubation plays a pathogenic role in human neurosis. Eysenck and Kelley (1987) subsequently hypothesized that neurohormones mediate incubation. The notion has recently been reiterated that, "Repeated reactivation and reconsolidation may further strengthen the memory trace and lead to persistence of trauma-related symptoms" (Charney 2004, p. 204). Although paradoxical enhancement lacks substantial supporting preclinical data, it has a possible neurophysiological basis in the decreased ratio of inhibitory (medial prefrontal) over excitatory (anterior limbic, amygdala) central nervous functions observed in PTSD (Shin et al. 2004). The concept of paradoxical enhancement offers an explanation for the hitherto unexplained, troublesome ability of psychological debriefing in the aftermath of trauma to exacerbate its psychopathological effect (Mayou et al. 2000).

Implications of the Model for the Prevention of Posttraumatic Disorder

If the model of PTSD pathogenesis presented herein is applicable, the possibility exists that the disorder can be prevented by pharmacologically intervening in the aftermath of a traumatic event to block potentiation of memory consolidation by stress hormones. Blocking consolidation would be distinct from, but potentially complemented by, preventive CBT, which is likely to act by facilitating extinction. However, the consideration that hormonal influences on memory consolidation are time-dependent processes raises the question as to how soon after the occurrence of a traumatic event a pharmacological agent would need to be administered to lower the risk of PTSD. The finding that injections of epinephrine administered to rats at intervals of 30 minutes following single-trial avoidance training are generally ineffective in strengthening memory (McGaugh 1990) would pessimistically suggest that pharmacological intervention might have to occur sooner

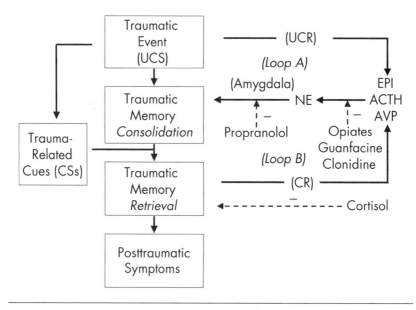

FIGURE 16–1. Conceptual model of the pathogenesis of posttraumatic stress disorder with points of opportunity for secondary preventive psychopharmacological agents.

ACTH = adrenocorticotropin; AVP = arginine vasopressin; EPI = epinephrine; CR = conditioned response; CS = conditioned stimulus; NE = norepinephrine; UCR = unconditioned response; UCS = unconditioned stimulus.

after traumatic exposure than would be practical. However, vasopressin given 3 hours posttraining has been found to produce a 45% increment in memory performance during subsequent testing (Kovacs and Telegdy 1982). The effect of vasopressin became insignificant after 6 hours, suggesting a wider but still limited window in which pharmacological agents could be administered. A study that employed positron emission tomography in humans found that it takes 6 hours to permanently store the memory of a newly learned skill in the brain (Shadmehr and Holcomb 1997). More recent studies in rats have indicated that there appear to exist several stages of memory consolidation involving different brain regions that may potentially be affected by pharmacological intervention for a number of days posttraining. For example, reversible inactivation of BLA by tetrodotoxin injection 2 days after a single-session acquisition paradigm impairs conditioned freezing responses when measured 48 hours postinjection. In the case of perirhinal cortex injection, the window of opportunity is a full 8 days (Sacchetti et al. 1999).

Importantly, rats are not humans and they do not develop the clinical syndrome of PTSD. One likely crucial difference between a single trial avoidance paradigm in rats and a traumatic event in humans is that humans may replay the traumatic event in their consciousness for variable periods of time after its occurrence (McFarlane et al. 2002). Indeed, this is one of the diagnostic features of acute stress disorder. Reexperiencing may produce sympathetic arousal (Pitman et al. 1987), and such recurrent arousal may further influence memory consolidation, as suggested in Figure 16–1, Loop B. Thus, there may be continuing hormonal influences on memory that persist for longer periods (i.e., days or weeks) following a traumatic event, which may be amenable to pharmacological intervention. Ultimately, the question of the window of opportunity for influencing the development of PTSD can only be resolved by clinical trial.

Anti-Adrenergic Agents

Based on the animal research to date, the most promising candidate drug for intervening in the aftermath of a traumatic event to block potentiation of the consolidation of its memory trace by stress hormones is propranolol, which as noted above acts to block postsynaptic beta-adrenergic receptors in the BLA. Support for the ability of posttrauma propranolol to attenuate the subsequent development of PTSD comes from two published but preliminary studies (Pitman et al. 1987, 2002). Pitman et al. (2002) recruited 41 patients who presented to a general hospital emergency room immediately following a traumatic event (mostly motor vehicle accidents). To be eligible, patients had to meet the current diagnostic criteria for PTSD. Patients also had to have a pulse rate of 80 beats/minute (bpm), presumably indicative of a hyperadrenergic state. The patients were randomized to receive a course of oral propranolol 40 mg or placebo four times daily for 10 days, followed by a 9-day medication taper period. The taper period ended about 12 days prior to the first outcome assessment, so that patients were fully withdrawn from the propranolol at the time of assessment. The first dose of study medication was administered an average of 4 hours after the traumatic event's occurrence. One month posttrauma, total scores on the Clinician-Administered PTSD Scale showed a trend to be lower in the 11 completers of the course of study medication who had received propranolol, compared with the 20 completers who had not. On the basis of their physiological responses during script-driven mental imagery of the traumatic event that had brought them to the emergency room 3 months earlier, 0 of 8 propranolol patients, but 8 of 14 placebo patients, were physiologically classified as PTSD ($P = 0.04$), which is consistent with a reduced conditioned fear response.

In a second, controlled, nonblind, nonrandomized preliminary study, Vaiva et al. (2003) recruited 19 patients with a heart rate of 90 bpm from two emergency departments in France 2–20 hours after a motor vehicle accident or a physical assault. All were offered propranolol 30 mg tid for 7 days followed by a taper period of 8–12 days. The investigators compared the 11 patients who agreed to take the propranolol with 8 patients who refused propranolol but agreed to participate in the study. The two groups did not differ on demographics, exposure characteristics, physical injury severity, or peritraumatic emotional responses. At 2 months posttrauma, levels of PTSD symptoms were significantly lower in the patients treated with propranolol. Eighty-six percent of the time, a patient who took propranolol had a score below that of a patient who did not ($P=0.04$). Both the American and the French groups are currently launching randomized clinical trials in larger samples in an attempt to obtain definitive results.

Finally, a single case study (Taylor and Cahill 2002) described a 44-year-old woman who had experienced several prior motor vehicle accidents, each followed by months of PTSD symptoms despite treatment with multiple drugs. Following yet another accident, severe PTSD symptoms again emerged, but these were rapidly and markedly reduced by propranolol started 48 hours after the event.

Another approach to blocking the potentiation of the consolidation of a traumatic memory would be to give pharmacological agents that act presynaptically to reduce norepinephrine release. Candidate drugs for this purpose include opioids and the α_2-adrenergic agonists clonidine and guanfacine. Saxe et al. (2001) performed an observational study of the relationship between the amounts of morphine given to severely burned children and the children's PTSD symptoms. The children who received higher doses of morphine had a greater reduction in PTSD symptoms over a 6-month hospital stay ($r=0.44$, $P<0.05$). However, an alternate explanation of this finding is that the analgesic properties of morphine reduced the intensity of repeated traumatic conditioned stimuli, such as painful dressing changes. Randomized controlled trials of the ability of opioids to prevent PTSD would appear to be indicated; however, because of the clinical bar to withholding opioids when severe pain is involved, and because of these agents' addictive potential, such trials will likely be difficult to implement. To date, there have been no reported studies of the use of α_2-adrenergic agonists to prevent PTSD.

This section should not conclude without mentioning gamma-aminobutyric acid (GABA) agents, which oppose norepinephrine action in the BLA. Some GABAergic drugs have been found to reduce the potentiation of memory by stress hormones (Introini-Collison et al. 1994). Benzodiazepines, however, are less effective in this regard when administered posttraining (rather than pretraining).

This limitation may account for the failure to find preventive value for PTSD of clonazepam or alprazolam administered in the acute aftermath of trauma (Gelpin et al. 1996). Nevertheless, given the ready availability of the benzodiazepines, and their current widespread use in psychologically traumatized persons, it would seem that further trials are indicated, either to search for some evidence of their preventive efficacy, or to establish the lack thereof and thereby alter practice patterns. Trials of newer GABAergic agents (e.g., gabapentin or tiagabine) that lack some of the undesirable effects of benzodiazepines are also indicated.

Cortisol

At first blush, the model of PTSD pathogenesis presented here would suggest that cortisol, which has also been found in animal research to potentiate memory consolidation when given posttraining, would be counterpreventive. The situation is complicated, however, by the fact that endogenous hypercortisolemia (Mauri et al. 1993) and exogenous glucocorticoid administration (Newcomer et al. 1999) have been found to impair human memory retrieval. Impaired performance in declarative memory tasks has been reported following a dose of hydrocortisone (cortisol) 10 mg (Kirschbaum et al. 1996).

The ability of cortisol to impair memory retrieval is indicated by an arrow in the bottom right of Figure 16–1. There it will be seen that such an effect has the capability to interrupt positive feedback Loop B. In other words, if PTSD patients' recall of their traumatic events could be reduced by cortisol, the hypothesized re-release of stress hormones that traumatic recall induces—and the resultant paradoxical enhancement of conditioned responding—might be reduced as well.

Cortisol could also work indirectly by containing an overshoot of epinephrine and other stress hormones. One function of cortisol is to shut down the adrenergic hormones of the "fight or flight" response, preventing their long-term elevation from damaging the body (Munck et al. 1984; Ursin and Olff 1993). Yehuda and colleagues (Yehuda and Harvey 1997; Yehuda et al. 1998) have suggested that during traumatic stress, catecholamine increases are likely to be exaggerated in the presence of a diminished regulatory influence of accompanying cortisol increase. In other words, lower cortisol levels at the time of the trauma may lead to a failure to contain the sympathetic stress response and to consequent prolonged availability of norepinephrine in the brain (Pacak et al. 1995). This may then lead to altered consolidation of memory of the traumatic incident (Yehuda 2002). In animals, low levels of cortisol have been shown to increase the memory-enhancing effects of catecholamines (Bohus 1984), and high doses of glucocorticoids to decrease these effects (Borrell et al. 1983).

Two observational studies (Delahanty et al. 2000; McFarlane et al. 1997) have found that lower posttrauma cortisol levels predict subsequent PTSD. Motor vehicle accident victims who subsequently were diagnosed with PTSD had lower plasma cortisol levels 30 minutes after the accident than victims who subsequently met criteria for major depression (McFarlane et al. 1997). Victims not meeting criteria for either diagnosis had intermediate cortisol levels. Delahanty et al. (2000) examined the relationship between initial urinary hormone levels and subsequent PTSD symptoms in 99 motor vehicle accident victims. In this study, motor vehicle accident victims were catheterized upon arrival to the trauma unit, and urine was collected for the next 15 hours. Victims who subsequently met acute PTSD diagnostic criteria 1 month after the accident had significantly lower cortisol excretion in the immediate aftermath of the accident than victims who did not meet diagnostic criteria. In addition, initial cortisol excretion was negatively correlated with subsequent symptoms of PTSD ($r = -0.46$, $P < 0.01$). Schelling et al. (1999) have found that exogenously administered stress doses of cortisol reduce the development of subsequent PTSD in medical-surgical patients. An initial retrospective case–control analysis revealed that septic shock patients who received hydrocortisone 100 mg bolus during the sepsis episode followed by 0.18 mg/kg/hour until shock reversal had a significantly lower subsequent incidence of PTSD than patients who received standard treatment for their septic shock. These findings were replicated in a randomized, double-blind study (Schelling et al. 2001). During a sepsis episode, 11 patients were randomly assigned to receive placebo, and 9 were assigned the above-mentioned dose of hydrocortisone for 6 days. Results revealed that only 1 of 9 from the hydrocortisone group but 7 of 11 from the placebo group ($P = 0.02$) met PTSD criteria assessed 31 months after discharge from the intensive care unit. However, interpretation of this finding is confounded by the observation that the placebo patients required higher amounts of norepinephrine for blood pressure support. Thus, the exogenous cortisol could have acted indirectly to prevent PTSD by reducing total exogenous norepinephrine requirement. More recently, Schelling et al. (2004) examined the efficacy of peri- and postoperative exogenous hydrocortisone in preventing PTSD symptoms in patients following cardiac surgery. Twenty-six patients received a loading dose of hydrocortisone 100 mg followed by a continuous infusion of 10 mg/hour during postoperative day 1. Patients received 5 mg/hour on postoperative day 2, and dosing was tapered to 20 mg tid on postoperative day 3 and 10 mg tid on postoperative day 4. Twenty-two comparison patients received standard treatment. Results revealed that the patients who received the hydrocortisone regimen reported significantly fewer PTSD symptoms than comparison patients ($P < 0.05$).

Other Candidate Agents for the Prevention of Posttraumatic Stress Disorder

In this review, emphasis has been given to possible preventive agents suggested by one translational model of PTSD pathogenesis highlighted here. However, at least two other models (Iancu et al. 2002; Sapolsky 1996, 2000) suggest other potential agents, although these will be mentioned only briefly. The neurophysiological kindling model of PTSD suggests that antikindling agents (i.e., antiepileptics), in addition to having some therapeutic value (Iancu et al. 2002), may also have preventive value. The stress- and cortisol-induced neurotoxicity model of PTSD (Sapolsky 1996, 2000) suggests that drugs that have been found to block stress-induced hippocampal damage—including antiepileptics (e.g., phenytoin [Zhang et al. 2003]) and selective serotonin reuptake inhibitors (e.g., tianeptine [Conrad et al. 1996]), and possibly even anticortisol drugs (e.g., mifepristone)—may also be useful in preventing PTSD.

EFFICACY VERSUS EFFECTIVENESS

This article has discussed several promising secondary preventive pharmacological interventions for PTSD, although their efficacy needs to be further tested in larger, randomized controlled trials. Even if the efficacy of one or more of these interventions becomes established through further research, this will not equate with effectiveness, which involves the application of the intervention in usual clinical settings. Obstacles to effectiveness include patients' psychological reluctance to accept acute posttraumatic psychiatric interventions, and their proneness to drop out before treatment is completed (Weisaeth 2001). However, this may be less problematic in clinical than in research settings. In research settings involving placebo-controlled trials, the investigator can only offer the patient the possibility of receiving a drug that may be efficacious. Once a drug has proven efficacious in clinical trials, however, the clinician can confidently offer a drug that is likely to be helpful. Another obstacle is posed by medical contraindications to the administration of even an efficacious drug. Propranolol, for example, may not be able to be safely administered to patients with asthma or heart block, or in situations in which it is clinically necessary to rely upon the sign of tachycardia to disclose the development of a medical complication such as hypovolemia or hypoglycemia. Cortisol may not be able to be given to patients with penetrating wounds that pose a risk of infection. It may turn out, however, that demonstration of the efficacy of one of these, or other, agents would spur the development of new drugs that retain efficacy with fewer contraindications. An example might be a beta-adrenergic blocker with the high capacity to cross the blood–brain barrier of propranolol but lacking in the latter's asthmagenic effect.

CONCLUSION

This review has highlighted a number of possible pharmacological interventions that could be implemented in the aftermath of traumatic events to prevent or reduce their potentially psychiatric consequences. A recent MEDLINE search on PTSD yielded 7,500 articles, only 5 (Gelpin et al. 1996; Pitman et al. 2002; Schelling et al. 2001, 2004; Vaiva et al. 2003) of which involved a prospective, controlled, preventive pharmacotherapeutic clinical trial. Moreover, these studies are properly regarded as preliminary. A recent review noted, "To date there is almost no empirical data on effective pharmacological interventions in the immediate aftermath of extreme psychological trauma. Controlled trials are essential given the limited information in this field" (Morgan et al. 2003, p. 841).

CLINICAL IMPLICATIONS

There have been few controlled trials of pharmacological prevention of PTSD. One model of the pathogenesis of PTSD implicates stress hormones in the over-consolidation of traumatic memories. Propranolol can block the memory-enhancing influence of stress hormones. Preliminary studies suggest that a 2- to 3-week course of propranolol begun in the aftermath of a traumatic event can reduce subsequent PTSD. Cortisol can enhance memory consolidation but diminish memory retrieval. Preliminary studies suggest that cortisol given to medical-surgical patients during their hospital stays can reduce subsequent PTSD.

REFERENCES

Blanchard EB, Hickling EJ, Mitnick N, et al: The impact of severity of physical injury and perception of life threat in the development of post-traumatic stress disorder in motor vehicle accident victims. Behav Res Ther 33:529–534, 1995

Blanchard EB, Hickling EJ, Taylor AE, et al: Who develops PTSD from motor vehicle accidents? Behav Res Ther 34:1–10, 1996

Blanchard EB, Hickling EJ, Galovski T, et al: Emergency room vital signs and PTSD in a treatment seeking sample of motor vehicle accident survivors. J Trauma Stress 15: 199–204, 2002

Bohus B: Endocrine influence on disease outcome: experimental findings and implications. J Psychosom Res 28:429–438, 1984

Borrell J, De Kloet ER, Versteeg DH, et al: Inhibitory avoidance deficit following short-term adrenalectomy in the rat: the role of adrenal catecholamines. Behav Neural Biol 39:241–258, 1983

Bryant RA, Harvey AG, Dang ST, et al: Treatment of acute stress disorder: a comparison of cognitive-behavioral therapy and supportive counseling. J Consult Clin Psychol 66:862–866, 1998

Bryant RA, Harvey AG, Guthrie RM, et al: A prospective study of psychophysiological arousal, acute stress disorder, and posttraumatic stress disorder. J Abnorm Psychol 109:341–344, 2000

Cahill L, Prins B, Weber M, et al: Beta-adrenergic activation and memory for emotional events. Nature 371:702–704, 1994

Cahill L, Pham CA, Setlow B: Impaired memory consolidation in rats produced with adrenergic blockade. Neurobiol Learn Mem 74:259–266, 2000

Charney DS: Psychobiological mechanisms of resilience and vulnerability: implications for successful adaptation to extreme stress. Am J Psychiatry 161:195–216, 2004

Conrad CD, Galea LA, Kuroda Y, et al: Chronic stress impairs rat spatial memory on the Y maze, and this effect is blocked by tianeptine pretreatment. Behav Neurosci 110:1321–1334, 1996

Croiset G, Nijsen MJ, Kamphuis PJ: Role of corticotropin-releasing factor, vasopressin and the autonomic nervous system in learning and memory. Eur J Pharmacol 405: 225–234, 2000

Davis M: Pharmacological and anatomical analysis of fear conditioning. NIDA Res Monogr 97:126–162, 1990

Delahanty DL, Raimonde AJ, Spoonster E: Initial posttraumatic urinary cortisol levels predict subsequent PTSD symptoms in motor vehicle accident victims. Biol Psychiatry 48:940–947, 2000

Eysenck HJ: A theory of the incubation of anxiety-fear responses. Behav Res Ther 6:309–321, 1968

Eysenck HJ, Kelley MJ: The interaction of neurohormones with Pavlovian A and Pavlovian B conditioning in the causation of neurosis, extinction, and incubation of anxiety, in Cognitive Processes and Pavlovian Conditioning in Humans. Edited by Davey G. Chichester, UK, John Wiley & Sons, 1987, pp 251–286

Gelpin E, Bonne O, Peri T, et al: Treatment of recent trauma survivors with benzodiazepines: a prospective study. J Clin Psychiatry 57:390–394, 1996

Gold PE, van Buskirk R: Facilitation of time-dependent memory processes with post-trial epinephrine injections. Behav Biol 13:145–153, 1975

Iancu I, Rosen Y, Moshe K: Antiepileptic drugs in posttraumatic stress disorder. Clin Neuropharmacol 25:225–229, 2002

Introini-Collison IB, Castellano C, McGaugh JL: Interaction of GABAergic and beta-noradrenergic drugs in the regulation of memory storage. Behav Neural Biol 61: 150–155, 1994

Kessler RC, Sonnega A, Bromet E, et al: Posttraumatic stress disorder in the National Comorbidity Survey. Arch Gen Psychiatry 52:1048–1060, 1995

Kirschbaum C, Wolf OT, May M, et al: Stress- and treatment-induced elevations of cortisol levels associated with impaired declarative memory in healthy adults. Life Sci 58:1475–1483, 1996

Kovacs GL, Telegdy G: Role of oxytocin in memory and amnesia. Pharmacol Ther 18: 375–395, 1982

Kulka RA, Schlenger WE, Fairbank JA, et al: Trauma and the Vietnam War Generation: Report of Findings From the National Vietnam Veterans Readjustment Study. New York, Brunner/Mazel, 1990

Larkin M: Can posttraumatic stress disorder be put on hold? Lancet 354:1008, 1999

LeDoux JE: The Emotional Brain: The Mysterious Underpinnings of Emotional Life. New York, Simon & Schuster, 1996

Liang KC, Juler RG, McGaugh JL: Modulating effects of posttraining epinephrine on memory: involvement of the amygdala noradrenergic system. Brain Res 368:125–133, 1986

Mauri M, Sinforiani E, Bono G, et al: Memory impairment in Cushing's disease. Acta Neurol Scand 87:52–55, 1993

Mayou RA, Ehlers A, Hobbs M: Psychological debriefing for road traffic accident victims: three-year follow-up of a randomised controlled trial. Br J Psychiatry 176: 589–593, 2000

McFarlane AC, Yehuda R: Clinical treatment of posttraumatic stress disorder: conceptual challenges raised by recent research. Aust N Z J Psychiatry 34:940–953, 2000

McFarlane AC, Atchison M, Yehuda R: The acute stress response following motor vehicle accidents and its relation to PTSD. Ann N Y Acad Sci 821:437–441, 1997

McFarlane AC, Yehuda R, Clark CR: Biologic models of traumatic memories and posttraumatic stress disorder. The role of neural networks. Psychiatr Clin North Am 25:253–270, 2002

McGaugh JL: Significance and remembrance: the role of neuromodulatory systems. Psychol Sci 1:15–25, 1990

McGaugh JL: Memory and Emotion: The Making of Lasting Memories. New York, Columbia University Press, 2003

McGaugh JL, Roozendaal B: Role of adrenal stress hormones in forming lasting memories in the brain. Curr Opin Neurobiol 12:205–210, 2002

McGaugh JL, McIntyre CK, Power AE: Amygdala modulation of memory consolidation: interaction with other brain systems. Neurobiol Learn Mem 78:539–552, 2002

McIntyre CK, Power AE, Roozendaal B, et al: Role of the basolateral amygdala in memory consolidation. Ann N Y Acad Sci 985:273–293, 2003

Morgan CA, Krystal JH, Southwick SM: Toward early pharmacological posttraumatic stress intervention. Biol Psychiatry 53:834–843, 2003

Munck A, Guyre PM, Holbrook NJ: Physiological functions of glucocorticoids in stress and their relation to pharmacological actions. Endocr Rev 5:25–44, 1984

National Highway Traffic Safety Administration: Traffic safety facts 1997: a compilation of motor vehicle crash data from the fatality analysis reporting system and the general estimates system. Washington, DC, National Center for Statistics and Analysis, U.S. Department of Transportation, 1998

Newcomer JW, Selke G, Melson AK, et al: Decreased memory performance in healthy humans induced by stress-level cortisol treatment. Arch Gen Psychiatry 56:527–533, 1999

Norris FH: Epidemiology of trauma: frequency and impact of different potentially traumatic events on different demographic groups. J Consult Clin Psychol 60:409–418, 1992

Pacak K, Palkovits M, Kopin IJ, et al: Stress-induced norepinephrine release in the hypothalamic paraventricular nucleus and pituitary-adrenocortical and sympathoadrenal activity: in vivo microdialysis studies. Front Neuroendocrinol 16:89–150, 1995

Parry G: Treatment choice in psychological therapies and counseling: evidence based clinical practice guideline [U.K. Department of Health web site]. 2001. Available at: http://www.doh.gov.uk/mentalhealth/treatmentguidelines. Accessed September 2004.

Pitman RK: Post-traumatic stress disorder, hormones, and memory. Biol Psychiatry 26:221–223, 1989

Pitman RK, Orr SP, Forgue DF, et al: Psychophysiologic assessment of posttraumatic stress disorder imagery in Vietnam combat veterans. Arch Gen Psychiatry 44:970–975, 1987

Pitman RK, Sanders KM, Zusman RM, et al: Pilot study of secondary prevention of posttraumatic stress disorder with propranolol. Biol Psychiatry 51:189–192, 2002

Radnitz CL, Hsu L, Tirch DD, et al: A comparison of posttraumatic stress disorder in veterans with and without spinal cord injury. J Abnorm Psychol 107:676–680, 1998

Resnick HS, Kilpatrick DG, Dansky BS, et al: Prevalence of civilian trauma and posttraumatic stress disorder in a representative national sample of women. J Consult Clin Psychol 61:984–991, 1993

Rose S, Bisson J, Wessely S: A systematic review of single-session psychological interventions ("debriefing") following trauma. Psychother Psychosom 72:176–184, 2003

Sacchetti B, Lorenzini CA, Baldi E, et al: Auditory thalamus, dorsal hippocampus, basolateral amygdala, and perirhinal cortex role in the consolidation of conditioned freezing to context and to acoustic conditioned stimulus in the rat. J Neurosci 19:9570–9578, 1999

Sapolsky RM: Why stress is bad for your brain. Science 273:749–750, 1996

Sapolsky RM: Glucocorticoids and hippocampal atrophy in neuropsychiatric disorders. Arch Gen Psychiatry 57:925–935, 2000

Saxe G, Stoddard F, Courtney D, et al: Relationship between acute morphine and the course of PTSD in children with burns. J Am Acad Child Adolesc Psychiatry 40:915–921, 2001

Schelling G, Stoll C, Kapfhammer HP, et al: The effect of stress doses of hydrocortisone during septic shock on posttraumatic stress disorder and health-related quality of life in survivors. Crit Care Med 27:2678–2683, 1999

Schelling G, Briegel J, Roozendaal B, et al: The effect of stress doses of hydrocortisone during septic shock on posttraumatic stress disorder in survivors. Biol Psychiatry 50:978–985, 2001

Schelling G, Kilger E, Roozendaal B: Stress doses of hydrocortisone, traumatic stress, and symptoms of posttraumatic stress disorder in patients after cardiac surgery: a randomized trial. Biol Psychiatry 55:627–633, 2004

Shadmehr R, Holcomb HH: Neural correlates of motor memory consolidation. Science 277:821–825, 1997

Shalev AY, Sahar T, Freedman S, et al: A prospective study of heart rate response following trauma and the subsequent development of posttraumatic stress disorder. Arch Gen Psychiatry 55:553–559, 1998

Shin LM, Orr SP, Carson MA, et al: Regional cerebral blood flow in the amygdala and medial prefrontal cortex during traumatic imagery in male and female Vietnam veterans with PTSD. Arch Gen Psychiatry 61:168–176, 2004

Sternberg DB, Isaacs KR, Gold PE, et al: Epinephrine facilitation of appetitive learning: attenuation with adrenergic receptor antagonists. Behav Neural Biol 44:447–453, 1985

Suzanna RO, Jonathan BI, Simon WE: Psychological debriefing for preventing posttraumatic stress disorder (PTSD). Cochrane Database Syst Rev (2):CD000560, 2002

Taylor F, Cahill L: Propranolol for reemergent posttraumatic stress disorder following an event of retraumatization: a case study. J Trauma Stress 15:433–437, 2002

Ursin H, Olff M: Psychobiology of coping and defense strategies. Neuropsychobiology 28:66–71, 1993

Vaiva G, Ducrocq F, Jezequel K, et al: Immediate treatment with propranolol decreases posttraumatic stress disorder two months after trauma. Biol Psychiatry 54:947–949, 2003 van Stegeren AH, Everaerd W, Cahill L, et al: Memory for emotional events: differential effects of centrally versus peripherally acting beta-blocking agents. Psychopharmacology (Berl) 138:305–310, 1998

Weisaeth L: Acute posttraumatic stress: nonacceptance of early intervention. J Clin Psychiatry 62 (suppl 17):35–40, 2001

Yehuda R: Posttraumatic stress disorder. N Engl J Med 346:108–114, 2002

Yehuda R, Harvey P: Relevance of neuroendocrine alterations in PTSD to memory related impairments of trauma survivors, in Recollection of Trauma. Edited by Read JD, Lindsay DS. New York, Plenum, 1997, pp 221–252

Yehuda R, McFarlane AC, Shalev AY: Predicting the development of posttraumatic stress disorder from the acute response to a traumatic event. Biol Psychiatry 44:1305–1313, 1998

Zatzick D, Russo J, Pitman RK, et al: Reevaluating the association between emergency department heart rate and the development of posttraumatic stress disorder: a public health approach. Biol Psychiatry 57:91–95, 2005

Zhang YM, Yang Q, Xu CT, et al: Effects of phenytoin on morphology and structure of hippocampal CA3 pyramidal neurons of rats in chronic stress. Acta Anaesthesiol Sin 24:403–407, 2003

Index

Page numbers printed in **boldface** type refer to tables or figures.

AA. *See* Alcoholics Anonymous
Abuse
    childhood, 78, 81, 98, 128
    sexual, 106
Acamprosate, for treatment of
    alcoholism, 311
ACTH. *See* Adrenocorticotropic
    hormone
Action for Mental Health (Joint
    Commission on Mental Illness
    and Health) 56
ADAMHA. *See* Alcohol, Drug Abuse,
    and Mental Health Administration
Adderall. *See* Dextroamphetamine
Addiction. *See* Alcohol abuse; Drugs;
    Substance abuse
    treatment, 265
ADH. *See* Alcohol dehydrogenase
ADHD. *See* Attention-deficit/
    hyperactivity disorder (ADHD)
Adolescents. *See also* Children; Puberty
    AIDS cases, **267**
    alcohol, hormones and, 307
    cognitive-behavioral therapy and,
        108–109
    drinking patterns, 303
    female, 307
    maturation, 88
    motivation for drinking, 304

    neural systems, 188
    neurodevelopment. *See* Neurodevel-
        opment, adolescent
    socialization theory, 127
    use of cannabis, 38–39
Adolescents Training and Learning
    to Avoid Steroids (ATLAS), 280
Adoption studies, 5, 213. *See also* Twin
    studies
Adrenarche, 194, 306
Adrenocorticotropic hormone
    (ACTH), 79
    adolescent neurodevelopment and,
        189, 194
    to facilitate memory, 373
    insufficiency in posttraumatic stress
        disorder, 80
ADS. *See* Alcohol dependence
    syndrome
"Affectionless control" pattern, 107
Afghanistan, 126
African Americans. *See also* Blacks
    Good-Behavior Game trial design
        and, 360–361
    low-income inner-city, 109
    HIV/AIDS rates in, 266
    psychiatric implications of cultural
        diversity, 67
    substance use disorders, 119

Age
    at first use of alcohol, nicotine, and
        cannabis, 301, **302**
    Good-Behavior Game trial, 362
    nonlinear effects on gray-matter
        density, **268–269**
    underage drinking, 301–304, **302**
Aggression. *See also* Behavior
    patterns, 364
    undersocialized, 348
Agoraphobia, **9**
AIDS, 286, 337. *See also* HIV
    drug abuse and, 265–266, **267**
Alaska, 65
Alcohol abuse, **10**. *See also* Alcoholism
    addiction, 263–296
    availability, 126
    consumption, 118–119
    costs, 264
    dopamine receptors and, 133
    efforts to increase consumption,
        125–126
    efforts to reduce availability and
        consumption, 121–125
    expectancies, 129
    heritability, 129
    laws and law enforcement, 123, **124**
    marketing and advertising, 125–126
    medical consequences, 263–296
    personality traits as predictor of,
        129–130
    political events and, 126
    pricing and taxation, 121
    "Rate the State" media campaign,
        125
    schizophrenia and, 23–24, **25**
    state distribution policies, 121, 123
    studies of alcohol and drug
        dependence, 130–136
    treating and preventing, 263–296,
        281
    vulnerability, 115–155

Alcohol, Drug Abuse, and Mental
        Health Administration
        (ADAMHA), 58–59
Alcohol dehydrogenase (ADH),
        131–132
Alcohol dependence syndrome (ADS),
        116, 330–331
Alcoholics Anonymous (AA), 284
Alcoholism, 297–316. *See also* Alcohol
        abuse
    age at first use, 301, **302**
    clinical implications, 312
    consumption, abuse, and
        dependence, 298–299
    genetic and environmental factors in
        development of alcohol
        dependence, 299
    prevention, 309–311
        adult drinking patterns and risks,
            310–311
        screening and interventions for
            alcohol use disorders, 309–310
    puberty, hormones, and sex
        differences in alcohol abuse and
        dependence, 305–309
        alcohol, hormones, and
            adolescents, 307
        hormonal changes associated with
            onset of puberty, 306–307
        neurosteroids, 308
        onset of substance use and abuse,
            305
        reproductive hormone changes
            effects on neural circuits
            associated with alcohol-
            seeking behavior, 307–308
        stress and gonadal hormones at
            puberty and gender
            differences in alcohol-seeking
            behavior, 309
        screening for high-risk drinking,
            311–312

use disorders, 299–304
    adolescent drinking patterns, 303
    adolescent motivation, 304
    development patterns of drinking, 300
    underage drinking
        biology and behavior, 303–304
        consequences, 301–303
        prevalence and problems, 300–301, **302**
Alcohol-seeking behavior, 307–308, 309
Alcohol Use Disorder and Associated Disabilities Interview Schedule—DSM-IV Version (AUDADIS-IV), 119
Alcohol use disorders (AUDS), 298, 299–304
    treatment, 311
Alcohol Use Disorders Identification Test (AUDIT-C), 310
Aldehyde dehydrogenase, 131–132
ALDH. *See* Aldehyde dehydrogenase
Allopregnanolone, 308
Alpha-adrenergic agonists
    for posttraumatic stress disorder, 378
    in response to stress, 82
Alzheimer's disease, **9**, 225, 246
    as a chronic disease, 319–322
    clinical implications, 326–327
    dementia, 320
    family history of, 320
    hormone therapy, 323–324, **325**
    neuropathology, 320
    NSAIDs and, 324–326
    postmenopausal hormone therapy and, 323
    prevention, 319–328
        preventive interventions, 320, **321**
    prodrome, 320
    treatment, 321
    trials data, 322–323
American Institutes for Research, 348

American Psychopathological Association, 54
The American Soldier (Stouffer et al.), 55–56
Americans View Their Mental Health (Gurin et al.), 56, 61
Amnesia, 83. *See also* Memory
Amphetamines
    contribution to psychosis, 28
    dopamine receptors and, 133
    mesolimbic transmission and, 35
    schizophrenia and, 24, **25**
    self-medication and, 27
Amygdala. *See also* Brain
    role in mediating fear and anxiety, 85–86
    role in posttraumatic stress disorder, 374
Animal studies, 190, 279, 304
Anorexia nervosa, **8**
Antabuse. *See* Disulfiram
Anticonvulsants, for treatment of alcoholism, 283
Antidepressants
    for normalization of HPA axis, 79
    prodromal schizophrenia and, 178
    for schizophrenia, 177
Anti-epileptics, for prevention of posttraumatic stress disorder, 381
Antipsychotics, 159
    for preventive intervention of psychotic disorders, 196–197
    prodromal schizophrenia and, 178
    for schizophrenia, 166, 176–177
    second-generation, 167, 176–177
    side effects of, 166
Antisocial personality disorder, **8**
Anxiety disorders
    "anticipatory," 86
    prefrontal modulation, 86–89
    prevention, 250–251

Anxiety disorders (continued)
  psychobiology of resilience to stress
      for prevention of, 77–96
  role of amygdala, 85–86
  self-medication and, 27
  socioeconomic class and, 63
  treatment, 246–247
Anxiolytics, for schizophrenia, 177
Apomorphine, 198
Archives of General Psychiatry, 61
Arginine vasopressin (AVP), to facilitate
    memory, 373
Aripiprazole, for treatment of
    alcoholism, 283
Asian Americans, 362
  psychiatric implications of cultural
      diversity, 67
  risk for alcohol use disorders, 130
Association studies
  in behavioral genetics, 15–17
  case–controls, 13
  haplotype risks, 13
  in molecular genetics, 12–13
Ataxia, 304
ATHENA. See Athletes Targeting
    Healthy Exercise and Nutrition
    Alternatives
Athletes Targeting Healthy Exercise and
    Nutrition Alternatives
    (ATHENA), 280
ATLAS. See Adolescents Training and
    Learning to Avoid Steroids
Attention-deficit/hyperactivity disorder
    (ADHD), 8, 286
  contribution to psychosis, 29
  prodromal schizophrenia and, 177
AUDADIS-IV. See Alcohol Use
    Disorder and Associated
    Disabilities Interview Schedule—
    DSM-IV Version
AUDIT-C. See Alcohol Use Disorders
    Identification Test

Australia, 305
  drug use prevalence in patients with
      schizophrenia, 25
Autism, 8, 11, 252–253
Avoidant personality disorder, 10
AVP. See Arginine vasopressin

BAC. See Blood alcohol content
Baclofen
  for treatment of alcoholism, 283
  for treatment of cocaine addiction,
      282
Baltimore City Public School System
    (BCPSS), 354, 362. See also Good-
    Behavior Game
Baltimore Prevention Program, 360
BCPSS. See Baltimore City Public
    School System
Beck's theory, 98–99
Behavior. See also Conduct disorder
  aggression, 352–353
  antisocial, 352–353
  clinical implications, 366
  community epidemiology, 349
  definitions, 356–357
  Good-Behavior Game intervention,
      353–364
  life course and social field theory,
      350–352
    psychological well-being, 352
    social adaptation, 350–351
  prevention of aggressive behavior
      through middle school,
      347–369
  theoretical framework, 349–350
    developmental epidemiology, 349
    life-course developmental
        perspective, 349
    randomized field trials, 349–350
"Behavioral high-risk design," 99
Behavioral therapies, for treatment of
    substance abuse, 284–285

Beijing, prevalence of mood disorders in, **67**

Benedict, Ruth, 55, 64

Benzodiazepines
  for posttraumatic stress disorder, 378–379
  schizophrenia and, 23–24, **25**

Beta-adrenergic antagonists, in response to stress, 82

Beta-blockers, in memory storage, 83

Bipolar disorder, **8,** 241–242
  linkage studies, 14–15
  prevention, 250

Blacks. *See also* African Americans
  psychiatric implications of cultural diversity, 67

Blazer, Dan, 61

Blood, for microarray analyses, 225–226

Blood alcohol content (BAC), 125

Borderline personality disorder, **8**

Brain. *See also* Amygdala
  in emotion regulation/models of stress resistance, 85–86
  Harvard Brain Tissue Resource Center, 230
  hormonal effects on, 194–195
  imaging studies, 85–86
  nonlinear effects of age on gray-matter density, **268–269**
  prefrontal modulation of fear and anxiety, 86–89
  stress and, 85–86
  structural abnormalities during pregnancy, 273

Bulimia nervosa, **9**

Bulletin of the World Health Organization, 330

Buprenorphine, for treatment of heroin addiction, 281

Burke, Jack, 61

Bush, President George H.W., 56

Cannabinoid receptor genes, 134, 283

Cannabis
  abuse, **8**
  adolescents' use, 38–39
  age at first use, 301, **302**
  contribution to psychosis, 29–31
  dose–response relationship, 29–30
  incidence, 338
  schizophrenia and, 24–25, 24–26

Carter, President Jimmy, 56

Carter Commission, 60, 61

CASIS cluster (Cognitive, Affective and Social Impairments, School decline and failure), 164, 165, 167, **168,** 180

Catechol-O-methyltransferase (COMT), 38–39, 214

Cathinone, contribution to psychosis, 29

CBT. *See* Cognitive-behavioral therapy

CDC. *See* Centers for Disease Control and Prevention

Centers for Disease Control and Prevention (CDC), 266

Child Behavior Checklist, 198

Children, 4. *See also* Adolescents; Adoption studies; Twin studies
  abuse in childhood, 78, 98, 106, 128
  adrenarche, 194, 306
  aggression in, 348
  childhood abuse, 81
  childhood stressors, 128
  cognitive vulnerability to depression, 105–106
  cultural differences and, 65
  lack of affection toward, 107
  neglect, 128
  prevention of aggressive behavior through middle school, 347–369
  propranolol trials, 85

Cholinesterase inhibitors, for symptomatic improvement of Alzheimer's disease, 321

CHR. *See* Clinical High-Risk (CHR) Project

Chromosomes
loci and genes in mental disorders, 14–17
association studies, 15–17
linkage studies, 14–15
meiosis, 12

Chronic pain, 286

CIDI. *See* Composite International Diagnostic Interview

Citalopram, 199

Clausen, John, 55–56

Clinical High-Risk (CHR) Project, 171

Clinician-Administered PTSD Scale, 85

Clonidine
for posttraumatic stress disorder, 378
in response to stress, 82

Clozapine, for preventive intervention of psychotic disorders, 197

Cocaine, abuse, **10**, 11, 330
contribution to psychosis, 28
dependence symptoms, 118
treatment, 281, 282
in utero, 271

COGA. *See* Collaborative Study on the Genetics of Alcoholism

Cognition
cognitive deficits, 216
cognitive vulnerability to depression, 97–113
flexibility, 78
negative cognitive styles as vulnerabilities for depression and suicidal behavior, 101–102
origins of cognitive vulnerability to depression, 105–108
reappraisal, 88–89
response styles theory, 103
role of stressful life events and, 103–105

rumination as vulnerability to depression, 102–103

Cognitive-behavioral therapy (CBT), 108–109, 244
for posttraumatic stress disorder, 372

Cognitive Style Questionnaire (CSQ), 100

Cognitive Vulnerability to Depression (CVD) Project, 98, 102, 108

Collaborative Cocaine Treatment Study, 284

Collaborative Psychiatric Epidemiology Surveys, 67

Collaborative Study on the Genetics of Alcoholism (COGA), 131

Colombia, prevalence of mood disorders in, **67**

Community Mental Health Centers program, 56

Composite International Diagnostic Interview (CIDI), 65

COMT. *See* Catechol-O-methyltransferase

Conduct disorder, **8**, 352–353. *See also* Behavior

Continuous Performance Task, 352

Coping, 78

CORGON algorithm, 228

Corticotropin-releasing factor (CRF), 78–79
role in stress response, 80

Corticotropin-releasing hormone (CRH), 78–79
adolescent neurodevelopment and, 189
to facilitate memory, 373

Cortisol (hydrocortisone), 188, **200, 201–203**, 380
adolescent neurodevelopment and, 190–191
adverse effects, 191
to facilitate memory, 373

functional abnormality in
 schizophrenia, 193
 for posttraumatic stress disorder,
 376, 379–380, 381–392
Counseling, genetic, 18
CRF. *See* Corticotropin-releasing factor
CRH. *See* Corticotropin-releasing
 hormone
CSQ. *See* Cognitive Style Questionnaire
Culture
 determinism, 64
 differences, 65–66
 historical changes, 66
 psychiatric implications of cultural
 diversity, 67
Cushing's syndrome, 188, 191
CVD. *See* Cognitive Vulnerability to
 Depression Project
CVG. *See* Gamma vinyl-GABA
Cytochrome P450, 132

DARE. *See* Drug Abuse Resistance
 Education
DAS. *See* Dysfunctional Attitudes Scale
Death, 242. *See also* Suicide
"Decade of the Brain," 56
Dehydroepiandrosterone (DHEA)
 adolescent neurodevelopment and,
 188
 stress and, 80
Delta-9-tetrahydrocannabinol, 34
Dementia, 320. *See also* Alzheimer's
 disease
 HIV-associated, 225
Dementia praecox, 160
Dependent personality disorder, **9**
Depression, 249–250
 abnormalities in noradrenergic
 function, 81
 "bluing of America," 67
 childhood maltreatment and,
 105–106

cognitive vulnerability, 97–113
 clinical implications, 108–109
 key findings, 100–108
 theories, 98–99
diathesis-stress model for
 development of, 249–250
hopelessness theory, 98–99
impaired HPA function and, 79
major, **9**
origins of cognitive vulnerability to,
 105–108
prodromal schizophrenia and, 177
rumination as vulnerability to,
 102–103
self-medication and, 27
socioeconomic class and, 63
Dexamethasone, impaired HPA
 function and, 79
Dexamphetamine, contribution to
 psychosis, 28–29
Dextroamphetamine (Adderall), 286
DHEA. *See* Dehydroepiandrosterone
*Diagnostic and Statistical Manual of Mental
 Disorders* (DSM-III), 59
Diagnostic Interview Schedule (DIS),
 61, 66
DIS. *See* Diagnostic Interview Schedule
Discordant twins, 196. *See also* Twin
 studies
Disinhibition, 130
Disrupted-in-schizophrenia 1 (DISC1),
 214
Disruptive behavioral disorders,
 248–249
Dissociative identity disorder, **9**
Disulfiram (Antabuse), for treatment of
 alcoholism and cocaine addictions,
 282, 311
D-amino acid oxidase (DAAO), 214
DNA. *See also* Genes
 coinheritance, 12

Dopamine, 13, 276–277
craving for drugs and, 34
hypothesis of schizophrenia and,
34–35
neurons, 275
sensitization as a shared
neurochemical mechanism,
35–37
Dopamine D_2-like receptor genes,
37–38
Dopamine receptors, 133
Driving under the influence (DUI), 123
Drug Abuse Resistance Education
(DARE), 340
Drugs. *See also individual drug names;*
Substance abuse
abuse, 21, 263–296
addiction, 263–296, 330
antipsychotic medication, 159
availability, 26
compliance with treatment, 26
costs of illicit, 264
definitions, **331**
dependence prevention, 329–346,
331
clinical course of drug
dependence, 336–338
clinical features, **333**
clinical implications, 343–344
facts, 338–342
phenotype as developmental
trajectory, 338
research and future directions,
342–343
social context, 336
efforts to reduce availability and
consumption, 123, 125
exposure, 270
gallons of ethanol consumed in the
United States, **124**
HIV/AIDS, 265–266, **267**

medical consequences, 263–296
metabolism and, 132
obstacles in the treatment of
addiction, 265
physical dependence, **331**
prevalence, **25**
psychic dependence, **331**
self-medication, 27
studies of alcohol and drug
dependence, 130–136
tolerance, 331
treatment, 265
trends in drug disorders by race/
ethnicity, **122**
use, 119
vulnerability to drug use disorders,
115–155
withdrawal, 331
DSM-III. *See Diagnostic and Statistical
Manual of Mental Disorders*
DTNBP1, 16
DUI. *See* Driving under the influence
DUP. *See* Duration of untreated
psychosis
Duration of untreated psychosis, 166
Dysbindin gene (*DTNBP1*), 214
Dysfunctional Attitudes Scale (DAS),
100
Dyslexia, **9**
Dysthymia, **10, 11**

Eaton, William, 61
Ebaugh, Frank, 54
ECA. *See* Epidemiologic Catchment
Area Program
Emory Study of At-Risk Adolescents,
198–204, **200–203**
Emotions
"affectionless control" pattern, 107
control of negative, 887
negative, 130

Enuresis, **10**, 11
Environment
 anxiety disorders and, 250–251
 depressive disorders and, 249–250
 determinants of psychosis, 21–51
  prenatal/perinatal factors, 22–27
  urbanicity, migration, and social
   factors, 23
 in the development of alcohol
  dependence, 299
 disruptive behavioral disorders and,
  248–249
 gene–environment interaction in
  psychosis development, 37–39,
  135–136
 neurodevelopmental disorders and,
  252–254
 social, 53–74
 substance abuse and, 277–278
 temporal changes, 66–67, **67**
 twins and, 5
Epidemiologic Catchment Area (ECA)
 Program, 61
Epinephrine
 to facilitate memory, 373–374
 in stress response, 80–81
Ethanol, 123, **124**
 pregnancy and, 271
Ethnicity, trends in drug disorders, **122**
Europe, Eastern, alcohol consumption,
 118–119
Europe, Western, alcohol consumption,
 118

Family planning, 18
Family studies
 general familial and genetic factors,
  6–7
 for risk factors for mental disorders, 4
 in studies of psychiatric disorders,
  8–10

FAS. *See* Fetal alcohol syndrome
FASD. *See* Fetal alcohol spectrum
 disorder
FDA. *See* U.S. Food and Drug
 Administration
Fear
 conditioned response, 377
 "instructed," 86
 prefrontal modulation, 86–89
 role of amygdala, 85–86
Felix, Robert, 54, 55
Fetal alcohol spectrum disorder
 (FASD), 274
Fetal alcohol syndrome (FAS), 271
Fetus. *See also* Pregnancy
 abnormal growth, 23
First-degree relatives, 4
fMRI. *See* Functional magnetic
 resonance imaging
France, drug use prevalence in patients
 with schizophrenia, **25**
Freud, Sigmund, 55
Frost, Wade Hampton, 337
Functional magnetic resonance imaging
 (fMRI), memory storage and, 84

GABA. *See* Gamma-aminobutyric acid
Gabapentin, for treatment of alcoholism,
 283
GAF. *See* Global Assessment of
 Functioning scale
Gambling, pathological, **9**
Gamma-aminobutyric acid (GABA),
 132, 214, 246–247, 304
 for posttraumatic stress disorder,
  378–379
Gamma receptor genes, 132–133
Gamma vinyl-GABA (CVG;
 vigabatrin), for treatment of cocaine
 addiction, 282
GBG. *See* Good-Behavior Game

Gender. *See also* Adolescents; Men;
Women
differences in alcohol abuse and
dependence, 305
Good-Behavior Game trial, 362
stress and gonadal hormones at
puberty, 309
Gender identity disorder, **8**
Gene mapping, 131, 245–246
Generalized anxiety disorder, **10**
Genes. *See also* DNA
cannabinoid receptor, 134
chromosomal loci in mental
disorders, 14–17
in the development of alcohol
dependence, 299
dopamine system, 13
familial and genetic factors, 6–11
family studies, 6–7
results of family, twin, linkage,
and association studies of
psychiatric disorders, **8–10**
twin studies, 7, 11
gene–environment interaction,
37–39, 135–136
in psychosis development, 37–39,
277–278
mu-opioid receptor, 134–135
neurotransmitter systems and, 132
risk factors for mental disorders,
3–20
behavioral genetic methods and
principles, 4–6
chromosomal loci and genes in
mental disorders, 14–17
clinical implications, 18–19
future research, 17–18
general familial and genetic
factors in mental disorders,
6–11
molecular genetic methods and
principles, 11–13

ROC curve analysis, **229**
"schizogene," 219–220
serotonin-related, 133–134
studies of alcohol and drug
dependence, 130–136
substance abuse and, 277–278
Genetic counseling, 18
Germany, drug use prevalence in
patients with schizophrenia, **25**
Global Assessment of Functioning
(GAF) scale, 221
Global Burden of Disease, 64–65
Glucocorticoid receptors, adolescent
neurodevelopment and, 189
Golden Fleece Awards, 59
Gonadarche, 306
Good-Behavior Game (GBG), 341,
353–364
analytic models, 357–360
randomized trial design, 358–359
unit of intervention assignment,
359–360
benefits, 355
description, 354
effects of intervention on aggressive
behavior, 362–364
hypotheses, 355–356
measures, 356–357
direct observation of classroom
behavior, 356–357
peer assessment inventory, 357
teacher observation of classroom
adaptation, 356
trial design, 360–362
Great Society, 58
Guanfacine
for posttraumatic stress disorder, 378
in response to stress, 82

Half-siblings, 4
Hallucinations, contribution to
psychosis, 28

Haloperidol, for preventive intervention
of psychotic disorders, 196–197
Haplotypes, of high-risk genes, 16
Harvard Brain Tissue Resource Center,
230
Helzer, John, 61
Hepatitis, 280, 286
HIV/AIDS and, 266
Heritability, 5–6
of drinking, 129
of psychiatric disorders, 14
Heroin, 119
production, 126
treatment, 281
Herpes simplex, 22
Hillside Recognition and Prevention
Program (RAP), 160, 164,
170–179, 180
clinical subgroups, 172–175, **174**
clinical trials, 170–171
description, 171–172
deterioration, 175
diagnostic procedures, 176
early treatment findings, 176–179
CHR-negative subgroup, 178
CHR-positive subgroup, 178–179
comorbidity, 177
SLP subgroup, 179
standard care, 177–178
treatment of prodromal
symptoms, 176–177
history, 171–172
initial selection strategy, 172
preliminary clinical outcome, 175–176
program developmental clinical
model, **174**
treatment conclusions, 179
Hippocampus
HPA function and, 189–191
schizophrenia and, 191–193
Hispanics, 362
substance use disorders, 119

Histrionic personality disorder, **8**
HIV, 280, 337. *See also* AIDS
dementia and, 225
drug abuse and, 265–266, **267**
hepatitis and, 268
Holland, 333
cannabis study and, 30
Hopelessness theory, 98–99, 102
Hormones, effects on the brain, 194–195
Hospitalization, for substance abuse and
schizophrenia, 26
HPA. *See* Hypothalamic-pituitary-
adrenal axis
Hydrocortisone. *See* Cortisol
Hyperalertness, 85
Hyperamnesia, 83. *See also* Memory
Hypothalamic-pituitary-adrenal axis
(HPA), 188
adolescent neurodevelopment and,
189
impaired function, 79–80
interaction of stress at puberty and,
309
in stress-induced depression and
stress resilience, 78–80
impaired HPA function, 79–80
normal functions, 78–79

Identity disorders
dissociative, **9**
gender, **8**
Immigrants, alcohol consumption, 119,
136
Impulsivity, 130
Infections, maternal viral, 22
Influenza, 22
Injection drug use (IDU), 265, **267**
Injuries, 375
The Inner American (Veroff et al.), 56–57,
61
Insomnia, **10,** 85
Institute of Medicine, 265

International HapMap Project, 246
Isolation, as factor of psychosis, 23
Israel
    alcohol consumption, 119, 136
    longitudinal studies of cannabis use
        and schizophrenia development,
        33
Italy, drug use prevalence in patients
    with schizophrenia, 25

Japan, 88
    alcohol consumption, 136
Jews, 130
    alcohol consumption, 136
Johnson, President Lyndon, 58
Joint Commission on Mental Illness and
    Health, 56

Katzman, Robert, 320
Kellam, Sheppard, 348
Kennedy, President John F., 56
Kessler, Ronald, 65
Khat
    contribution to psychosis, 29
    schizophrenia and, 24
Klerman, Gerald, 58
Koreans, risk for alcohol use disorders, 130
K-SADS. See Schedule for Affective
    Disorders and Schizophrenia for
    School-Age Children—
    Epidemiologic Version

"The Latent Structure of Substance Use
    Disorders: Results from the
    National Longitudinal Alcohol
    Epidemiologic Survey (NLAES)"
    (Blanco et al.), 116, 118
Latinos, psychiatric implications of
    cultural diversity, 67
Lebanon, prevalence of mood disorders
    in, 67

Leighton, Alexander, 55
Lemkau, Paul, 55
LES. See Life Events Scale
Less developed countries, prevalence of
    mood disorders in, 65, 67
Lewis, Sir Aubrey, 330, 334
Life Events and Difficulties Schedule,
    104
Life Events Scale (LES), 103–104
Lifestyles, 64
    optimism and, 78
LIFT. See Linking the Interests of
    Families and Teachers trial
Linkage studies
    for bipolar disorder, 14–15
    "crossing over," 11–12
    in molecular genetics, 11–12
    outcomes, 12
    for schizophrenia, 14
Linking the Interests of Families and
    Teachers (LIFT) trial, 360
Lundby Study, 66

MADCAP algorithm, 228
MADD. See Mothers Against Drunk
    Driving (MADD)
Magnetic resonance imaging (MRI),
    274, 276–277
    adolescent neurodevelopment and,
        190–191
    during pregnancy, 273
Major depression. See Depression
Malnutrition, 22
Marijuana
    new users, 119, 120
    peer influence, 127
Mastery Learning (ML), 353–354
Matrix model, 285
Mead, Margaret, 55, 64
Measurement and Prediction (Stouffer et
    al.), 55–56

Medicaid, 242
Medicare, 242
Meiosis, chromosomal, 12
Memantine, for symptomatic
improvement of Alzheimer's
disease, 321
Memory. *See also* Amnesia
changes in performance on a memory
test, **222**
emotional memories and memory
storage, 83–84
influence of stress hormones on
memory consolidation, 372–374
Men
disinhibitory psychopathology, 304
HIV/AIDS, 266
lack of affection to children, 107
prevalence of posttraumatic stress
disorder, 78
substance use disorders, 119, 121
Menninger, Karl, 55
Mental disorders. *See also* Mental illness;
Psychiatric disorders
family studies, 4
genetic risk factors, 3–20
twin studies. *See* Twin studies
Mental health. *See also* Mental illness;
Psychiatric disorders
Mental Health in America (Veroff et al.),
56–57, 61
"Mental Hygiene and Socio-
Environmental Factors"
(Felix and Bowers), 54
Mental illness. *See also* Mental disorders;
Psychiatric disorders
clinical implications, 256–257
comorbidity with drugs and alcohol,
278–279
future research, 255–256
indicated preventive interventions,
244
prevention, definition, 243

selective preventive interventions, 244
universal, definition, 243–244
Mesocorticolimbic system, 31, 34
Metabotropic glutamate receptor 3 gene
(GRM3), 214
Methamphetamines
during pregnancy, 273
schizophrenia and, 24, **25**
treatment, 281
Methylphenidate (Ritalin)
contribution to psychosis, 28–29
for narcolepsy, 29
for preventive intervention of
psychotic disorders, 198
for treatment of ADHD, 286
Mexico
alcohol consumption, 119
prevalence of mood disorders in,
67
Meyer, Adolf, 54
Michigan Survey Research Center, 56
Midtown Manhattan Study, 55, 57, 62
Mifepristone, for prevention of
posttraumatic stress disorder, 381
Migration
as factor of psychosis, 23
rates of schizophrenia, 23
social environment and psychiatric
disorders, 59
Mineralocorticoid receptors, adolescent
neurodevelopment and, 189
Mirtazapine, for preventive intervention
of psychotic disorders, 197
ML. *See* Mastery Learning
Modafinil, for treatment of cocaine and
methamphetamine dependence,
281
Molecular genetics, methods and
principles, 11–13
association studies, 12–13
linkage studies, 11–12
Monitoring the Future (MTF), 264

Mood disorders, 278
cultural differences and, 65–66,
67
impaired HPA function and, 79
treatments, 246–247
Mood stabilizers, for schizophrenia,
177
Mothers Against Drunk Driving
(MADD), 125
Motor vehicle accidents, 372
MRI. See Magnetic resonance imaging
MTF. See Monitoring the Future
Multiple sclerosis, 225
Mu-opioid receptor genes, 134–135

NAA. See N-acetylaspartate
NAc. See Nucleus accumbens
N-acetylaspartate (NAA), 191
Naltrexone, for treatment of alcoholism,
282, 311
NAPLS. See North American
Prodromal Longitudinal Study
Narcissistic personality disorder, 8
Narcolepsy, 9
methylphenidate and, 29
Narcotics Anonymous, 284
NAS/NRC. See National Academy of
Sciences/National Research
Council
National Academy of Sciences/National
Research Council (NAS/NRC),
338
National Comorbidity Survey (NCS),
62, 337, 371–372
National Epidemiologic Survey on
Alcohol and Related Conditions
(NESARC), 119, 121, 122, 278,
300
National Institute of Child Health and
Human Development (NICHD),
270

National Institute of Mental Health
(NIMH), 270
Epidemiologic Catchment Area
Program, 61
establishment, 53
goals for prevention research, 244
history, 53–54, 58–59
Intramural Program, 55–56
Laboratories of Social Environmental
Studies, Psychiatry, Psychology,
and Clinical Sciences, 56
prevention of mental illness and,
243
role, 53–56
National Institute of Neurological
Disorders and Stroke (NINDS),
270
National Institute on Alcohol Abuse
and Alcoholism (NIAAA), 270,
274, 300, 311
National Institute on Drug Abuse
(NIDA), 119, 266, 270, 273–274,
280, 285, 340, 348
National Institutes of Health Magnetic
Resonance Imaging Study of
Normal Brain Development, 270
National Institutes of Health
Neuroscience Blueprint and
Roadmap initiatives, 287
National Longitudinal Alcohol
Epidemiological Survey (NLAES),
300–301
National Science Foundation (NSF),
59–60
National Survey on Drug Use and
Health, 264, 305
National Youth Anti-Drug Media
Campaign, 339
Native Americans, 362
risk for alcohol use disorders, 130
NCS. See National Comorbidity Survey

Neglect, 78
Neuregulin (*NRG1*), 214
Neuroactive steroids, 308
Neurocognitive deficits
    attenuated negative features, 162, 164
    schizophrenia and, 161–162
Neurodevelopment, adolescent,
    187–211
    clinical implications, 205
    as a critical period, 193–195
    Emory Study of At-Risk
        Adolescents, 198–204, **200–203**
    hippocampus and
        HPA function, 189–191
        schizophrenia, 191–193
    HPA axis and, 189
    preventive intervention, 196–198
    sensitivity to adverse effects of stress,
        195–196
Neurodevelopment disorders, 252–254.
    See also Autism; Schizophrenia
Neuropeptide Y (NPY)
    modulation of sympathetic response,
        82
    in response to stress, 82
    for treatment of alcoholism, 283
Neuropsychological functions, 216, **217**
Neuroscience, for prevention of mental
    illness, 244–248
Neurosteroids, alcoholism and, 308
Neuroticism, 130
Neurotransmitter systems, genes and, 132
New York High-Risk Project
    (NYHRP), 162, 170
New Zealand, 247
    longitudinal studies of cannabis use
        and schizophrenia development,
        32–33
NIAAA. *See* National Institute on
    Alcohol Abuse and Alcoholism
NICHD. *See* National Institute of Child
    Health and Human Development

Nicotine
    age at first use, 301, **302**
    costs, 264
    dependence, **9**
    during pregnancy, 64
    schizophrenia and, 24, **25**
NIDA. *See* National Institute on Drug
    Abuse
NIDA Clinical Trials network, 21
Nigeria, 65
    prevalence of mood disorders, **67**
Nightmare disorder, **9**, 85
NIMH. *See* National Institute of Mental
    Health
NINDS. *See* National Institute of
    Neurological Disorders and Stroke
Nixon, President Richard, 327
NLAES. *See* National Longitudinal
    Alcohol Epidemiological Survey;
    "The Latent Structure of Substance
    Use Disorders: Results from the
    National Longitudinal Alcohol
    Epidemiologic Survey"
NMDA. *See* N-methyl-D-aspartate
N-methyl-D-aspartate (NMDA),
    304
Nonsteroidal anti-inflammatory
    treatments (NSAIDS),
    Alzheimer's disease and, 324–326
Noradrenergic function, abnormalities,
    81
Norepinephrine
    in stress-induced depression, 79
    in stress response, 80–81
North American Prodromal
    Longitudinal Study (NAPLS),
    253, 254
North Shore–Long Island Jewish
    Health System, 171
NPY. *See* Neuropeptide Y
NRG1, 16
NSF. *See* National Science Foundation

Nucleus accumbens, 31, 34
NYHRP. *See* New York High-Risk
    Project

Obesity, psychiatric disorders and, 64
"Obsessional Illness" (Lewis), 334
Obsessive-compulsive disorder, 8
Obsessive-compulsive personality
    disorder, **8**
    prodromal schizophrenia and, 177
Office of the Surgeon General, 242
Oklahoma, 274
Olanzapine
    for preventive intervention of
        psychotic disorders, 196–197
    prodromal schizophrenia and, 178
Opiates, abuse, **9**
    dopamine receptors and, 133
    schizophrenia and, 23–24, **25**
    treatment, 281
Opioid receptors, 277
Oppositional defiant disorder, **9**
    prodromal schizophrenia and, 177

PAI. *See* Peer Assessment Inventory
Pain, 286
Panic disorder, **9**
Paranoid personality disorder, **10**
Pardes, Herbert, 59
Parents, 4
    negative parenting, 98
    parental inferential feedback,
        106–107
    parental modeling of substance use,
        126
    parenting practices of substance
        abuse, 126
    parenting styles, 107–108
    separation, 128
Peer Assessment Inventory (PAI), 357
Penn Optimism Project, 108–109

Personality disorders, 11
    antisocial, **8**
    avoidant, **10**
    borderline, **8**
    dependent, **9**
    histrionic, **8**
    narcissistic, **8**
    obsessive-compulsive, **8**
    paranoid, **10**
    personality traits in substance use
        disorders, 129–130
    schizoid, **10**
    schizotypal, 7, **10**
PET. *See* Positron emission tomography
Pharmacotherapies. *See also individual*
    drug names
    for drugs and alcohol, 281–284
Phenotype, 4
Phenytoin, for prevention of
    posttraumatic stress disorder, 381
Phobias, **10**
Physical Anhedonia Scale, 221
Polk, Frank, 336–337
Positron emission tomography (PET),
    274, **276–277**
    for evaluation of schizophrenia, 34
    in regulation of stress resistance,
        86
    of third trimester, **272**
Postpartum psychosis, **9**
Posttraumatic stress disorder (PTSD),
    9, 77
    adrenocortical insufficiency and, 80
    amygdala and, 374
    anti-adrenergic agents and, 377–379
    cortisol and, 379–380
    efficacy vs. effectiveness, 381–382
    inclusion in DSM-III, 60–61
    influence of stress hormones on
        memory consolidation,
        373–374

pathogenesis, 374–375, **376**
prevention, 84–85, 247, 251,
 375–377
  primary, 372
  secondary, 372, **376**
  tertiary, 372
significance of remembrance,
 372–381
Prazosin, in response to stress, 82
Preeclampsia, maternal, 22
Pregnancy. *See also* Women
 abnormal fetal growth, 23
 cocaine use, in utero, 271
 complications of delivery, 23
 material viral infection, 22
 maternal preeclampsia, 22
 maternal toxoplasmosis, 22
 neurobiological effects of substance
  abuse, 270–274, **272**
 nicotine during, 64
 obstetric complications, 22
 premature rupture of membranes,
  22
 smoking in, 270–271
 structural brain abnormalities
  during, 273
 substance abuse in, 270–274, **272**
President's Commission on Mental
 Health, 56, 58–59, 61, 62, 241
"Preventing Violence and Related
 Health-Risking Social Behaviors in
 Adolescents" (National Institutes of
 Health), 249
Probands, 4
"Problems of Obsessional Illness"
 (Lewis), 334
"Procedures for Classroom Observation
 of Teachers and Children" (O'Leary
 et al.), 357
Project MATCH (Matching
 Alcoholism Treatments to Client
 Heterogeneity), 284–285

Project on Human Development in
 Chicago Neighborhoods, 64
Propranolol
 to facilitate memory, 373–374
 memory and, 83, 84
 for posttraumatic stress disorder,
  377–378, 381–382
 in response to stress, 82
 in secondary prevention of
  posttraumatic stress disorder,
  84–85
 treatment trials, 85
Psychiatric disorders. *See also* Mental
 disorders; Mental illness
 in an environmental context,
  248–254
 antidiagnostic approach, 55
 clinical implications, 256–257
 etiology, 55
 evolution for prevention of mental
  illness, 243–244
 future research to predict and prevent
  mental illness, 255–256
 heritable, **10**, 14
 neuroscientific perspectives on
  prevention, 244–248
 "new cross-cultural," 64
 prevention, 241–261
 social environment and, 53–74
 translational research priorities,
  254–255
Psychiatric Disorders in America (Robins
 and Regier), 61
Psychobiology, resilience to stress, 77–96
Psychobiology of Depression Study, 66
Psychological well-being, 352
Psychoses. *See also* Schizophrenia
 causal factors, 27
 clinical implications of substance
  abuse, 39
 dopamine and mechanisms of drug
  reward, 31, 34

Psychoses (*continued*)
  duration of untreated, 166
  environmental determinants, 21–51
  florid, 160
  gene–environment interaction, 37–39
  increased risk of substance abuse and,
    26–27
  mechanisms of substance misuse and,
    31–37
  mood-incongruency and, 29
  neurobiological mechanisms
    underlying, 31–34, **32–33**
  not otherwise specified, 7
  substance misuse and, 23–24, **25,**
    28–31
Psychostimulants
  dopamine receptors and, 133
  dose–response relationship, 28
  hallucinations, 28
  prescribed, 29
  schizophrenia and, 24
  substance misuse and, 28–29
Psychotropic medications, 205
PTSD. *See* Posttraumatic stress disorder
Puberty. *See also* Adolescents
  hormonal changes with onset of,
    306–307
  hormones and sex differences in
    alcohol abuse and dependence,
    305–309
PWB. *See* Psychological well-being

QRT-PCR. *See* Quantitative reverse
    transcriptase polymerase chain
    reaction
Quantitative reverse transcriptase
    polymerase chain reaction
    (QRT-PCR), 228

Race, trends in drug disorders, **122**
Radioligand imaging studies, 35

RAP. *See* Hillside Recognition and
    Prevention Program
"Rate the State," 125
Reagan, President Ronald, 60
Receiver operating characteristic
    (ROC), 228, **229**
Receptors, 13
Regier, Darrel, 61
Regulator of G-protein signaling
    (RGS4), 214
Relatives
  first-degree, 4
  second-degree, 4
Religion, 78
Religiosity, substance use/dependence
    and, 128–129
Rennie, Thomas A.C., 55
Research. *See also* Adoption studies;
    Family studies; Twin studies
  "chain of psychiatric genetic,"
    15–16
  challenges, 2887
  clinical implications for risk factor
    genes, 18–19
  "cohort effect," 66
  current prevalence, 66
  for drug dependence prevention,
    342–343
  gene-based versus genome-based,
    224–230, **229**
  of genes as basis for genetic risk
    factors for mental disorders,
    17–18
  history, 60–61
  integrative approaches, 63–64
  on mental illness, 255–256
  NIMH goals for prevention research,
    244
  quality, 60
  retrospective incidence, 66
  on schizophrenia, 231, **232**

for substance abuse, 279–286
   behavioral therapies, 284–285
   clinical implications, 288
   comorbidity treatment, 286
   pharmacotherapies, 281–284
   prevention, 279–281
   translational priorities, 254–255
Resuscitation, 22
Risperidone
   changes in performance on a memory
      test, **222**
   changes in SANS, **223**
   for preventive intervention of
      psychotic disorders, 196–197
   prodromal schizophrenia and, 178
Ritalin. *See* Methylphenidate
Robins, Lee N., 61, 337
ROC. *See* Receiver operating
   characteristic
Rofecoxib, 326
Rotterdam Study, 326
Russia, alcohol consumption, 118–119,
   123

SADS-L. *See* Schedule for Affective
   Disorders and Schizophrenia—
   Lifetime Version
SAMHSA. *See* Substance Abuse and
   Mental Health Services
   Administration
SANS. *See* Schedule for the Assessment
   of Negative Symptoms
SAS. *See* Social adaptational status
SAS-SR. *See* Social Adjustment Scale—
   Self-Report
Schedule for Affective Disorders and
   Schizophrenia for School-Age
   Children—Epidemiologic Version
   (K-SADS), 172
Schedule for Affective Disorders and
   Schizophrenia—Lifetime Version
   (SADS-L), 100

Schedule for the Assessment of Negative
   Symptoms (SANS), 220, **223**
Schedule of Prodromal Symptoms
   (SOPS), 172
Schizoaffective disorder, 7, **8,** 213
"Schizogene," 219–220
Schizoid personality disorder, **10**
Schizophrenia, **8,** 246
   alcohol and, 23–24, **25**
   benzodiazepines and, 23–24, **25**
   cannabis and, 24–26
   causal risk factors, 161–165
   clinical implications, 180–181, 231,
      233
   coherence of cognitive and clinical
      deficits in relatives into a
      syndrome of liability, 219–224,
      222–223
   developmental abnormalities, 161
   dopamine hypothesis, 34–35
   drug use prevalence in patients, **25**
   future directions, 231, **232**
   gene-based versus genome-based
      research, 224–230, **229**
   gene expression profiles from
      peripheral blood, 227–230, **229**
   genetic and phenotypic heterogeneity
      model, 214–218, **215, 217**
   Hillside Recognition and Prevention
      Program, 170–179
   hippocampus and, 191–193
   incidence, 7
   linkage studies, 14
   in migrants, 23
   neurodevelopmental hypothesis,
      160–161
   neurodevelopmental model, **163, 168**
   neuropathology, 27
   neuropsychological profiles, **217**
   nicotine use and, 24
   opiates and, 23–24, **25**
   pharmaco-intervention, 166–170

Schizophrenia (*continued*)
  prevalence of stimulant use and, 24
  prevention, 213–237, 253–254
  prodromal indicators, 164–165
  psychostimulants and, 24
  substance use and, 26
  treatment, 159–185
    benefits of early, 166
    developmental concerns, 169–170
    heterogeneity of the prodrome, 167, 169
    second-generation antipsychotic medications, 166
    type of medication, 167
Schizophrenia-like psychosis (SLP), 173
Schizotaxia, 219–220, 224
Schizotypal personality disorder (SPD), 7, **10**, 237
Schneider Children's Hospital, 172
SCID. *See* Structured Clinical Interview for Axis I DSM-IV Disorders
SCL-90-R. *See* Symptom Checklist–90—Revised
Seasonal affective disorder, **10**
Second-degree relatives, 4
Sedatives, 304
  abuse, **9**
Selective serotonin reuptake inhibitors (SSRIs)
  for prevention of posttraumatic stress disorder, 381
  for schizophrenia, 177
Senator Proxmire's Golden Fleece Awards, 59
Sense of humor, 78
Serotonin, 133–134, 135
SES. *See* Socioeconomic status
Sexual abuse, depression and, 106
Sexually transmitted diseases (STDs), 280
Shanghai, prevalence of mood disorders in, **67**

SI. *See* Stress Interview
Siblings, 4. *See also* Twin studies
SIDP-IV. *See* Structured Interview for DSM-IV Personality Disorders
Simple phobia, **10**
Single photon emission computed tomography (SPECT), in regulation of stress resistance, 86
SIPS. *See* Structured Interview for Prodromal Symptoms
Sleepwalking, **9**
SLP. *See* Schizophrenia-like psychosis
Smoking
  in pregnancy, 270–271
  psychiatric disorders and, 64
SNS. *See* Sympathetic nervous system
Social adaptational status (SAS), 350–351
Social Adjustment Scale—Self-Report (SAS-SR), 221
Social defeat, as factor of psychosis, 23
Social environment, psychiatric disorders and, 53–74
  attitudes toward substance abuse, 121
  challenges to psychosocial research, 59–60
  clinical implications, 68
  cultural determinism, 64
  definition, 54
  history
    changes, 66–67
    significance, 56–57
  integrative research, 63–64
  National Institute of Mental Health, developments at, 58–59
  role of, 53–56
  "new cross-cultural psychiatry," 64
  nonepidemiological social models, 57–58
  recent research, 60–62
  social class and, 62–63
  socialization theory, 127

Social factors, psychosis and, 23

Social functioning, for substance abuse and schizophrenia, 26

Social impairment, 304

Social networks, 78

Social phobia, **10**
  prodromal schizophrenia and, 177

Socioeconomic status (SES), 55

SOPS. *See* Schedule of Prodromal Symptoms

Southeast Asia, psychostimulants and, 24

SPD. *See* Schizotypal personality disorder

SPECT. *See* Single photon emission computed tomography

Spectrum conditions, 4

Spirituality, 78

SSRIs. *See* Selective serotonin reuptake inhibitors

STAART. *See* Studies to Advance Autism Research and Treatment

Startle, 85

STDs. *See* Sexually transmitted diseases

Stimulants, 177

Stirling County Study, 55, 63, 65, 66

Stress, 64
  α-adrenergic agonists and, 82
  β-adrenergic antagonists and, 82
  brain regions in resistance to, 85–86
  clinical implications, 89
  cognitive vulnerability and role of stressful live events, 103–105
  emotional memories and memory storage, 83–84
  exposure, 188
  gender differences in alcohol-seeking behavior, 309
  gonadal hormones at puberty, 309
  hypothalamic-pituitary-adrenal axis, 78–80

neuropeptide Y modulation of sympathetic response, 82

noradrenergic response to, 80–82

pharmacological secondary prevention of PTSD, 84–85

physical, 195

prefrontal modulation of fear and anxiety, 86–89

psychobiology of resilience to, 77–96

treatment with propranolol, 84–85

vulnerability to alcohol and drug use disorders, 127–128

Stress Interview (SI), 104

Striatal function, 36

Structured Clinical Interview for Axis I DSM-IV Disorders (SCID), 198

Structured Interview for DSM-IV Personality Disorders (SIDP-IV), 172, 198

Structured Interview for Prodromal Symptoms (SIPS), 172

Studies to Advance Autism Research and Treatment (STAART), 252, 254

Stuttering, **8**

Substance abuse
  causal factors, 27
  clinical implications, 136–137, 288
  comorbidy treatment, 286
  dependence, 116–118
  disorders, 119, 121, **122**
  epidemiology, 118–121
  increased risk with psychosis, 26–27
  macro/external factors, **117**, 121–129
  micro/internal factors, **117**, 129–136
  neural substrates, 274–277, **276–277**
  neurobiological effects, 21, **268–269**, 269–279
    comorbidity with mental illness, 278–279
    developmental aspects, **268–269**, 269–270

Substance abuse *(continued)*
  neurobiological effects *(continued)*
    genes, environment, and their
        interactions, 277–278
    neural substrates, 274–277,
        276–277
    in pregnancy, 270–274, **272**
  onset, 305
  parental influences, 126
  peer influence, 127
  prevalence, trends, and costs, 23–24,
      25, 264–265
  primary addiction model, 27
  psychostimulants and, 28–31
  research
    behavioral therapies, 284–285
    challenges, 287
    comorbidity treatment, 286
    pharmacotherapies, 281–284
    prevention, 279–281
  social attitudes toward, 121
  strategies for scientific research,
      279–286
  vulnerability to alcohol and drug use
      disorders, 115–155
Substance Abuse and Mental Health
    Services Administration
    (SAMHSA), 119, **120**, 287
Suicide, **9**, 242. *See also* Death
  ideation, 102
  negative cognitive styles as
      vulnerabilities for, 101–102
Surgeon General, 242
Survival school, 82
Sweden, 66
  longitudinal studies of cannabis use
      and schizophrenia development,
      32
Switzerland, drug use prevalence in
    patients with schizophrenia, **25**
Sympathetic nervous system (SNS)
  response to stress, 80–82

Symptom Checklist–90—Revised
    (SCL-90-R), 221
Synaptic pruning, 161

"Taking Stock of Risk Factors for Child/
    Youth Externalizing Behavior
    Problems" (Hann), 248–249
Tardive dyskinesia, 166
Teacher Observation of Classroom
    Adaptation—Revised (TOCA-R),
    356
  TOCA-R Likeability/Rejection
      subscale, 356, 357
Tetrahydrocannabinol (THC),
    contribution to psychosis, 29
Tetrodotoxin, 376
THC. *See* Tetrahydrocannabinol
The Netherlands, 22, 192
  longitudinal studies of cannabis use
      and schizophrenia development,
      32
Tianeptine, for prevention of
    posttraumatic stress disorder, 381
Tobacco. *See also* Nicotine; Smoking
  dependence, 64
TOCA-R. *See* Teacher Observation of
    Classroom Adaptation—
    Revised
Topiramate
  for treatment of alcohol and opiate
      addiction, 281
  for treatment of alcoholism, 283
Tourette's disorder, **8**
Toxoplasmosis, maternal, 22
Transporters, 13
Trauma, 371–387. *See also* Posttraumatic
    stress disorder
Truman, President Harry S., 53
12-Step programs, 284
Twin studies, 213. *See also* Siblings
  alcoholism and, 307
  association studies method, 15–16

concordant, 5, 7, 11

discordant, 5

environment and, 5

fraternal, 5

gene–environment interaction, 135–136

general familial and genetic factors, 7, 11

hippocampal reductions in schizophrenia, 192

identical, 5

peer influence of alcohol and drug use, 127

religiosity and, 129

for risk factors for mental disorders, 5–6

studies of alcohol and drug dependence, 130–131

in studies of psychiatric disorders, **8–10**

Ukraine

alcohol consumption, 118–119

prevalence of mood disorders, 67

Undersocialized aggression, 348. *See also* Behavior

United Kingdom, drug use prevalence in patients with schizophrenia, **25**

United States, drug use prevalence in patients with schizophrenia, **25**

Urbanicity, as factor of psychosis, 23

U.S. Army, 82

U.S. Constitution, 18th Amendment, 123

U.S. Food and Drug Administration (FDA), 254, 321

U.S. Navy, 82

U.S. Preventive Services Task Force, 242

Valproate, for treatment of alcoholism, 283

Velocardiofacial syndrome, 38

Ventral tegmental area (VTA), 31, 34

Vietnam, 371–372

Vigabatrin. *See* Gamma vinyl-GABA

Vlahov, David, 337

VTA. *See* Ventral tegmental area

Weissman, Myrna, 61

WHO. *See* World Health Organization

Women. *See also* Pregnancy

postmenopausal hormone therapy and Alzheimer's disease, 323

postpartum psychosis, **9**

posttraumatic stress disorder, 87–88

prevalence of posttraumatic stress disorder, 78

Women's Health Initiative Memory Study (WHIMS), 323–324, **325**

Workgroup Report on Prevention from the National Advisory Mental Health Council, 243, 256–257

World Health Organization (WHO), 64–65, 241

definitions for drug dependence, **331**

Expert Committee on Addiction-Producing Drugs, 330

WHO Expert Committee on Drug Dependence, 330

World Mental Health Initiative, 65, 66

World War II, 54, 55–56

Yolles, Stanley, 58

Youth. *See* Adolescents

"Youth Violence: A Report of the Surgeon General" (U.S. Public Health Service), 249

Zucker Hillside Hospital, 171